SOUL OF THE ORGANON - II
APHORISM IN DETAIL

DR. JYOTI JOSHI

INDIA • SINGAPORE • MALAYSIA

Notion Press

Old No. 38, New No. 6
McNichols Road, Chetpet
Chennai - 600 031

First Published by Notion Press 2020
Copyright © Dr. Jyoti Joshi 2020
All Rights Reserved.

ISBN 978-1-64850-906-3

This book has been published with all efforts taken to make the material error-free after the consent of the author. However, the author and the publisher do not assume and hereby disclaim any liability to any party for any loss, damage, or disruption caused by errors or omissions, whether such errors or omissions result from negligence, accident, or any other cause.

While every effort has been made to avoid any mistake or omission, this publication is being sold on the condition and understanding that neither the author nor the publishers or printers would be liable in any manner to any person by reason of any mistake or omission in this publication or for any action taken or omitted to be taken or advice rendered or accepted on the basis of this work. For any defect in printing or binding the publishers will be liable only to replace the defective copy by another copy of this work then available.

DEDICATED & SPECIAL THANKS TO

PARENTS, GOD

&

SPECIALLY THANKS TO

Dr. Meenakshi Pandey [M.B.B.S / LMO]

*'Believe in yourself. You are braver than you think,
more talented than you know, and capable of more than you imagine.'*

Important Note:

THE VITAL FORCE HAS MANY NAMES IN HOMOEOPATHIC HISTORY LIKE:

* DR. HAHNEMANN GAVE THE NAME – "VITAL FORCE."
* DR. KENT TERMED – "SIMPLE SUBSTANCES."
* I HAVE GIVEN IT THE TERM – "SOUL OF THE ORGANON."

Never stop trying. Never stop believing. Never give up. Your day will come.

PREFACE

I **Dr. JYOTI JOSHI**, is very happy regarding publishing of my second Book ....

- ✦ I have worked hard to write the content in a simpler and easy to understand way.
  I have tried to bring a new outlook to it, so that the matter becomes interesting to read and understand.
- ✦ You would feel this yourself while reading it.
- ✦ Till now we have read aphorisms in form of titles or through our Seniors or Teachers through their explanation.
- ✦ None of the books have explained them but this book explains what Hahnemann wants to say through each aphorism in the most easy and correct way.
- ✦ I am very thankful to Master Hahnemann for gifting us with this invaluable knowledge of permanent cure, that is, Homoeopathy and Organon form the basis of Homeopathic treatment.
- ✦ I feel very happy that I am able to convey this knowledge and have been able to enlighten this knowledge in an easy way.

Dr. JYOTI JOSHI

I have not failed. I've just found 10,000 ways that won't work

ACKNOWLEDGEMENTS

Hello Medical Students & Teachers:-

I am glad to say that "This book basically contains the aphorisms in detail and in easy to understand language.

The Organon developed out of Hahnemann's research and experimentation over a period of time.
It has six editions. This book contains all the aphorisms of latest edition.
All measure have been taken to convey the message in a reader friendly manner.

1. Font & size making it a pleasure to read.
2. Footnote which were earlier given at the bottom and spread over different Aphorism were difficult to find and read.
   In this new book we have incorporated them under the appropriate aphorisms at one place. This makes the reading and understanding of Organon in a more easy way.
3. This book is an effort to reach every student and practitioner and enlighten them with the knowledge of Homoeopathy.
4. The knowledge of Organon is available to the reader in the most simple words.
5. Knowledge of Organon is basis of Homoepathic mode of cure.
6. A must have book for all students/teachers.

Success is what comes after you stop making excuses.

MESSAGE FOR THE STUDENTS/TEACHERS & PROFESSORS

We are Doctors, it doesn't matter which medical field we belong to. The mode of treatment does not classify a doctor, as the sole mission of all Doctors is to cure the patient.

Organon is not only for Homeopathic doctors but every doctor of all medical field can study it because it's like Geeta /Bible/Quran/Guru granth sahib which teach us that all are the same, they teach us what life is and what is humanity and our duties.

In the same way Organon teaches us how to cure the patient, what is our sole aim, mode of treatment and whether we are on the right path to cure or not.

Every doctor can read this book because a true physician has the final target of curing the sick.

This book contains answers to all the questions like how and when to treat the patient, are we following the right way, can it be treated & Hahnemann's principle of treatment Etc.

Always remember you are a Doctor and you have a big responsibility, so follow this book and do your duty well.

In your life -Never give up, spread happiness and remember everything that happens is for a good reason.

Whoever is reading this message he/she should fell proud that we are doctors, not just a Homeopathic / Allopathic /Ayurvedic doctor, these and many such are just pathy names.

We are Doctors and our duty is curing and saving the lives and serving the humankind.

Dr. JYOTI JOSHI

You are the only one who can limit your greatness

THE COMMENTS OF STUDENTS/TEACHERS/PROFESSORS ON THE FIRST BOOK "SOUL OF THE ORGANON"

Respected Mam, I am a final year medical student. I am reading this book now. Thank you again for writing such a nice concise book, it is helping me a lot and almost all of my classmates.

— **Komal [B. H. M. S final year]**

Mam, your book is very useful for university examination and also for solving Entrance MCQs…, proves its excellence and perfection.

— **Praneet, Bhopal**

Mam…big fan of your book, saved my life in second year, simple & rich. Everything in the book. Thanks a lot Mam, my personal favourite book. I still read it once in a while.

— **Pooja, Kerala**

Very informative book & kudos to Dr. Jyoti Joshi for bringing up this book which will be a great help to understand the soul of Homeopathy for students as well as, it works as a guiding principle for practitioners as well.

— **Dr. Kalyani sharma**

Best approach of organon for students & the way the topics are explained is very easy to understand…thanks again.

— **Dr. Neha**

Amazing book, well done, complete booster to my knowledge.

— **Dr. Akanksha jain**

I find it so helpful & comprehensive to study with, one can easily gain the proper knowledge of subject of organon of medicine by this. I would like

To thanks & congratulate the AUTHOR.

— **Dr. Mohd faisal {Student}**

ORGANON OF MEDICINE

Organon of Medicine is the compilation of doctrine principles of Homeopathic medicine as invented by Dr. Samuel Hahnemann... The Organon of Medicine by Samuel Hahnemann is popular as "Organon by Hahnemann" or "Hahnemann's Organon" or "Organon Medicine" or "Homeopathy Organon" or "Organon of homeopathic medicine". This is "the homeopathy Bible"

An aphorism is an original thought, spoken or written in a laconic (concise) and memorable form. Aphorism literally means a "distinction" or "definition". The term was first used in the **Aphorism of Hippocrates**. The term was later applied to maxims of physical science, then statements of all kinds of philosophical, moral, or literary principles. In modern usage an aphorism is generally understood to be a concise statement containing a subjective truth or observation cleverly and pithily written.

Aphorism is a statement of truth or opinion expressed in a concise and witty manner. The term is often applied to philosophical, moral, and literary principles. To qualify as an A**phorism**, it is necessary for a statement to contain a truth revealed in a terse manner.

Organon of Medicine Editions

Hahnemann first experienced the effect of Peruvian Bark Cinchona in 1790, and then after six years, in 1796, he published an article under the title "Essay on a New Principle." And, in 1805 he published an article 'Medicine of Experience'.

After conducting personal observation and experiment, Hahnemann collected his new theory of homeopathy into book form in 1810. The original title of the book was Organon of Rational Art of Healing.

In 1819, the second edition was published, with the revised title Organon of Healing Art. The third edition (1824) and fourth edition (1829) kept this new title, while the latter introduced Hahnemann's "Theory of Chronic Diseases."

The fifth edition was published in 1833, and included the doctrine of vital force and drug-dynamization. The sixth edition, written in 1842, a year before his death, was retitled Organon of Medicine and not published until 1921. Published editions of homoeopathy books on organon of medicine and homoeopathic philosophy

Year	Edition
1920	Organon of medicine 6th edition
1833	Organon of medicine 5th edition
1829	Organon of medicine 4th edition
1824	Organon of medicine 3rd edition
1819	Organon of medicine 2nd edition
1810	Organon of medicine 1st edition

APHROSIM 1 TO 294

§ 1

The physician's high and only mission is to restore the sick to health, to cure, as it is termed.[1]

1. His mission is not, however, to construct so-called systems, by interweaving empty speculations and hypotheses concerning the internal essential nature of the vital processes and the mode in which diseases originate in the interior of the organism, (whereon so many physicians have hitherto ambitiously wasted their talents and their time); nor is it to attempt to give countless explanations regarding the phenomena in diseases and their proximate cause (which must ever remain concealed), wrapped in unintelligible words and an inflated abstract mode of expression, which should sound very learned in order to astonish the ignorant – whilst sick humanity sighs in vain for aid. Of such learned reveries (to which the name of theoretic medicine is given, and for which special professorships are instituted) we have had quite enough, and it is now high time that all who call themselves physicians should at length cease to deceive suffering mankind with mere talk, and begin now, instead, for once to act, that is, really to help and to cure.

§ 2

The highest ideal of cure is rapid, gentle and permanent restoration of the health, or removal and annihilation of the disease in its whole extent, in the shortest, most reliable, and most harmless way, on easily comprehensible principles.

§ 3

If the physician clearly perceives what is to be cured in diseases, that is to say, in every individual case of disease (knowledge of disease, indication), if he clearly perceives what is curative in medicines, that is to say, in each individual medicine (knowledge of medical powers), and if he knows how to adapt, according to clearly defined principles, what is curative in medicines to what he has discovered to be undoubtedly morbid in the patient, so that the recovery must ensue – to adapt it, as well in respect to the suitability of the medicine most appropriate according to its mode of action to the case before him (choice of the remedy, the medicine indicated), as also in respect to the exact mode of preparation and quantity of it required (proper dose),

and the proper period for repeating the dose; – if, finally, he knows the obstacles to recovery in each case and is aware how to remove them, so that the restoration may be permanent, then he understands how to treat judiciously and rationally, and he is a true practitioner of the healing art.

§ 4

He is likewise a preserver of health if he knows the things that derange health and cause disease, and how to remove them from persons in health.

§ 5

Useful to the physician in assisting him to cure are the particulars of the most probable exciting cause of the acute disease, as also the most significant points in the whole history of the chronic disease, to enable him to discover its fundamental cause, which is generally due to a chronic miasm. In these investigations, the ascertainable physical constitution of the patient (especially when the disease is chronic), his moral and intellectual character, his occupation, mode of living and habits, his social and domestic relations, his age, sexual function, etc., are to be taken into consideration.

§ 6 FIFTH EDITION

The unprejudiced observer – well aware of the futility of transcendental speculations which can receive no confirmation from experience – be his powers of penetration ever so great, takes note of nothing in every individual disease, except the changes in the health of the body and of the mind (morbid phenomena, accidents, symptoms) which can be perceived externally by means of the senses; that is to say, he notices only the deviations from the former healthy state of the now diseased individual, which are felt by the patient himself, remarked by those around him and observed by the physician. All these perceptible signs represent the disease in its whole extent, that is, together they form the true and only conceivable portrait of the disease.[1]

Is not, then, that which is cognizable by the senses in diseases through the phenomena it displays, the disease itself in the eyes of the physician, since he never can see the spiritual being that produces the disease, the vital force? nor is it necessary that he should see it, but only that he should ascertain its morbid actions, in order that he may thereby be enabled to cure the disease. What else will the old school search for in the hidden interior of the organism, as a prima causa morbi, whilst they reject as an object of cure and contemptuously despise the sensible and manifest representation of the disease, the symptoms, that so plainly address themselves to us? What else do they wish to cure in disease but these?[2]

1. I know not, therefore, how it was possible for physicians at the sick-bed to allow themselves to suppose that, without most carefully attending to the symptoms and being guided by them in the treatment, they ought to seek and could discover, only in the hidden and unknown interior, what there was to be cured in the disease, arrogantly and ludicrously pretending that they could, without paying much attention to the symptoms, discover the alteration that had occurred in the invisible interior, and set it to rights with (unknown!) medicines, and that such a procedure as this could alone be called radical and rational treatment.
2. The physician whose researches are directed towards the hidden relations in the interior of the organism, may daily err; but the homoeopathist who grasps with requisite carefulness the whole group of symptoms, possesses a sure guide; and if he succeed in removing the whole group of symptoms he has likewise most assuredly destroyed the internal, hidden cause of the disease.

§ 6 SIXTH EDITION

The unprejudiced observer – well aware of the futility of transcendental speculations which can receive no confirmation from experience – be his powers of penetration ever so great, takes note of nothing in every individual disease, except the changes in the health of the body and of the mind (morbid phenomena, accidents, symptoms) which can be perceived externally by means of the senses; that is to say, he notices only the deviations from the former healthy state of the now diseased individual, which are felt by the patient himself, remarked by those around him and observed by the physician. All these perceptible signs represent the disease in its whole extent, that is, together they form the true and only conceivable portrait of the disease.[1]

1. I know not, therefore, how it was possible for physicians at the sick-bed to allow themselves to suppose that, without most carefully attending to the symptoms and being guided by them in the treatment, they ought to seek and could discover, only in the hidden and unknown interior, what there was to be cured in the disease, arrogantly and ludicrously pretending that they could, without paying much attention to the symptoms, discover the alteration that had occurred in the invisible interior, and set it to rights with (unknown!) medicines, and that such a procedure as this could alone be called radical and rational treatment.

Is not, then, that which is cognizable by the senses in diseases through the phenomena it displays, the disease itself in the eyes of the physician, since he never can see the spiritual being that produces the disease, the vital force? nor is it necessary that he should see it, but only that he should ascertain its morbid actions, in order that he may thereby be enabled to cure the disease. What else will the old school search for in the hidden interior of the organism, as a prima causa morbi, whilst they reject as an object of cure and contemptuously despise the sensible and manifest representation of the disease, the symptoms, that so plainly address themselves to us? What else do they wish to cure in disease but these?

§ 7

Now, as in a disease, from which no manifest exciting or maintaining cause (causa occasionalis) has to be removed1, we can perceive nothing but the morbid symptoms, it must (regard being had to the possibility of a miasm, and attention paid to the accessory circumstances, § 5) be the symptoms alone by which the disease demands and points to the remedy suited to relieve it – and, moreover, the totality of these its symptoms, of this outwardly reflected picture of the internal essence of the disease, that is, of the affection of the vital force, must be the principal, or the sole means, whereby the disease can make known what remedy it requires – the only thing that can determine the choice of the most appropriate remedy – and thus, in a word, the totality2 of the symptoms must be the principal, indeed the only thing the physician has to take note of in every case of disease and to remove by means of his art, in order that it shall be cured and transformed into health.

§ 8

It is not conceivable, not can it be proved by any experience in the world, that, after removal of all the symptoms of the disease and of the entire collection of the perceptible phenomena, there should or could remain anything else besides health, or that the morbid alteration in the interior could remain uneradicated.[1]

1. When a patient has been cured of his disease by a true physician, in such a manner that no trace of the disease, no morbid symptom, remains, and all the signs of health have permanently returned, how can anyone, without offering an insult to common sense, affirm in such an individual the whole bodily disease still remains interior? And yet the chief of the old school, Hufeland, asserts this in the following words: "Homoeopathy can remove symptoms, but the disease remains." (Vide Homoopathie, p.27, 1, 19.) This he maintains partly from mortification at the progress made by homoeopathy to the benefits of mankind, partly because he still holds thoroughly material notions respecting disease, which he is still unable to regard as a state of being of the organism wherein it is dynamically altered by the morbidly deranged vital force, as an altered state of health, but he views the disease as a something material, which after the cure is completed, may still remain lurking in some corner in the interior of the body, in order, some day during the most vigorous health, to burst forth at its pleasure with its material presence! So dreadful is still the blindness of the old pathology! No wonder that it could only produce a system of therapeutics which is solely occupied with scouring out the poor patient.]

§ 9

In the healthy condition of man, the spiritual vital force (autocracy), the dynamis that animates the material body (organism), rules with unbounded sway, and retains all the parts of the organism in admirable, harmonious, vital operation, as regards both sensations and functions, so that our indwelling, reason-gifted mind can freely employ this living, healthy instrument for the higher purpose of our existence.

§ 10 FIFTH EDITION

The material organism, without the vital force, is capable of no sensation, no function, no self-preservation1, it derives all sensation and performs all the functions of life solely by means of the immaterial being (the vital force) which animates the material organism in health and in disease.

1. It is dead, and only subject to the power of the external physical world; it decays, and is again resolved into its chemical constituents.

§ 10 SIXTH EDITION

The material organism, without the vital force, is capable of no sensation, no function, no self-preservation1, it derives all sensation and performs all the functions of life solely by means of the immaterial being (the vital principle) which animates the material organism in health and in disease.

1. It is dead, and only subject to the power of the external physical world; it decays, and is again resolved into its chemical constituents.

§ 11 FIFTH EDITION

When a person falls ill, it is only this spiritual, self acting (automatic) vital force, everywhere present in his organism, that is primarily deranged by the dynamic1 influence upon it of a morbific agent inimical to life; it is only the vital force, deranged to such an abnormal state, that can furnish the organism with its disagreeable sensations, and incline it to the irregular processes which we call disease; for, as a power invisible in itself, and only cognizable by its effects on the organism, its morbid derangement only makes itself known by the manifestation of disease in the sensations and functions of those parts of the organism exposed to the senses of the observer and physician, that is, by morbid symptoms, and in no other way can it make itself known.

1. Materia peccans!

§ 11 SIXTH EDITION

When a person falls ill, it is only this spiritual, self acting (automatic) vital force, everywhere present in his organism, that is primarily deranged by the dynamic1 influence upon it of a

morbific agent inimical to life; it is only the vital force, deranged to such an abnormal state, that can furnish the organism with its disagreeable sensations, and incline it to the irregular processes which we call disease; for, as a power invisible in itself, and only cognizable by its effects on the organism, its morbid derangement only makes itself known by the manifestation of disease in the sensations and functions of those parts of the organism exposed to the senses of the observer and physician, that is, by morbid symptoms, and in no other way can it make itself known.2

1. Materia peccans!

2. What is dynamic influence, – dynamic power? Our earth, by virtue of a hidden invisible energy, carries the moon around her in twenty-eight days and several hours, and the moon alternately, in definite fixed hours (deducting certain differences which occur with the full and new moon) raises our northern seas to flood tide and again correspondingly lowers them to ebb. Apparently this takes place not through material agencies, not through mechanical contrivances, as are used for products of human labor; and so we see numerous other events about us as results of the action of one substance on another substance without being able to recognize a sensible connection between cause and effect. Only the cultured, practised in comparison and deduction, can form for himself a kind of supra-sensual idea sufficient to keep all that is material or mechanical in his thoughts from such concepts. He calls such effects dynamic, virtual, that is, such as result from absolute, specific, pure energy and action of he one substance upon the other substance.

For instance, the dynamic effect of the sick-making influences upon healthy man, as well as the dynamic energy of the medicines upon the principle of life in the restoration of health is nothing else than infection and so not in any way material, not in any way mechanical. Just as the energy of a magnet attracting a piece of iron or steel is not material, not mechanical. One sees that the piece of iron is attracted by one pole of the magnet, but how it is done is not seen. This invisible energy of the magnet does not require mechanical (material) auxiliary means, hook or lever, to attract the iron. The magnet draws to itself and this acts upon the piece of iron or upon a steel needle by means of a purely immaterial invisible, conceptual, inherent energy, that is, dynamically, and communicates to the steel needle the magnetic energy equally invisibly (dynamically). The steel needle becomes itself magnetic, even at a distance when the magnet does not touch it, and magnetises other steel needles with the same magnetic property (dynamically) with which it had been endowed previously by the magnetic rod, just as a child with small-pox or measles communicates to a near, untouched healthy child in an invisible manner (dynamically) the small-pox or measles, that is, infects it at a distance without anything material from the infective child going or capable of going to the one to be infected. A purely specific conceptual influence communicated to the near child small-pox or measles in the same way as the magnet communicated to the near needle the magnetic property.

In a similar way, the effect of medicines upon living man is to be judged. Substances, which are used as medicines, are medicines only in so far as they possess each its own specific energy to alter the well-being of man through dynamic, conceptual influence, by means of the living sensory fibre, upon the conceptual controlling principle of life. The medicinal property of those material substances which we call medicines proper, relates only to their energy to call out alterations in the well-being of animal life. Only upon this conceptual principle of life, depends their medicinal health-altering, conceptual (dynamic) influence. Just as the nearness of a magnetic pole can communicate only magnetic energy to the steel (namely, by a kind of infection) but cannot communicate other properties (for instance, more hardness or ductility, etc.). And thus every special medicinal substance alters through a kind of infection, that well-being of man in a peculiar manner exclusively its own and not in a manner peculiar to another medicine, as certainly as the nearness of the child ill with small-pox will communicate to a healthy child only small-pox and not measles. These medicines act upon our well-being wholly without communication of material parts of the medicinal substances, thus dynamically, as if through infection. Far more healing energy is expressed in a case in point by the smallest dose of the best dynamized medicines, in which there can be, according to calculation, only so little of material substance that its minuteness cannot be thought and conceived by the best arithmetical mind, than by large doses of the same medicine in substance. That smallest dose can therefore contain almost entirely only the pure, freely-developed, conceptual medicinal energy, and bring about only dynamically such great effects as can never be reached by the crude medicinal substances itself taken in large doses.

It is not in the corporal atoms of these highly dynamized medicines, nor their physical or mathematical surfaces (with which the higher energies of the dynamized medicines are being interpreted but vainly as still sufficiently material) that the medicinal energy is found. More likely, there lies invisible in the moistened globule or in its solution, an unveiled, liberated, specific, medicinal force contained in the medicinal substance which acts dynamically by contact with the living animal fibre upon the whole organism (without communicating to it anything material however highly attenuated) and acts more strongly the more free and more immaterial the energy has become through the dynamization.

Is it then so utterly impossible for our age celebrated for its wealth in clear thinkers to think of dynamic energy as something non-corporeal, since we see daily phenomena which cannot be explained in any other manner? If one looks upon something nauseous and becomes inclined to vomit, did a material emetic come into his stomach which compels him to this anti-peristaltic movement? Was it not solely the dynamic effect of the nauseating aspect upon his imagination? And if one raises his arm, does it occur through a material visible instrument? a lever? Is it not solely the conceptual dynamic energy of his will which raises it?

§ 12 FIFTH EDITION

It is the morbidly affected vital force alone that produces disease1, so that the morbid phenomena perceptible to our senses express at the same time all the internal change, that is to say, the whole morbid derangement of the internal dynamis; in a word, they reveal the whole disease; consequently, also, the disappearance under treatment of all the morbid phenomena and of all the morbid alterations that differ from the healthy vital operations, certainly affects and necessarily implies the restoration of the integrity of the vital force and, therefore, the recovered health of the whole organism.

1. How the vital force causes the organism to display morbid phenomena, that is, how it produces disease, it would be of no practical utility to the physician to know, and will forever remain concealed from him; only what it is necessary for him to know of the disease and what is fully sufficient for enabling him to cure it, has the Lord of life revealed to his senses

§ 12 SIXTH EDITION

It is the morbidly affected vital energy alone that produces disease1, so that the morbid phenomena perceptible to our senses express at the same time all the internal change, that is to say, the whole morbid derangement of the internal dynamis; in a word, they reveal the whole disease; consequently, also, the disappearance under treatment of all the morbid phenomena and of all the morbid alterations that differ from the healthy vital operations, certainly affects and necessarily implies the restoration of the integrity of the vital force and, therefore, the recovered health of the whole organism.

1. How the vital force causes the organism to display morbid phenomena, that is, how it produces disease, it would be of no practical utility to the physician to know, and will forever remain concealed from him; only what it is necessary for him to know of the disease and what is fully sufficient for enabling him to cure it, has the Lord of life revealed to his senses

§ 13

Therefore disease (that does not come within the province of manual surgery) considered, as it is by the allopathists, as a thing separate from the living whole, from the organism and its animating vital force, and hidden in the interior, be it ever so subtle a character, is an absurdity, that could only be imagined by minds of a materialistic stamp, and has for thousands of years given to the prevailing system of medicine all those pernicious impulses that have made it a truly mischievous (non-healing) art.

§ 14

There is, in the interior of man, nothing morbid that is curable and no invisible morbid alteration that is curable which does not make itself known to the accurately observing physicians by means of morbid signs and symptoms – an arrangement in perfect conformity with the infinite goodness of the all-wise Preserver of human life.

§ 15 FIFTH EDITION

The affection of the morbidly deranged, spirit-like dynamis (vital force) that animates our body in the invisible interior, and the totality of the outwardly cognizable symptoms produced by it in the organism and representing the existing malady, constitute a whole; they are one and the same. The organism is indeed the material instrument of the life, but it is not conceivable without the animation imparted to it by the instinctively perceiving and regulating vital force (just as the vital force is not conceivable without the organism), consequently the two together constitute a unity, although in thought our mind separates this unity into two distinct conceptions for the sake of facilitating the comprehension of it.

§ 15 SIXTH EDITION

The affection of the morbidly deranged, spirit-like dynamis (vital force) that animates our body in the invisible interior, and the totality of the outwardly cognizable symptoms produced by it in the organism and representing the existing malady, constitute a whole; they are one and the same. The organism is indeed the material instrument of the life, but it is not conceivable without the animation imparted to it by the instinctively perceiving and regulating dynamis, just as the vital force is not conceivable without the organism, consequently the two together constitute a unity, although in thought our mind separates this unity into two distinct conceptions for the sake of easy comprehension.

§ 16 FIFTH EDITION

Our vital force, as a spirit-like dynamis, cannot be attacked and affected by injurious influences on the healthy organism caused by the external inimical forces that disturb the harmonious play of life, otherwise than in a spirit-like (dynamic) way, and in like manner, all such morbid derangements (diseases) cannot be removed from it by the physician in any other way than by the spirit-like (dynamic1, virtual) alterative powers of the serviceable medicines acting upon our spirit-like vital force, which perceives them through the medium of the sentient faculty of the nerves everywhere present in the organism, so that it is only by their dynamic action on the vital force that remedies are able to re-establish and do actually re-establish health and vital harmony, after the changes in the health of the patient cognizable by our senses (the totality of the symptoms) have revealed the disease to the carefully observing and investigating physician as fully as was requisite in order to enable him to cure it.

1. Most severe disease may be produced by sufficient disturbance of the vital force through the imagination and also cured by the same means.

§ 16 SIXTH EDITION

Our vital force, as a spirit-like dynamis, cannot be attacked and affected by injurious influences on the healthy organism caused by the external inimical forces that disturb the harmonious play of life, otherwise than in a spirit-like (dynamic) way, and in like manner, all such morbid derangements (diseases) cannot be removed from it by the physician in any other way than by the spirit-like (dynamic1, virtual) alterative powers of the serviceable medicines acting upon our spirit-like vital force, which perceives them through the medium of the sentient faculty of the nerves everywhere present in the organism, so that it is only by their dynamic action on the vital force that remedies are able to re-establish and do actually re-establish health and vital harmony, after the changes in the health of the patient cognizable by our senses (the totality of the symptoms) have revealed the disease to the carefully observing and investigating physician as fully as was requisite in order to enable him to cure it.

1. Most severe disease may be produced by sufficient disturbance of the vital force through the imagination and also cured by the same means.

§ 17 FIFTH EDITION

Now, as in the cure effected by the removal of the whole of the perceptible signs and symptoms of the disease the internal alteration of the vital force to which the disease is due – consequently the whole of the disease – is at the same time removed,1 it follows that the physician has only to remove the whole of the symptoms in order, at the same time, to abrogate and annihilate the internal change, that is to say, the morbid derangement of the vital force – consequently the totality of the disease, the disease itself.2 But when the disease is annihilated the health is restored, and this is the highest, the sole aim of the physician who knows the true object of his mission, which consists not in learned – sounding prating, but in giving aid to the sick.

1. A warning dream, a superstitious fancy, or a solemn prediction that death would occur at a certain day or at a certain hour, has not unfrequently produced all the signs of commencing and increasing disease, of approaching death and death itself at the hour announced, which could not happen without the simultaneous production of the inward change (corresponding to the state observed internally); and hence in such cases all the morbid signs indicative of approaching death have frequently been dissipated by an identical cause, by some cunning deception or persuasion to a belief in the contrary, and health suddenly restored, which could not have happened without the removal, by means of this mortal remedy, of the internal and external morbid change that threatened death.
2. It is only thus that God the preserver of mankind, could reveal His wisdom and goodness in reference to the cure of the disease to which man is liable here below, by showing to the physician what he had to remove in disease in order to annihilate them and thus re-establish health. But what would we think of His wisdom and goodness if He has shrouded in mysterious obscurity that which was to be cured in diseases (as is asserted by the dominant school of medicine, which affects to possess a supernatural insight into the nature of things), and shut it up in the hidden interior, and thus rendered it impossible for man to know the malady accurately, consequently impossible for him to cure it?

§ 17 SIXTH EDITION

Now, as in the cure effected by the removal of the whole of the perceptible signs and symptoms of the disease the internal alteration of the vital principle to which the disease is due – consequently the whole of the disease – is at the same time removed,1 it follows that the physician has only to remove the whole of the symptoms in order, at the same time, to abrogate and annihilate the internal change, that is to say, the morbid derangement of the vital force – consequently the totality of the disease, the disease itself.2 But when the disease is annihilated the health is restored, and this is the highest, the sole aim of the physician who knows the true object of his mission, which consists not in learned – sounding prating, but in giving aid to the sick.

1. A warning dream, a superstitious fancy, or a solemn prediction that death would occur at a certain day or at a certain hour, has not unfrequently produced all the signs of commencing and increasing disease, of approaching death and death itself at the hour announced, which could not happen without the simultaneous production of the inward change (corresponding to the state observed internally); and hence in such cases all the morbid signs indicative of approaching death have frequently been dissipated by an identical cause, by some cunning deception or persuasion to a belief in the contrary, and health suddenly restored, which could not have happened without the removal, by means of this mortal remedy, of the internal and external morbid change that threatened death.
2. It is only thus that God the preserver of mankind, could reveal His wisdom and goodness in reference to the cure of the disease to which man is liable here below, by showing to the physician what he had to remove in disease in order to annihilate them and thus re-establish health. But what would we think of His wisdom and goodness if He has shrouded in mysterious obscurity that which was to be cured in diseases (as is asserted by the dominant school of medicine, which affects to possess a supernatural insight into the nature of things), and shut it up in the hidden interior, and thus rendered it impossible for man to know the malady accurately, consequently impossible for him to cure it?

§ 18 FIFTH EDITION

From this indubitable truth, that besides the totality of the symptoms nothing can by any means be discovered in disease wherewith they could express their need of aid, it follows undeniably that the sum of all the symptoms in each individual case of disease must be the sole indication, the sole guide to direct us in the choice of a remedy.

§ 18 SIXTH EDITION

From this indubitable truth, that besides the totality of the symptoms with consideration of the accompanying modalities (§ 5) nothing can by any means be discovered in disease wherewith they could express their need of aid, it follows undeniably that the sum of all the symptoms and conditions in each individual case of disease must be the sole indication, the sole guide to direct us in the choice of a remedy.

§ 19

Now, as diseases are nothing more than alterations in the state of health of the healthy individual which express themselves by morbid signs, and the cure is also only possible by a change to the healthy condition of the state of health of the diseased individual, it is very evident that medicines could never cure disease if they did not possess the power of altering man's state of health which depends on sensations and functions; indeed, that their curative power must be owing solely to this power they possess of altering man's state of health.

§ 20 FIFTH EDITION

This spirit-like power to alter man's state of health (and hence to cure diseases) which lies hidden in the inner nature of medicines can never be discovered by us by a mere effort of reason; it is only by experience of the phenomena it displays when acting on the state of health of man that we can become clearly cognizant of it.

§ 20 SIXTH EDITION

This spirit-like power to alter man's state of health (and hence to cure diseases) which lies hidden in the inner nature of medicines can in itself never be discovered by us by a mere effort of reason; it is only by experience of the phenomena it displays when acting on the state of health of man that we can become clearly cognizant of it.

§ 21

Now, as it is undeniable that the curative principle in medicines is not in itself perceptible, and as in pure experiments with medicines conducted by the most accurate observers, nothing can be observed that can constitute them medicines or remedies except that power of causing distinct alterations in the state of health of the human body, and particularly in that of the healthy individual, and of exciting in him various definite morbid symptoms; so it follows that when medicines act as remedies, they can only bring their curative property into play by means of this their power of altering man's state of health by the production of peculiar symptoms; and that, therefore, we have only to rely on the morbid phenomena which the medicines produce in the healthy body as the sole possible revelation of their in-dwelling curative power, in order to learn what disease-producing power, and at the same time what disease-curing power, each individual medicine possesses.

§ 22 FIFTH EDITION

But as nothing is to be observed in diseases that must be removed in order to change them into health besides the totality of their signs and symptoms, and likewise medicines can show nothing curative besides their tendency to produce morbid symptoms in healthy persons and to remove them in diseased persons; it follows, on the one hand, that medicines only become remedies and capable of annihilating disease, because the medicinal substance, by exciting certain effects and symptoms, that is to say, by producing a certain artificial morbid state, removes and abrogates the symptoms already present, to wit, the natural morbid state we wish to cure. On the other hand, it follows that, for the totality of the symptoms of the disease to be cured, a medicine must be sought which (according as experience shall prove whether the morbid symptoms are most readily, certainly, and permanently removed and changed into health by similar or opposite medicinal symptoms1) has a tendency to produce similar or opposite symptoms.

1. The other possible mode of employing medicines for diseases besides these two is the allopathic method, in which medicines are given, whose symptoms have no direct pathological relation to the morbid state, neither similar nor opposite, but quite heterogeneous to the symptoms of the disease, is, as shown above, in the introduction (Review of the therapeutics, allopathy and palliative treatment that have hitherto been practiced in the old school of medicine), merely instinctive vital force, which, when made ill by noxious agents, strives to save itself at whatever sacrifice by the production and continuance of morbid irritation in the organism – an imitation, consequently, of the crude vital force which was implanted in our organism in order to preserve our life in health, in the most beautiful harmony; but when deranged by disease, was so constituted as to admit of being again changed to health (homoeopathically) by the intelligent physician, but not to cure itself, for which the little power it possesses is so far from being a pattern to be copied, that all the changes and symptoms it produces in the (morbidly deranged) organism are just the disease itself. But this injudicious system of therapeutics of the old school of medicine can no more be passed by unnoticed that can history omit to record the thousands of years of opposition to which mankind has been subjected under the irrational, despotic Governments.

§ 22 SIXTH EDITION

But as nothing is to be observed in diseases that must be removed in order to change them into health besides the totality of their signs and symptoms, and likewise medicines can show nothing curative besides their tendency to produce morbid symptoms in healthy persons and to remove them in diseased persons; it follows, on the one hand, that medicines only become remedies and capable of annihilating disease, because the medicinal substance, by exciting certain effects and symptoms, that is to say, by producing a certain artificial morbid state, removes and abrogates the symptoms already present, to wit, the natural morbid state we wish to cure. On the other hand, it follows that, for the totality of the symptoms of the disease to be cured, a medicine must be sought which (according as experience shall prove whether the morbid symptoms are most

readily, certainly, and permanently removed and changed into health by similar or opposite medicinal symptoms1) have the greatest tendency to produce similar or opposite symptoms.**

1. The other possible mode of employing medicines for diseases besides these two is the allopathic method, in which medicines are given, whose symptoms have no direct pathological relation to the morbid state, neither similar nor opposite, but quite heterogeneous to the symptoms of the disease. This procedure plays, as I have shown elsewhere, an irresponsible murderous game with the life of the patient by means of dangerous, violent medicines, whose action is unknown and which are chosen on mere conjectures and given in large and frequent doses. Again, by means of painful operations, intended to lead the disease to other regions and taking the strength and vital juices of the patient, through evacuations above and below, sweat or salivation, but especially through squandering the irreplaceable blood, as is done by the reigning routine practice, used blindly and relentlessly, usually with the pretext that the physician should imitate and further the sick nature in its efforts to help itself, without considering how irrational it is, to imitate and further these very imperfect, mostly inappropriate efforts of the instinctive unintelligent vital energy which is implanted in our organism, so long as it is healthy to carry on life in harmonious development, but not to heal itself in disease. For, were it possessed of such a model ability, it would never have allowed the organism to get sick. When made ill by noxious agents, our life principle cannot do anything else than express its depression caused by disturbance of the regularity of its life, by symptoms, by means of which the intelligent physician is ask for aid. If this is not given, it strives to save by increasing the ailment, especially through violent evacuations, no matter what this entails, often with the largest sacrifices or destruction of life itself.

For the purpose of cure, the morbidly depressed vital energy possesses so little ability worthy of imitation since all changes and symptoms produced by it in the organism are the disease itself. What intelligent physician would want to imitate it with the intention to heal if he did not thereby sacrifice his patient?

§ 23

All pure experience, however, and all accurate research convince us that persistent symptoms of disease are far from being removed and annihilated by opposite symptoms of medicines (as in the antipathic, enantiopathic or palliative method), that, on the contrary, after transient, apparent alleviation, they break forth again, only with increased intensity, and become manifestly aggravated (see § 58 – 62 and 69).

§ 24

There remains, therefore, no other mode of employing medicines in diseases that promises to be of service besides the homoeopathic, by means of which we seek, for the totality of the symptoms of the case of disease, a medicine which among all medicines (whose pathogenetic effects are

known from having been tested in healthy individuals) has the power and the tendency to produce an artificial morbid state most similar to that of the case of disease in question.

§ 25

Now, however, in all careful trials, pure experience,1 the sole and infallible oracle of the healing art, teaches us that actually that medicine which, in its action on the healthy human body, has demonstrated its power of producing the greatest number of symptoms similar to those observable in the case of disease under treatment, does also, in doses of suitable potency and attenuation, rapidly, radically and permanently remove the totality of the symptoms of this morbid state, that is to say (§ 6 – 16), the whole disease present, and change it into health; and that all medicines cure, without exception, those diseases whose symptoms most nearly resemble their own, and leave none of them uncured.

1. I do not mean that sort of experience of which the ordinary practitioners of the old school boast, after they have for years worked away with a lot of complex prescriptions on a number of diseases which they never carefully investigate, but which, faithful to their school, they consider as already described in works of systematic pathology, and dreamed that they could detect in them some imaginary morbific matter, or ascribe to them some other hypothetical internal abnormality. They always saw something in them, but knew not what it was they saw, and they got results, from the complex forces acting on an unknown object, that no human being but only a God could have unravelled – results from which nothing can be learned, no experience gained. Fifty years' experience of this sort is like fifty years of looking into a kaleidoscope filled with unknown colored objects, and perpetually turning round; thousands of ever changing figures and no accounting for them!

§ 26

This depends on the following homoeopathic law of nature which was sometimes, indeed, vaguely surmised but not hitherto fully recognized, and to which is due every real cure that has ever taken place:

A weaker dynamic affection is permanently extinguished in the living organism by a stronger one, if the latter (whilst differing in kind) is very similar to the former in its manifestations.1

1. Thus are cured both physical affections and moral maladies. How is it that in the early dawn the brilliant Jupiter vanishes from the gaze of the beholder? By a stronger very similar power acting on his optic nerve, the brightness of approaching day! – In situations replete with foetid odors, wherewith is it usual to soothe effectually the offended olfactory nerves? With snuff, that affects the sense of smell in a similar but stronger manner! No music, no sugared cake, which act on the nerves of other senses, can cure this olfactory disgust. How does the soldier cunningly stifle the piteous cries of him who runs the gauntlet from the ears of the compassionate bystanders? By the

shrill notes of the fife commingled with the roll of the noisy drum! And the distant roar of the enemy's cannon that inspires his army with fear? By the loud boom of the big drum! For neither the one nor the other would the distribution of a brilliant piece of uniform nor a reprimand to the regiment suffice. In like manner, mourning and sorrow will be effaced from the mind by the account of another and still greater cause for sorrow happening to another, even though it be a mere fiction. The injurious consequences of too great joy will be removed by drinking coffee, which produces an excessive joyous state of mind. Nations like the Germans, who have for centuries been gradually sinking deeper and deeper in soulless apathy and degrading serfdom, must first be trodden still deeper in the dust by the Western Conqueror, until their situation became intolerable; their mean opinion of themselves was thereby over-strained and removed; they again became alive to their dignity as men, and then, for the first time, they raised their heads as Germans.

§ 27

The curative power of medicines, therefore, depends on their symptoms, similar to the disease but superior to it in strength (§ 12 – 26), so that each individual case of disease is most surely, radically, rapidly and permanently annihilated and removed only by a medicine capable of producing (in the human system) in the most similar and complete manner the totality of its symptoms, which at the same time are stronger than the disease.

§ 28

As this natural law of cure manifests itself in every pure experiment and every true observation in the world, the fact is consequently established; it matters little what may be scientific explanation of how it takes place; and I do not attach much importance to the attempts made to explain it. But the following view seems to commend itself as the most probable one, as it is founded on premises derived from experience.

§ 29 FIFTH EDITION

As every disease (not strictly belonging to the domain of surgery) depends only on a peculiar morbid derangement of our vital force in sensations and functions, when a homoeopathic cure of the vital force deranged by natural disease is accomplished by the administration of a medicinal agent selected on account of an accurate similarity of symptoms, a somewhat stronger, similar, artificial morbid affection is brought into contact with and, as it were, pushed into the place of the weaker, similar, natural morbid irritation, against which the instinctive vital force, now merely (though in a stronger degree) medicinally diseased, is then compelled to direct an increased amount of energy, but, on account of the shorter duration of the action1 of the medicinal agent that now morbidly affects it, the vital force soon overcomes this, and as it was in the first instance relieved from the natural morbid affection, so it is now at last freed from the substituted artificial (medicinal) one, and hence is enable again to carry on healthily the vital operations of the organism. This highly probable explanation of the process rests on the following axioms.

1. The short duration of the action of the artificial morbific forces, which we term medicines, makes it possible that, although they are stronger than the natural diseases, they can yet be much more easily overcome by the vital force than can the weaker natural diseases, which solely in consequence of the longer, generally lifelong, duration of their action (psora, syphilis, sycosis), can never be vanquished and extinguished by it alone, until the physician affects the vital force in a stronger manner by an agent that produces a disease very similar, but stronger to wit a homoeopathic medicine, which, when taken (or smelt), is as it were, forced upon the unintelligent, instinctive vital force, and substituted in the place of the former natural morbid affection, by which means the vital force, and substituted in the place of the former natural morbid affection, by which means the vital force then remains merely medicinally ill, but only for a short time, because the action of the medicine (the time in which the medicinal disease excited by it run its course) does not last long. The cures of diseases of many years' duration (§ 46), by the occurrence of smallpox and measles (both of which run a course of only a few weeks), are processes of a similar character.

§ 29 SIXTH EDITION

As every disease (not entirely surgical) consists only in a special, morbid, dynamic alteration of our vital energy (of the principle of life) manifested in sensation and motion, so in every homoeopathic cure this principle of life dynamically altered by natural disease is seized through the administration of medicinal potency selected exactly according to symptom-similarity by a somewhat stronger, similar artificial disease-manifestation. By this the feeling of the natural (weaker) dynamic disease-manifestation ceases and disappears. This disease-manifestation no longer exists for the principle of life which is now occupied and governed merely by the stronger, artificial disease-manifestation. This artificial disease-manifestation has soon spent its force and leaves the patient free from disease, cured. The dynamis, thus freed, can now continue to carry life on in health. This most highly probable process rests upon the following propositions.

§ 30 FIFTH EDITION

The human body appears to admit of being much more powerfully affected in its health by medicines (partly because we have the regulation of the dose in our own power) than by natural morbid stimuli – for natural diseases are cured and overcome by suitable medicines.

§ 30 SIXTH EDITION

The human body appears to admit of being much more powerfully affected in its health by medicines (partly because we have the regulation of the dose in our own power) than by natural morbid stimuli – for natural diseases are cured and overcome by suitable medicines.1

1. The short duration of the action of the artificial morbific forces, which we term medicines, makes it possible that, although they are stronger than the natural diseases, they can yet be much more easily overcome by the vital force than can the weaker natural diseases, which solely in consequence of the longer, generally lifelong, duration of their action (psora, syphilis, sycosis), can never be vanquished and extinguished by it alone, until the physician affects the vital force in a stronger manner by an agent that produces a disease very similar, but stronger to wit a homoeopathic medicine. The cures of diseases of many years' duration (§ 46), by the occurrence of smallpox and measles (both of which run a course of only a few weeks), are processes of a similar character.

§ 31

The inimical forces, partly psychical, partly physical, to which our terrestrial existence is exposed, which are termed morbific noxious agents, do not possess the power of morbidly deranging the health of man unconditionally1; but we are made ill by them only when our organism is sufficiently disposed and susceptible to attack of the morbific cause that may be present, and to be altered in its health, deranged and made to undergo abnormal sensations and functions – hence they do not produce disease in every one nor at all times.

1. When I call a disease a derangement of man's state of health, I am far from wishing thereby to give a hyperphysical explanation of the internal nature of disease generally, or of any case of disease in particular. It is only intended by this expression to intimate, what it can be proved diseases are not and cannot be, that they are not mechanical or chemical alterations of material substance of the body, and not dependant on a material morbific substance, but that they are merely spirit-like (conceptual) dynamic derangements of the life.

§ 32

But it is quite otherwise with the artificial morbific agents which we term medicines. Every real medicine, namely, acts at all times, under all circumstances, on every living human being, and produces in him its peculiar symptoms (distinctly perceptible, if the dose be large enough), so that evidently every living human organism is liable to be affected, and, as it were, inoculated with the medicinal disease at all times, and absolutely (unconditionally), which, as before said, is by no means the case with the natural diseases.

§ 33

In accordance with this fact, it is undeniably shown by all experience1 that the living organism is much more disposed and has a greater liability to be acted on, and to have its health deranged by medicinal powers, than by morbific noxious agents and infectious miasms, or, in order words, that the morbific noxious agents possess a power of morbidly deranging man's health that is subordinate and conditional, often very conditional; whilst medicinal agents have an absolute unconditional power, greatly superior to the former.

1. A striking fact in corroboration of this is, that whilst previously to the year 1801, when the smooth scarlatina of Sydenham still occasionally prevailed epidemically among children, it attacked without exception all children who had escaped it in a former epidemic; in a similar epidemic which I witnessed in Konigslutter, on the contrary, all the children who took in time a very small dose of belladonna remained unaffected by this highly infectious infantile disease. If medicines can protect from a disease that is raging around, they must possess a vastly superior power of affecting our vital force.

§ 34 FIFTH EDITION

The greater strength of the artificial diseases producible by medicines is, however, not the sole cause of their power to cure natural disease. In order that they may effect a cure, it is before all things requisite that they should be capable of producing in the human body an artificial disease as similar as possible to the disease to be cured, in order, by means of this similarity, conjoined with its somewhat greater strength, to substitute themselves for the natural morbid affection, and thereby deprive the latter of all influence upon the vital force. This is so true, that no previously existing disease can be cured, even by Nature herself, by the accession of a new dissimilar disease, be it ever so strong, and just as little can it be cured by medical treatment with drugs which are incapable of producing a similar morbid condition in the healthy body.

§ 34 SIXTH EDITION

The greater strength of the artificial diseases producible by medicines is, however, not the sole cause of their power to cure natural disease. In order that they may effect a cure, it is before all things requisite that they should be capable of producing in the human body an artificial disease as similar as possible to the disease to be cured, which, with somewhat increased power, transforms to a very similar morbid state the instinctive life principle, which in itself is incapable of any reflection or act of memory. It not only obscures, but extinguishes and thereby annihilates the derangement caused by the natural disease. This is so true, that no previously existing disease can be cured, even by Nature herself, by the accession of a new dissimilar disease, be it ever so strong, and just as little can it be cured by medical treatment with drugs which are incapable of producing a similar morbid condition in the healthy body.

§ 35

In order to illustrate this, we shall consider in three different cases, as well what happens in nature when two dissimilar natural diseases meet to in one person, as also the result of the ordinary medical treatment of diseases with unsuitable allopathic drugs, which are incapable of producing an artificial morbid condition similar to the disease to be cured, whereby it will appear that even Nature herself is unable to remove a dissimilar disease already present by one that is unhomoeopathic, even though it be stronger, and just as little is the unhomoeopathic employment of even the strongest medicines ever capable of curing any disease whatsoever.

§ 36

I. If the two dissimilar diseases meeting together in the human being be of equal strength, or still more if the older one be the stronger, the new disease will be repelled by the old one from the body and not allowed to affect it. A patient suffering from a severe chronic disease will not be infected by a moderate autumnal dysentery or other epidemic disease. The plague of the Levant, according to Larry,1 does not break out where scurvy is prevalent, and persons suffering from eczema are not infected by it. Rachitis, Jenner alleges, prevents vaccination from taking effect. Those suffering from pulmonary consumption are not liable to be attacked by epidemic fevers of a not very violent character, according to Von Hildenbrand.

1. "Memoires et Observations," in the Description de l' Egpte, tom. i.

§ 37 FIFTH EDITION

So, also under ordinary medical treatment, an old chronic disease remains uncured and unaltered if it is treated according to the common allopathic method, that is to say, with medicines that are incapable of producing in healthy individuals a state of health similar to the disease, even though the treatment should last for years and is not of too violent character. This is daily witnessed in practice, it is therefore unnecessary to give any illustrative examples.

§ 37 SIXTH EDITION

So, also under ordinary medical treatment, an old chronic disease remains uncured and unaltered if it is treated according to the common allopathic method, that is to say, with medicines that are incapable of producing in healthy individuals a state of health similar to the disease, even though the treatment should last for years and is not of too violent character.1 This is daily witnessed in practice, it is therefore unnecessary to give any illustrative examples.

1. But if treated with violent allopathic remedies, other diseases will be formed in its place which are more difficult and dangerous to life.

§ 38

II. Or the new dissimilar disease is the stronger. In this case the disease under which the patient originally labored, being the weaker, will be kept back and suspended by the accession of the stronger one, until the latter shall have run its course or been cured, and then the old one reappears uncured. Two children affected with a kind of epilepsy remained free from epileptic attacks after infection with ringworm (tinea) but as soon as the eruption on the head was gone the epilepsy returned just as before, as Tulpius1 observed. The itch, as Schopf2 saw, disappeared on the occurrence of the scurvy, but after the cure of the latter it again broke out. So, also the pulmonary phthisis remained stationary when the patient was attacked by a violent typhus, but went on again after the latter had run its course.3 If mania occur in a consumptive patient, the phthisis with all its symptoms is removed by the former; but if that go off, the phthisis returns immediately and proves fatal.4 When measles and smallpox are prevalent at the same time, and both attack the same child, the measles that had already broken out is generally checked by the smallpox that came somewhat later; nor does the measles resume its course until after the cure of the smallpox; but it not infrequently happens that the inoculated smallpox is suspended for four days by the supervention of the measles, as observed by Manget,5 after the desquamation of which the smallpox completes its course. Even when the inoculation of the smallpox had taken effect for six days, and the measles then broke out, the inflammation of the inoculation remained stationary and the smallpox did not ensue until the measles had completed its regular course of seven days.6 In an epidemic of measles, that disease attacked many individuals on the fourth or fifth day after the inoculation of smallpox and prevented the development of the smallpox until it had completed its own course, whereupon the smallpox appeared and proceeded regularly to its termination.7 The true, smooth, erysipelatous-looking scarlatina of Sydenham, with sore throat, was checked on the fourth day by the eruption of cow-pox, which ran its regular course, and not till it was ended did the scarlatina again establish itself; but on another occasion, as both diseases seem to be of equal strength, the cow-pox was suspended on the eighth day by the supervention of the true, smooth scarlatina of Sydenham,8 and the red areola of the former disappeared until the scarlatina was gone, wherein the cow-pox immediately resumed its course, and went on its regular termination.9 The measles suspended the cow-pox; on the eighth day, when the cow-pox had nearly attained its climax, the measles broke out; the cow-pox now remained stationary, and did not resume and complete its course until the desquamation of the measles, had taken place, so that on the sixteenth day it presented the appearance it otherwise would have shown on the tenth day, as Kortum10 observed.

Even after the measles had broken out the cow-pox inoculation took effect, but did not run its course until these measles had disappeared, as Kortum likewise witnessed.11

I myself saw the mumps (angina parotidea) immediately disappear when the cow-pox inoculation had taken effect and had nearly attained its height; it was not until the complete termination of the cow-pox and the disappearance of its red areola that this febrile tumefaction of the parotid and submaxillary glands, that is caused by a peculiar miasm, reappeared and ran its regular course of seven days.

And thus it is with all dissimilar disease; the stronger suspends the weaker (when they do not complicate one another, which is seldom the case with acute disease), but they never cure one another.

1. Obs., lib. I, obs. 8.
2. In Hufeland's Journal, xv, 2.
3. Chevalier, in Hufeland's Neuesten Annalen der franzosichen Heikunde, ii, p.192.
4. Mania phthisi superveniens eam cum omnibus suis phaenomenis auffert, verum mox redit phthisis et occidit, abeunte mania. Reil Memorab., fasc. iii, v, p.171.
5. In the Edinb. Med. Comment., pt. i, 1.
6. John Hunter, On the veneral Disease, p.5.
7. Rainey, in the Edinb. Med. Comment., iii, p.480.
8. Very accurately described by Withering and Plenciz, but differing greatly from the purpura (or Roodvonk), which is often erroneously denominated scarlet fever. It is only of late year that the two, which were originally very different diseases, have come to resemble each other in their symptoms.
9. Jenner, in Medicinische Annalen, August, 1800, p.747.
10. In Hufeland's Journal der praktischen Arzneikunde, xx, 3, p.50.
11. Loc. cit.

§ 39

Now the adherents of the ordinary school of medicine saw all this for so many centuries; they saw that Nature herself cannot cure any disease by the accession of another, be it ever so strong, if the new disease be dissimilar to that already present in the body. What shall we think of them, that they nevertheless went on treating chronic disease with allopathic remedies, namely, with medicines and prescriptions capable of producing God knows what morbid state – almost invariably, however, one dissimilar to the disease to be cured? And even though physicians did not hitherto observe nature attentively, the miserable results of their treatment should have taught them that they were pursuing an inappropriate, a false path. Did they not perceive when they employed, as was their custom, and aggressive allopathic treatment in a chronic disease, that thereby they only created an artificial disease dissimilar to the original one, which, as long as it was kept up, merely held in abeyance, merely suppressed, merely suspended the original disease, which latter, however, always returned, and must return, as soon as the diminished strength of the patient no longer admitted of a continuance of the allopathic attacks on the life? Thus the itch exanthema certainly disappears very soon from the skin under the employment of violent purgatives, frequently repeated; but when the patient can no longer stand the factitious (dissimilar) disease of the bowels, and can take no more purgatives, then either the cutaneous eruption breaks out as before, or the internal psora displays itself in some bad symptom, and the patient, in addition to his undiminished original disease, has to endure the misery of a painful ruined digestion and impaired strength to boot. So, also, when the ordinary physicians keep up artificial ulcerations of the skin and issues on the exterior of the body, with the view of thereby eradicating a chronic disease, they can NEVER cure them by that means, as such artificial cutaneous ulcers are quite alien and allopathic to the internal affection; but inasmuch as the irritation produced by several tissues is at least sometimes a stronger (dissimilar) disease than the indwelling malady, the latter is thereby sometimes silenced and suspended for a week or two. But it is only suspended, and that for a very short time, while the patient's powers are gradually worn out. Epilepsy, suppressed for many years by means of issues, invariably recurred, and in an aggravated form, when they were allowed to heal up, as Pechlin[1] and others testify. But purgatives for itch, and issues for epilepsy, cannot be more heterogeneous, more dissimilar deranging agents – cannot be more allopathic, more exhausting modes of treatment – than are the customary prescriptions, composed of unknown ingredients, used in ordinary practice for the other nameless, innumerable forms of disease. These likewise do nothing but debilitate, and only suppress or suspend the malady for a short time without being able to cure it, and when used for a long time always add a new morbid state to the old disease.

1. Obs. phys. med., lib. ii, obs, 30.

§ 40

III. Or the new disease, after having long acted on the organism, at length joins the old one that is dissimilar to it, and forms with it a complex disease, so that each of them occupies a particular locality in the organism, namely, the organs peculiarly adapted for it, and, as it were, only the place specially belonging to it, while it leaves the rest to the other disease that is dissimilar to it. Thus a syphilitic patient may become psoric, and vice versa. As two disease dissimilar to each other, they cannot remove, cannot cure one another. At first the venereal symptoms are kept in abeyance and suspended when the psoric eruption begins to appear; in course of time, however (as the syphilis is at least as strong as the psora), the two join together,[1] that is, each involves those parts of the organism only which are most adapted for it, and the patient is thereby rendered more diseased and more difficult to cure.

When two dissimilar acute infectious diseases meet, as, for example, smallpox and measles, the one usually suspends the other, as has been before observed; yet there have also been severe epidemics of this kind, where, in rare cases, two dissimilar acute diseases occurred simultaneously in one and the same body, and for a short time combined, as it were, with each other. During an epidemic, in which smallpox and measles were prevalent at the same time, among three hundred cases (in which these diseases avoided or suspended one another, and measles attacked patients twenty days after the smallpox broke out, the smallpox, however, from seventeen to eighteen days after the appearance of the measles, so that the first disease had previously completed its regular course) there was yet one single case in which P. Russell[2] met with both these dissimilar diseases in one person at the same time. Rainey3 witnessed the simultaneous occurrence of smallpox and measles in two girls. J. Maurice4, in his whole practice, only observed two such cases. Similar cases are to be found in Ettmuller's5 works, and in the writings of a few others.

Zencker6 saw cow-pox run its regular course along with measles and along with purpura.

The cow-pox went on its course undisturbed during a mercurial treatment for syphilis, as Jenner saw.

1. From careful experiments and cures of complex diseases of this kind, I am now firmly convinced that no real amalgamation of the two takes place, but that in such cases the one exists in the organism besides the other only, each in pairs that are adapted for it, and their cure will be completely effected by a judicious alternation of the best mercurial preparation, with the remedies specific for the psora, each given in the most suitable dose and form

§ 41 FIFTH EDITION

Much more frequent than the natural diseases associating with and complicating one another in the same body are the morbid complication resulting from the art of the ordinary practitioner, which the inappropriate medical treatment (the allopathic method) is apt to produce by the long-continued employment of unsuitable drugs. To the natural disease, which it is proposed to cure, there are then added, by the constant repetition of the unsuitable medical agent, the new, often very tedious, morbid conditions which might be anticipated from the peculiar powers of the drug; these gradually coalesce with and complicate the chronic malady which is dissimilar to them (which they were unable to cure by similarity of action, that is, homoeopathically), adding to the old disease a new, dissimilar, artificial malady of a chronic nature, and thus give the patient a double in place of a single disease, that is to say, render him much worse and more difficult to cure, often quite incurable. Many of the cases for which advice is asked in medical journals, as also the records of other cases in medical writings, attest the truth of this. Of a similar character are the frequent cases in which the venereal chancrous disease, complicated especially with psora or with the venereal chancrous disease, complicated especially with psora or with dyscrasia of condylomatous gonorrhoea, is not cured by long-continued or frequently repeated treatment with large doses of unsuitable mercurial preparations, but assumes its place in the organism beside the chronic mercurial affection1 that has been in the meantime gradually developed, and thus along with it often forms a hideous monster of complicated disease (under the general name of masked venereal disease), which then, when not quite incurable, can only be transformed into health with the greatest difficulty.

1. For mercury, besides the morbid symptoms which by virtue of similarity can cure the venereal disease homoeopathically, has among its effects many others unlike those of syphilis, for instance, swelling and ulceration of bones, which, if it be employed in large doses, causes new maladies and commit great ravages in the body, especially when complicated with psora, as is so frequently the case.

§ 41 SIXTH EDITION

Much more frequent than the natural diseases associating with and complicating one another in the same body are the morbid complication resulting from the art of the ordinary practitioner, which the inappropriate medical treatment (the allopathic method) is apt to produce by the long-continued employment of unsuitable drugs. To the natural disease, which it is proposed to cure, there are then added, by the constant repetition of the unsuitable medical agent, the new, often very tedious, morbid conditions corresponding to the nature of this agent; these gradually coalesce with and complicate the chronic malady which is dissimilar to them (which they were unable to cure by similarity of action, that is, homoeopathically), adding to the old disease a new, dissimilar, artificial malady of a chronic nature, and thus give the patient a double in place of a single disease, that is to say, render him much worse and more difficult to cure, often quite incurable. Many of the cases for which advice is asked in medical journals, as also the records of other cases in medical writings, attest the truth of this. Of a similar character are the frequent cases in which the venereal chancrous disease, complicated especially with psora or with the venereal chancrous disease, complicated especially with psora or with dyscrasia of condylomatous gonorrhoea, is not cured by long-continued or frequently repeated treatment with large doses of unsuitable mercurial preparations, but assumes its place in the organism beside the chronic mercurial affection1 that has been in the meantime gradually developed, and thus along with it often forms a hideous monster of complicated disease (under the general name of masked venereal disease), which then, when not quite incurable, can only be transformed into health with the greatest difficulty.

1. For mercury, besides the morbid symptoms which by virtue of similarity can cure the venereal disease homoeopathically, has among its effects many others unlike those of syphilis, for instance, swelling and ulceration of bones, which, if it be employed in large doses, causes new maladies and commit great ravages in the body, especially when complicated with psora, as is so frequently the case.

§ 42

Nature herself permits, as has been stated, in some cases, the simultaneous occurrence of two (indeed, of three) natural disease in one and the same body. This complication, however, it must be remarked, happens only in the case of two dissimilar disease, which according to the eternal laws of nature do not remove, do not annihilate and cannot cure one another, but, as it seems, both (or all three) remain, as it were, separate in the organism, and each takes possession of the parts and systems peculiarly appropriate to it, which, on account of the want of resemblance of these maladies to each other, can very well happen without disparagement to the unity of life.

§ 43

Totally different, however, is the result when two similar disease meet together in the organism, that is to say, when to the disease already present a stronger similar one is added. In such cases we see how a cure can be effected by the operations of nature, and we get a lesson as to how man ought to cure.

§ 44 FIFTH EDITION

Two diseases similar to each other can neither (as is asserted of dissimilar disease in I) repel one another, nor (as has been shown of dissimilar disease in II) suspend on another, so that the old one shall return after the new one has run its course; and just as little can two similar disease (as has been demonstrated in III respecting dissimilar affections) exist beside each other in the same organism, or together form a double complex disease.

§ 44 SIXTH EDITION

Similar diseases can neither (as is asserted of dissimilar disease in I) repel one another, nor (as has been shown of dissimilar disease in II) suspend on another, so that the old one shall return after the new one has run its course; and just as little can two similar disease (as has been demonstrated in III respecting dissimilar affections) exist beside each other in the same organism, or together form a double complex disease.

§ 45 FIFTH EDITION

No! Two diseases, differing, it is true, in kind1 but very similar in their phenomena and effects and in the sufferings and symptoms they severally produce, invariably annihilate one another whenever they meet together in the organism; the stronger disease namely, annihilates the weaker, and that for this simple reason, because the stronger morbific power when it invades the system, by reason of its similarity of action involves precisely the same part of the organism that were previously affected by the weaker morbid irritation, which, consequently, can no longer act on these parts, but is extinguished2, or (in other words) because, whenever the vital force, deranged by the primary disease, is more strongly attacked by the new, very similar, but stronger dynamic morbific power, it therefore now remains affected by the latter alone, whereby the original, similar but weaker disease must, as a mere dynamic power without material substratum, cease to exercise any further morbid influence on the vital force, consequently it must cease to exist.

1. Vide, supra, § 26, note.
2. Just as the image of a lamp's flame is rapidly overpowered and effaced from our retina by the stronger sunbeam impinging on the eye.

§ 45 SIXTH EDITION

No! Two diseases, differing, it is true, in kind[1] but very similar in their phenomena and effects and in the sufferings and symptoms they severally produce, invariably annihilate one another whenever they meet together in the organism; the stronger disease namely, annihilates the weaker, and that for this simple reason, because the stronger morbific power when it invades the system, by reason of its similarity of action involves precisely the same part of the organism that were previously affected by the weaker morbid irritation, which, consequently, can no longer act on these parts, but is extinguished[2], or (in other words), the new similar but stronger morbific potency controls the feelings of the patient and hence the life principle on account of its peculiarity, can no longer feel the weaker similar which becomes extinguished – exists no longer – for it was never anything material, but a dynamic – spirit-like – (conceptual) affection. The life principle henceforth is affected only and this but temporarily by the new, similar but stronger morbific potency.

1. Vide, supra, § 26, note.
2. Just as the image of a lamp's flame is rapidly overpowered and effaced from our retina by the stronger sunbeam impinging on the eye.

§ 46

Many examples might be adduced of disease which, in the course of nature, have been homoeopathically cured by other diseases presenting similar symptoms, were it not necessary, as our object is to speak about something determinate and indubitable, to confine our attention solely to those (few) disease which are invariably the same, arise from a fixed miasm, and hence merit a distinct name.

Among these the smallpox, so dreaded on account of the great number of its serious symptoms, occupies a prominent position, and it has removed and cured a number of maladies with similar symptoms.

How frequently does smallpox produce violent ophthalmia, sometimes even causing blindness! And see! By its inoculation Dezoteux[1] cured a chronic ophthalmia permanently, and Leroy[2] another.

An amaurosis of two years' duration, consequent on suppressed scald head, was perfectly cured by it, according to Klein.[3]

How often does smallpox cause deafness and dyspnoea! And both these chronic diseases it removed on reaching its acme, as J. Fr. Closs[4] observed.

Swelling of the testicle, even of a very severe character, is a frequent symptom of small-pox, and on this account it was enabled, as Klein[5] observed, to cure, by virtue of similarity, a large hard swelling of the left testicle, consequently on a bruise. And another observer[6] saw a similar swelling of the testicle cured by it.

Among the troublesome symptoms of small-pox is a dysenteric state of the bowels; and it subdued, as Fr. Wendt[7] observed, a case of dysentery, as a similar morbific agent.

Smallpox coming on after vaccination, as well on account of its greater strength as its great similarity, at once removes entirely the cow-pox homoeopathically, and does not permit it to come to maturity; but, on the other hand, the cow-pox when near maturity does, on account of its great similarity, homoeopathically diminish very much the supervening smallpox and make it much milder[8], as Muhry[9] and many others testify.

The inoculated cow-pox, whose lymph, besides the protective matter, contains the contagion of a general cutaneous eruption of another nature, consisting of usually small, dry (rarely large, pustular) pimples, resting on a small red areola, frequently conjoined with round red cutaneous spots and often accompanied by the most violent itching, which rash appears in not a few children several days before, more frequently, however, after the red areola of the cow-pock, and goes off in a few days, leaving behind small, red, hard spots on the skin; – the inoculated cow-pox, I say, after it has taken, cures perfectly and permanently, in a homoeopathic manner, by the similarity of this accessory miasm, analogous cutaneous eruptions of children, often of very long standing and of a very troublesome character, as a number of observers assert.[10]

The cow-pox, a peculiar symptom of which is to cause tumefaction of the arm[11], cured, after it broke out, a swollen half-paralyzed arm.[12]

The fever accompanying cow-pox, which occurs at the time of the production of the red areola, cured homoeopathically intermittent fever in two individuals, as the younger Hardege[13] reports, confirming what J. Hunter[14] had already observed, that two fevers (similar diseases) cannot co-exist in the same body.

The measles bear a strong resemblance in the character of its fever and cough to the whooping-cough, and hence it was that Bosquillon[15] noticed, in an epidemic where both these affections prevailed, that many children who then took measles remained free from whooping-cough during that epidemic. They would all have been protected from, and rendered incapable of being infected by, the whooping-cough in that and all subsequent epidemics, by the measles, if the whooping-cough were not a disease that has only a partial similarity to the measles, that is to say, if it had also a cutaneous eruption similar to what the latter possesses. As it is, however, the measles can but preserve a large number from whooping-cough homoeopathically, and that only in the epidemic prevailing at the time.

If, however, the measles come in contact with a disease resembling it in its chief symptom, the eruption, it can indisputably remove, and effect a homoeopathic cure of the latter. Thus a chronic herpetic eruption was entirely and permanently (homoeopathically) cured[16] by the breaking out of the measles, as Kortum[17] observed. An excessively burning miliary rash on the face, neck, and arms, that had lasted six years, and was aggravated by every change of weather, on the invasion of measles assumed the form of a swelling of the surface of the skin; after the measles had run its course the exanthema was cured, and returned no more.[18]

1. Traite de l'inoculation, p.189.
2. Heilkunde fur Mutter, p.384.
3. Interpres clinicus, p.293.
4. Neue Heilart der Kinderpocken. Ulm, 1769, p.68; and Specim., obs. No. 18.

5. Op. cit.
6. Nov. Act. Nat. cur., vol, I, obs. 22.
7. Nachricht Von dem Krankeninstitut zu Erlangen, 1783.
8. A new footnote is added here in the Sixth Edition, as follows:
    This seems to be the reason for this beneficial remarkable fact namely that since the general distribution of Janner's Cow-pox vaccination, human small-pox never again appeared as epidemically or virulently as 40-45 years before when one city visited lost at least one-half and often three-quarters of its children by death of this miserable pestilence.
9. Willian, Ueber die Kuhpockenimpfung, aus dem Engl., mit Zusatzen G. P. Muhry, Gottingen, 1808.
10. Especially Clavier, Hurel and Desmormeaux, in the Bulletin des sciencs medicales, publie par les membres de l' Eure, 1808, also in the Journal de medicine continue, vol. xv, p.206.
11. Balhorn, in Hufeland's Journal, 10, ii.
12. Stevenson, in Duncan's Annals of Medicine, lustr. 2, vol. I, pt. 2, No. 9.
13. In Hufeland's Journal, xxiii.
14. On the Veneral Disease, p.4.
15. Cullen's Elements of Practical Medicine, pt. 2, I, 3, ch. vii.
16. Or at least that symptom was removed.
17. In Hufeland's Journal, xx, 3, p.50.
18. Rau, Ueber d. Werth des hom. Heidelb., 1824, p.85.

§ 47

Nothing could teach the physician in a plainer and more convincing manner than the above what kind of artificial morbific agent (medicine) he ought to choose in order to cure in a sure, rapid and permanent manner, conformably with the process that takes place in nature.

§ 48

Neither in the course of nature, as we see from all the above examples, nor by the physician's art, can an existing affection or malady in any one instance be removed by a dissimilar morbific agent, be it ever so strong, but solely by one that is similar in symptoms and is somewhat stronger, according to eternal, irrevocable laws of nature, which have not hitherto been recognized.

§ 49

We should have been able to meet with many more real, natural homoeopathic cures of this kind if, on the one hand, the attention of observers had been more directed to them, and, on the other hand, if nature had not been so deficient in helpful homoeopathic diseases.

§ 50

Mighty Nature herself has, as we see, at her command, as instruments for effecting homoeopathic cures, little besides the miasmatic diseases of constant character, (the itch) measles and smallpox[1], morbific agents which[2], as remedies, are either more dangerous to life and more to be dreaded than the disease they are to cure, they themselves require curing, in order to be eradicated in their turn – both circumstances that make their employment, as homoeopathic remedies, difficult, uncertain and dangerous. And how few diseases are there to which man is subject that find their similar remedy in smallpox, measles or itch! Hence, in the course of nature, very few maladies can be cured by these uncertain and hazardous homoeopathic remedies, and the cure by their instrumentality is also attended with danger and much difficulty, for this reason that the doses of these morbific powers cannot be diminished according to circumstances, as doses of medicine can; but the patient afflicted with an analogous malady of long standing must be subjected to the entire dangerous and tedious disease, to the entire disease of smallpox, measles (or itch), which in its turn has to be cured. And yet, as is seen, we can point to some striking homoeopathic cures effected by this lucky concurrence, all so many incontrovertible proofs of the great, the sole therapeutic law of nature that obtains in them: Cure by symptoms similarity!

1. And the exanthematous contagious principle present in the cow-pox lymph.
2. Namely, small-pox and measles.

§ 51

This therapeutic law is rendered obvious to all intelligent minds by these instances, and they are amply sufficient for this end. But, on the other hand, see what advantages man has over crude Nature in her happy-go-lucky operations. How many thousands more of homoeopathic morbific agents has not man at his disposal for the relief of his suffering fellow-creatures in the medicinal substances universally distributed throughout creation! In them he has producers of disease of all possible varieties of action, for all the innumerable, for all conceivable and inconceivable natural diseases, to which they can render homoeopathic aid – morbific agents (medicinal substances), whose power, when their remedial employment is completed, being overcome by the vital force, disappears spontaneously without requiring a second course of treatment for its extirpation, like the itch – artificial morbific agents, which the physician can attenuate, subdivide and potentize almost to an infinite extent, and the dose of which he can diminish to such a degree that they shall remain only slightly stronger than the similar natural disease they are employed to cure; so that in this incomparable method of cure, there is no necessity for any violent attack upon the organism for the eradication of even an inveterate disease of old standing; the cure by this method takes place by only a gentle, imperceptible and yet often rapid transition from the tormenting natural disease to the desired state of permanent health.

§ 52 FIFTH EDITION

Surely no intelligent physician, after these examples as clear as daylight, can still go on in the old ordinary system of medicine, attacking the body, as has hitherto been done, in its least diseased parts with (allopathic) medicines that have no direct pathological (homoeopathic) relation to the disease to be cured, with purgatives, counter-irritants, derivatives, etc.1, and thus at a sacrifice of the patient's strength, inducing a morbid state quite heterogeneous and dissimilar to the original one, to the ruin of his constitution, by large doses of mixtures of medicines generally of unknown qualities, the employment of which can have no other result, as is demonstrated by the eternal laws of nature in the above and all other cases in the world in which a dissimilar disease is added to the other in the human organism, for a cure is never thereby effected in disease, but an aggravation is the invariable consequence, – therefore it can have no other result than that either (because, according to the process of nature described in I, the older disease in the body repels the dissimilar one wherewith the patient is assailed) the natural disease remains as it was, under mild allopathic treatment, be it ever so long continued, the patient being thereby weakened; or (because, according to the process of nature described in II, the new and stronger disease merely obscures and suspends for a short time the original weaker dissimilar one), by the violent attack on the body with strong allopathic drugs, the original disease seems to yield for a time, to return in at least all its former strength; or (because, according to the process of nature described in III, two dissimilar diseases, when both are of a chronic character and of equal strength, take up a position when beside one another in the organism and complicate each other) in those cases in which the physician employs for a long time morbific agents opposite and dissimilar to the natural chronic disease and allopathic medicines in large doses, such allopathic treatment, without ever being able to remove and to cure the original (dissimilar) chronic disease, only develops new artificial diseases beside it; and, as daily experience shows, only renders the patient much worse and more incurable than before.

1. Vide supra in the Introduction: A review of the Therapeutics, etc., and my book, Die Alloopathie, ein Wort der Warnung fur Kranke jeder Art, Leipzig, bei Baumgartner (translated in Hahnemann's Lesser Writings.)

§ 52 SIXTH EDITION

There are but two principle methods of cure: the one based only on accurate observation of nature, on careful experimentation and pure experience, the homoeopathic (before we never designedly used) and a second which does not do this, the heteropathic or allopathic. Each opposes the other, and only he who does not know either can hold the delusion that they can ever approach each other or even become united, or to make himself so ridiculous as to practice at one time homoeopathically at another allopathically, according to the pleasure of the patient; a practice which may be called criminal treason against divine homoeopathy.

§ 53 FIFTH EDITION

True, mild cures take place, as we see, only in a homoeopathic way – a way which, as we have also shown above (§§ 7-25) in a different manner, by experience and deductions, is also the true and only one whereby diseases may be most surely, rapidly and permanently extinguished by art; for this mode of cure is founded on an eternal, infallible law of nature.

§ 53 SIXTH EDITION

The true mild cures take place only according to the homoeopathic method, which, as we have found (§§ 7-25) by experience and deduction, is unquestionably the proper one by which through art the quickest, most certain and most permanent cures are obtained since this healing art rests upon an eternal infallible law of nature.

The pure homoeopathic healing art is the only correct method, the one possible to human art, the straightest way to cure, as certain as that there is but one straight line between two given points.

§ 54 FIFTH EDITION

This, the homoeopathic way, must, moreover, as observed above (§§ 43-49) be the only proper one, because, of the three possible modes of employing medicines in diseases, it is the only direct way to a mild, sure, permanent cure without doing injury in another direction, and without weakening the patient. The pure homoeopathic mode of cure is the only proper way, the only direct way, the only way possible to human skill, as certainly as only one straight line can be drawn betwixt two given points.

§ 54 SIXTH EDITION

The allopathic method of treatment utilized many things against disease, but usually only improper ones (alloea) and ruled for ages in different forms called systems. Every one of these, following each other from time to time and differing greatly each from the other, honored itself with the name of Rational Medicine1.

Every builder of such a system cherished the haughty estimation of himself that he was able to penetrate into the inner nature of life of the healthy as well as of the sick and clearly to recognize it and accordingly gave the prescription which noxious matter2 should be banished from the sick man, and how to banish it in order to restore him to health, all this according to empty assumptions and arbitrary suppositions without honestly questioning nature and listening without prejudice to the voice of experience. Diseases were held to be conditions that reappeared pretty much in the same manner. Most systems gave, therefore, names to their imagined disease pictures and classified them, every system differently. To medicines were ascribed actions which were supposed to cure these abnormal conditions. (Hence the numerous text books on Materia Medica.3)

1. As if the establishment of a science, based only on observation of nature and pure experiment and experience idle speculation and scholastic vaporings could have a place.
2. Up to the most recent times what is curable in sickness was supposed to be material that had to be removed since no one could conceive of a dynamic effect (§ 11 note) of morbific agencies, such as medicines exercise upon the life of the animal organism.
3. To fill the measure of self infatuation to overflowing here were mixed (very learnedly) constantly more, indeed, many different medicines in so-called prescriptions to be administered in frequent and large doses and thereby the precious, easily-destroyed human life was endangered in the hands of these perverted ones. Especially so with seton, venesection, emetics, purgatives, plasters, fontanelles and cauterization.

§ 55 FIFTH EDITION

The second mode of employing medicines in diseases, the allopathic or homoeopathic, which, without any pathological relation to what is actually diseased in the body, attacks the parts most exempt from the disease, in order to draw away the disease through them and thus to expel it, as is imagined, has hitherto been the most general method. I have treated of it above in the Introduction1, and shall not dwell longer on it.

1. Review of the Therapeutics, etc.

§ 55 SIXTH EDITION

Soon, however, the public became convinced that the sufferings of the sick increased and heightened with the introduction of every one of these systems and methods of cure if followed exactly. Long ago these allopathic physicians would have been left had it not been for the palliative relief obtained at times from empirically discovered remedies whose almost instantaneous flattering action is apparent to the patient and this to some extent served to keep up their credit.

§ 56 FIFTH EDITION

The third and only remaining method1 of employing medicines in diseases, which, besides the other two just alluded to, is the only other possible one, is the antipathic (enantiopathic) or palliative method, wherewith the physician could hitherto appear to be most useful, and hoped most certainly to gain his patient's confidence by deluding him with momentary amelioration. But I shall now proceed to show how inefficacious and how injurious this third and sole remaining way was, in diseases of a not very rapid course. It is certainly the only one of the modes of treatment adopted by the allopaths that had any manifest relation to a portion of the sufferings caused by the natural disease; but what kind of relation? Of a truth the very one (the exact contrary of the right one) that ought most to be avoided if we would not delude and make a mockery of the patient affected with a chronic disease.

1. A fourth mode of employing medicines in diseases has been attempted to be created by means of Isopathy, as it is called – that is to say, a method of curing a given disease by the same contagious particle that produces it. But even granting this could be done, which would certainly be a valuable discovery, yet, after all, seeing that the virus is given to the patient highly potentized, and thereby, consequently, to a certain degree in an altered condition, the cure is effected only by opposing a simillimum to a simillimum.

§ 56 SIXTH EDITION

By means of this palliative (antipathic, enantiopathic) method, introduced according to Galen's teaching "Contraria contrariis" for seventeen centuries, the physicians hitherto could hope to win confidence while they deluded with almost instantaneous amelioration. But how fundamentally unhelpful and hurtful this method of treatment is (in diseases not running a rapid course) we shall see in what follows. It is certainly the only one of the modes of treatment adopted by the allopaths that had any manifest relation to a portion of the sufferings caused by the natural disease; but what kind of relation? Of a truth the very one (the exact contrary of the right one) that ought carefully to be avoided if we would not delude and make a mockery of the patient affected with a chronic disease1.

1. A third mode of employing medicines in diseases has been attempted to be created by means of Isopathy, as it is called – that is to say, a method of curing a given disease by the same contagious principle that produces it. But even granting this could be done, yet, after all, seeing that the virus is given to the patient highly potentized, and consequently, in an altered condition, the cure is effected only by opposing a simillimum to a simillimum.

To attempt to cure by means of the very same morbific potency (per Idem) contradicts all normal human understanding and hence all experience. Those who first brought Isopathy to notice, probably thought of the benefit which mankind received from cowpox vaccination by which the vaccinated individual is protected against future cowpox infection and as it were cured in advance. But both, cowpox and smallpox are only similar, in no way the same disease. In many respects they differ, namely in the more rapid course and mildness of cowpox and especially in this, that is never contagious to man by more nearness. Universal vaccination put an end to all epidemics of that deadly fearful smallpox to such an extent that the present generation does no longer possess a clear conception of the former frightful smallpox plague.

Moreover, in this way, undoubtedly, certain diseases peculiar to animals may give us remedies and thus happily enlarge our stock of homoeopathic remedies.

But to use a human morbific matter (a Psorin taken from the itch in man) as a remedy for the same itch or for evils arisen therefrom is –?

Nothing can result from this but trouble and aggravation of the disease.

§ 57

In order to carry into practice this antipathic method, the ordinary physician gives, for a single troublesome symptom from among the many other symptoms of the disease which he passes by unheeded, a medicine concerning which it is known that it produces the exact opposite of the morbid symptom sought to be subdued, from which, agreeably to the fifteen – centuries – old traditional rule of the antiquated medical school (contraria contrariis) he can expect the speediest (palliative) relief. He gives large doses of opium for pains of all sorts, because this drug soon benumbs the sensibility, and administers the same remedy for diarrhoeas, because it speedily puts a stop to the peristaltic motion of the intestinal canal and makes it insensible; and also for sleeplessness, because opium rapidly produces a stupefied, comatose sleep; he gives purgatives when the patient has suffered long from constipation and costiveness; he causes the burnt hand to be plunged into cold water, which, from its low degree of temperature, seems instantaneously to remove the burning pain, as if by magic; he puts the patient who complains of chilliness and deficiency of vital heat into warm baths, which warm him immediately; he makes him who is suffering from prolonged debility drink wine, whereby he is instantly enlivened and refreshed; and in like manner he employs other opposite (antipathic) remedial means, but he has very few besides those just mentioned, as it is only of very few substances that some peculiar (primary) action is known to the ordinary medical school.

§ 58

If, in estimating the value of this mode of employing medicines, we should even pass over the circumstance that it is an extremely faulty symptomatic treatment (v. note to § 7), wherein the practitioner devotes his attention in a merely one-sided manner to a single symptom, consequently to only a small part of the whole, whereby relief for the totality of the disease, which is what the patient desires, cannot evidently be expected, – we must, on the other hand, demand of experience if, in one single case where such antipathic employment of medicine was made use of in a chronic or persisting affection, after the transient amelioration there did not ensue an increased aggravation of the symptom which was subdued at first in a palliative manner, an aggravation, indeed, of the whole disease? And every attentive observer will agree that, after such short antipathic amelioration, aggravation follows in every case without exception, although the ordinary physician is in the habit of giving his patient another explanation of this subsequent aggravation, and ascribes it to malignancy of the original disease, now for the first time showing itself, or to the occurrence of quite a new disease1.

1. Little as physicians have hitherto been in the habit of observing accurately, the aggravation that so certainly follows such palliative treatment could not altogether escape their notice. A striking example of this is to be found in J. H. Schulze's Diss. qua corporis humani momentanearum alterationum specimina quoedam expenduntur, Hale, 1741, § 28. Willis bears testimony to something similar (Pharm. rat., § 7, cap. I, p.298): "Opiata dolores atroscissimos plerumque sedant atque indolentiam – procurant, camque – aliquamdiu et pro stato quodam tempore continuant, quo spatio elapso dolores mox recrusescunt et brevi ad sol itam ferociam augentur." And also at page 295: "Exactis opii viribus illico redeunt tormina, nec atrocitatem suam remittunt, nisi dum ab eodem pharmaco rursus incantuntur." In like manner J. Hunter (On the Venereal Disease, p.13) says that wine and cordials given to the weak increase the action without giving real strength, and the powers of the body are afterwards sunk proportionally as they have been raised, by which nothing can be gained, but a great deal may be lost.

§ 59

Important symptoms of persistent diseases have never yet been treated with such palliative, antagonistic remedies, without the opposite state, a relapse – indeed, a palpable aggravation of the malady – occurring a few hours afterwards. For a persistent tendency to sleepiness during the day the physician prescribed coffee, whose primary action is to enliven; and when it had exhausted its action the day – somnolence increased; – for frequent waking at night he gave in the evening, without heeding the other symptoms of the disease, opium, which by virtue of its primary action produced the same night (stupefied, dull) sleep, but the subsequent nights were still more sleepless than before; – to chronic diarrhoeas he opposed, without regarding the other morbid signs, the same opium, whose primary action is to constipate the bowels, and after a transient stoppage of the diarrhoea it subsequently became all the worse; – violent and frequently recurring pains of all kinds he could suppress with opium for but a short time; they then always returned in greater, often intolerable severity, or some much worse affection came in their stead. For nocturnal cough of long standing the ordinary physician knew no better than to administer opium, whose primary action is to suppress every irritation; the cough would then perhaps cease the first night, but during the subsequent nights it would be still more severe, and if it were again and again suppressed by this palliative in increased doses, fever and nocturnal perspiration were added to the disease; – weakness of the bladder, with consequent retention of urine, was sought to be conquered by the antipathic work of cantharides to stimulate the urinary passages whereby evacuation of the urine was certainly at first effected but thereafter the bladder becomes less capable of stimulation and less able to contract, and paralysis of the bladder is imminent; – with large doses of purgative drugs and laxative salts, which excite the bowels to frequent evacuation, it was sought to remove a chronic tendency to constipation, but in the secondary action the bowels became still more confined; – the ordinary physician seeks to remove chronic debility by the administration of wine, which, however, stimulates only in its primary action, and hence the forces sink all the lower in the secondary its primary action, and hence the forces sink all the lower in the secondary action; – by bitter substances and heating

condiments he tries to strengthen and warm the chronically weak and cold stomach, but in the secondary action of these palliatives, which are stimulating in their primary action only, the stomach becomes yet more inactive; – long standing deficiency of vital heat and chilly disposition ought surely to yield to prescriptions of warm baths, but still more weak, cold, and chilly do the patients subsequently become; – severely burnt parts feel instantaneous alleviation from the application of cold water, but the burning pain afterwards increases to an incredible degree, and the inflammation spreads and rises to a still greater height;[1] – by means of the sternutatory remedies that provoke a secretion of mucus, coryza with stoppage of the nose of long standing is sought to be removed, but it escapes observation that the disease is aggravated all the more by these antagonistic remedies (in their secondary action), and the nose becomes still more stopped; – by electricity and galvanism, with in their primary action greatly stimulate muscular action, chronically weak and almost paralytic limbs were soon excited to more active movements, but the consequence (the secondary action) was complete deadening of all muscular irritability and complete paralysis; – by venesections it was attempted to remove chronic determination of blood to the head, but they were always followed by greater congestion; – ordinary medical practitioners know nothing better with which to treat the paralytic torpor of the corporeal and mental organs, conjoined with unconsciousness, which prevails in many kinds of typhus, than with large doses of valerian, because this is one of the most powerful medicinal agents for causing animation and increasing the motor faculty; in their ignorance, however, they knew not that this action is only a primary action, and that the organism, after that is passed, most certainly falls back, in the secondary (antagonistic) action, into still greater stupor and immobility, that is to say, into paralysis of the mental and corporeal organs (and death); they did not see, that the very diseases they supplied most plentifully with valerian, which is in such cases an oppositely acting, antipathic remedy, most infallibly terminated fatally. The old school physician rejoices[2] that he is able to reduce for several hours the velocity of the small rapid pulse in cachectic patients with the very first dose of uncombined purple foxglove (which in its primary action makes the pulse slower); its rapidity, however, soon returns; repeated, and now increased doses effect an ever smaller diminution of its rapidity, and at length none at all – indeed – in the secondary action the pulse becomes uncountable; sleep, appetite and strength depart, and a speedy death is invariably the result, or else insanity ensues. How often, in one word, the disease is aggravated, or something even worse is effected by the secondary action of such antagonistic (antipathic) remedies, the old school with its false theories does not perceive, but experience teaches it in a terrible manner.

1. Vide Introduction.
2. Vide Hufeland, in his pamphlet, Die Homoopathie, p.20.

§ 60 FIFTH EDITION

If these ill-effects are produced, as may very naturally be expected from the antipathic employment of medicines, the ordinary physician imagines he can get over the difficulty by giving, at each renewed aggravation, a stronger dose of the remedy, whereby an equally transient suppression is

effected; and as there then is a still greater necessity for giving ever-increasing quantities of the palliative there ensues either another more serious disease or frequently even danger to life and death itself, but never a cure of a disease of considerable or of long standing.

§ 60 SIXTH EDITION

If these ill-effects are produced, as may very naturally be expected from the antipathic employment of medicines, the ordinary physician imagines he can get over the difficulty by giving, at each renewed aggravation, a stronger dose of the remedy, whereby an equally transient suppression1 is effected; and as there then is a still greater necessity for giving ever – increasing quantities of the palliative there ensues either another more serious disease or frequently even danger to life and death itself, but never a cure of a disease of considerable or of long standing.

1. All usual palliatives given for the suffering of the sick have (as is seen here) as after-effects an increase of the same suffering and the older physicians had to repeat them in ever stronger doses in order to achieve a similar modification, which however, was never permanent and never sufficient to prevent an increased recurrence of the ailment. But Brousseau, who twenty-five years before contended against the senseless mixing of different drugs in prescription and thereby ending its reign in France, (for which mankind is grateful to him) introduced his so-called physiological system (without taking note of the homoeopathic method then already established), a method of treatment, while effectively lessening and permanently preventing the return of all the sufferings, was applicable to all diseases of mankind; a thing that the palliatives then in use were not capable of affecting.

Being able to heal disease with mild innocent remedies and thus establish health, Brousseau found the easier way to quiet the sufferings of patients more and more at the cost of their life and at last to extinguish life wholly – a method of treatment that, alas, seemed sufficient to his contemporaries. In the degree that the patient retains his strength will his ailments be apparent and the more intensely will he feel his pains. He moans and groans and cries out and calls for help more and more vociferously so that the physician cannot come any too soon to give relief. Brousseau needed only to depress the vital force, to lessen it more and more and behold, the more frequently the patient was bled, the more leeches and cupping glasses sucked out the vital fluid (for the innocent irreplaceable blood was according to him responsible for almost all ailments). In the same proportion the patient lost strength to feel pain or to express his aggravated condition by violent complaint and gestures. The patient appears more quiet in proportion as he grows weaker, the bystanders rejoice in his apparent improvement, ready to return to the same measures on the renewal of his sufferings – be they spasms, suffocation, fears or pain, for they had so beautifully quieted him before and gave promise of further ease. In disease of long duration and when the patient retained some strength, he was deprived of food, put on a "hunger diet," in order to depress life so much more successfully and inhibit the restless states. The debilitated patient feels unable to protest against further similar measures of blood-letting leeches, vesication, warm baths and so forth to refuse their employment. That death must follow such frequently repeated reduction and exhaustion of the vital energy is not noticed by the patient, already robbed of all consciousness, and the relatives, blinded by the improvements even of the last sufferings of the patient by means of blood letting and warm baths, cannot understand and are surprised when the patient quietly slips away.

"But God knows the patient on his bed of sickness was not treated with violence, for the prick of a small lancet is not really painful and the gum Arabic solution (Eau de Gourme, almost the only medicine that Brousseau used) was mild in taste and without apparent action – the bite of the leeches insignificant and the blood letting by the physician done quietly while the luke warm baths could only soothe, hence the disease from the very start must have been fatal, so that the patient, notwithstanding all efforts of the physician, had to leave the earth." In this way the relatives, and especially the heirs of the dear departed, consoled themselves.

The physicians in Europe and elsewhere accepted this convenient treatment of all disease according to a single rule, since it saved them from all further thinking (the most laborious of all work under the sun). They only had to take care "to assuage the pangs of conscience and console themselves that they were not the originators of this system and this method of treatment, that all the other thousands of Brousseauists did the same and that possibly everything would cease with death anyway as was taught by their master." In this way many thousand physicians were miserably misled to shed (with cold heart) the warm blood of their patients that were capable of cure and thereby rob millions of men gradually of their life, according to Brousseau's method, more than fell on Napoleon's battlefields. Was it perhaps necessary by the disposition of God for that system of Brousseau which destroyed medically the life of curable patients to precede homoeopathy in order to open the eyes of the world to the only true science and art of medicine, homoeopathy, in which curable patients find health and new life when this most difficult of all arts is practised by an indefatigable discriminating physician in a pure and conscientious manner?

§ 61

Had physicians been capable of reflecting on the sad results of the antagonistic employment of medicines, they had long since discovered the grand truth, THAT THE TRUE RADICAL HEALING ART MUST BE FOUND IN THE EXACT OPPOSITE OF SUCH AN ANTIPATHIC TREATMENT OF THE SYMPTOMS OF DISEASE; they would have become convinced, that as a medicinal action antagonistic to the symptoms of the disease (an antipathically employed medicine) is followed by only transient relief, and after that is passed, by invariable aggravation, the converse of that procedure, the homoeopathic employment of medicines according to similarity of symptoms, must effect a permanent and perfect cure, if at the same time the opposite of their large doses, the most minute doses, are exhibited. But neither the obvious aggravation that ensued from their antipathic treatment, nor the fact that no physician ever effected a permanent cure of disease of considerable or of long standing unless some homoeopathic medicinal agent was accidentally a chief ingredient in his prescription, nor yet the circumstances that all the rapid and perfect cures that nature ever performed (§ 46), were always effected by the supervention upon the old disease of one of a similar character, ever taught them, during such a long series of centuries, this truth, the knowledge of which can alone conduce to the benefit of the sick.

§ 62

But on what this pernicious result of the palliative, antipathic treatment and the efficacy of the reverse, the homoeopathic treatment, depend, is explained by the following facts, deduced from manifold observations, which no one before me perceived, though they are so very palpable and so very evident, and are of such infinite importance to the healing art.

§ 63

Every agent that acts upon the vitality, every medicine, deranges more or less the vital force, and causes a certain alteration in the health of the individual for a longer or a shorter period. This is termed primary action. Although a product of the medicinal and vital powers conjointly, it is principally due to the former power. To its action our vital force endeavors to oppose its own energy. This resistant action is a property, is indeed an automatic action of our life-preserving power, which goes by the name of secondary action or counteraction.

§ 64

During the primary action of the artificial morbific agents (medicines) on our healthy body, as seen in the following examples, our vital force seems to conduct itself merely in a passive (receptive) manners, and appears, so to say, compelled to permit the impressions of the artificial power acting from without to take place in it and thereby after its state of health; it then, however, appears to rouse itself again, as it were, and to develop (A) the exact opposite condition of health (counteraction, secondary action) to this effect (primary action) produced upon it, if there be such an opposite, and that in as great a degree as was the effect (primary action) of the artificial morbific agent on it, and proportionate to its own energy; – or (B) if there be not in nature a state exactly the opposite of the primary action, it appears to endeavor to indifferentiate itself, that is, to make its superior power available in the extinction of the change wrought in it from without (by the medicine), in the place of which it substitutes its normal state (secondary action, curative action).

§ 65

Examples of (A) are familiar to all. A hand bathed in hot water is at first much warmer than the other hand that has not been so treated (primary action); but when it is withdrawn from the hot water and again thoroughly dried, it becomes in a short time cold, and at length much colder than the other (secondary action). A person heated by violent exercise (primary action) is afterwards affected with chilliness and shivering (secondary action). To one who was yesterday heated by drinking much wine (primary action), today every breath of air feels too cold (counteraction of the organism, secondary action). An arm that has been kept long in very cold water is at first much paler and colder (primary action) than the other; but removed from the cold water and dried, it subsequently becomes not only warmer than the other, but even hot, red and inflamed (secondary action, reaction of the vital force). Excessive vivacity follows the use of strong coffee (primary action), but sluggishness and drowsiness remain for a long time afterwards (reaction, secondary action), if this be not always again removed for a short time by imbibing fresh supplies of coffee (palliative). After the profound stupefied sleep caused by opium (primary action), the following night will be all the more sleepless (reaction, secondary action). After the constipation produced by opium (primary action), diarrhoea ensues (secondary action); and after purgation with medicines that irritate the bowels, constipation of several days' duration ensues (secondary action). And in like manner it always happens, after the primary action of a medicine that produces in large doses a great change in the health of a healthy person, that its exact opposite, when, as has been observed, there is actually such a thing, is produced in the secondary action by our vital force.

§ 66

An obvious antagonistic secondary action, however, is, as may readily be conceived, not to be noticed from the action of quite minute homoeopathic doses of the deranging agents on the healthy body. A small dose of every one of them certainly produces a primary action that is perceptible to a sufficiently attentive; but the living organism employs against it only so much reaction (secondary action) as is necessary for the restoration of the normal condition.

§ 67 FIFTH EDITION

These incontrovertible truths, which spontaneously offer themselves to our notice and experience, explain to us the beneficial action that takes place under homoeopathic treatment; while, on the other hand, they demonstrate the perversity of the antipathic and palliative treatment of diseases with antagonistically acting medicines.1

1. Only in the most urgent cases, where danger to life and imminent death allow no time for the action of a homoeopathic remedy – not hours, sometimes not even quarter-hours, and scarcely minutes – in sudden accidents occurring to previously healthy individuals – for example, in asphyxia and suspended animation from lightning, from suffocation, freezing, drowning, etc. – is it admissible and judicious, at all events as a preliminary measure to stimulate the irritability and sensibility (the physical life) with a palliative, as for instance, with gentle electrical shocks, with clysters of strong coffee, with a stimulating odor, gradual application of heat, etc. When this stimulation is effected, the play of the vital organs again goes on in its former healthy manner, for there is here no disease* to be removed, but merely an obstruction and suppression of the healthy vital force. To this category belong various antidotes to sudden poisoning: alkalies from mineral acids, hepar sulphuris for metallic poisons, coffee and camphora (and ipecacuanha) for poisoning by opium, etc.

It does not follow that a homoeopathic medicine has been ill selected for a case of disease because some of the medicinal symptoms are only antipathic to some of the less important and minor symptoms of the disease; if only the others, the stronger well-marked (characteristic), and peculiar symptoms of the disease are covered and matched by the same medicine with similarity of symptoms – that is to say, overpowered, destroyed and extinguished; the few opposite symptoms also disappear of themselves after the expiry of the term of action of the medicament, without retarding the cure in the least.

* And yet the new sect that mixes the two systems appeals (though in vain) to this observation, in order that they may have an excuse for encountering everywhere such exceptions to the general rule in diseases, and to justify their convenient employment of allopathic palliatives, and of other injurious allopathic trash besides, solely for the sake of sparing themselves the trouble of seeking for the suitable homoeopathic remedy for each case of disease – I might almost say for the sake of sparing themselves the trouble of being homoeopathic physicians, and yet wishing to appear as such. But their performances are on a par with the system they pursue; they are nothing to boast of.

§ 67 SIXTH EDITION

These incontrovertible truths, which spontaneously offer themselves to our notice and experience, explain to us the beneficial action that takes place under homoeopathic treatment; while, on the other hand, they demonstrate the perversity of the antipathic and palliative treatment of diseases with antagonistically acting medicines.1

1. Only in the most urgent cases, where danger to life and imminent death allow no time for the action of a homoeopathic remedy – not hours, sometimes not even quarter-hours, and scarcely minutes – in sudden accidents occurring to previously healthy individuals – for example, in asphyxia and suspended animation from lightning, from suffocation, freezing, drowning, etc. – is it admissible and judicious, at all events as a preliminary measure to stimulate the irritability and sensibility (the physical life) with a palliative, as for instance, with gentle electrical shocks, with clysters of strong coffee, with a stimulating odor, gradual application of heat, etc. When this stimulation is effected, the play of the vital organs again goes on in its former healthy manner, for there is here no disease* to be removed, but merely an obstruction and suppression of the healthy vital force. To this category belong various antidotes to sudden poisoning: alkalies from mineral acids, hepar sulphuris for metallic poisons, coffee and camphora (and ipecacuanha) for poisoning by opium, etc.

It does not follow that a homoeopathic medicine has been ill selected for a case of disease because some of the medicinal symptoms are only antipathic to some of the less important and minor symptoms of the disease; if only the others, the stronger well-marked (characteristic), and peculiar symptoms of the disease are covered and matched by the same medicine with similarity of symptoms – that is to say, overpowered, destroyed and extinguished; the few opposite symptoms also disappear of themselves after the expiry of the term of action of the medicament, without retarding the cure in the least.

* And yet the new sect that mixes the two systems appeals (though in vain) to this observation, in order that they may have an excuse for encountering everywhere such exceptions to the general rule

in diseases, and to justify their convenient employment of allopathic palliatives, and of other injurious allopathic trash besides, solely for the sake of sparing themselves the trouble of seeking for the suitable homoeopathic remedy for each case of disease – and thus conveniently appear as homoeopathic physicians, without being such. But their performances are on a par with the system they pursue; they are corrupting.

§ 68 FIFTH EDITION

In homoeopathic cures they show us that from the uncommonly small doses of medicine (§§ 275 – 287) required in this method of treatment, which are just sufficient, by the similarity of their symptoms, to overpower and remove the similar nature disease, there certainly remains, after the destruction of the latter, at first a certain amount of medicinal disease alone in the organism, but, on account of the extraordinary minuteness of the dose, it is so transient, so slight, and disappears so rapidly of its own accord, that the vital force has no need to employ, against this small artificial derangement of its health, any more considerable reaction than will suffice to elevate its present state of health up to the healthy point – that is, than will suffice to effect complete recovery, for which after the extinction of the previous morbid derangement but little effort is required (§ 64, B).

§ 68 SIXTH EDITION

In homoeopathic cures they show us that from the uncommonly small doses of medicine (§§ 275 – 287) required in this method of treatment, which are just sufficient, by the similarity of their symptoms, to overpower and remove from the sensation of the life principle the similar natural disease there certainly remains, after the destruction of the latter, at first a certain amount of medicinal disease alone in the organism, but, on account of the extraordinary minuteness of the dose, it is so transient, so slight, and disappears so rapidly of its own accord, that the vital force has no need to employ, against this small artificial derangement of its health, any more considerable reaction than will suffice to elevate its present state of health up to the healthy point – that is, than will suffice to effect complete recovery, for which after the extinction of the previous morbid derangement but little effort is required (§ 64, B).

§ 69 FIFTH EDITION

In the antipathic (palliative) mode of treatment, however precisely the reverse of this takes place. The medicinal symptom which the physician opposes to the disease symptom (for example, the insensibility and stupefaction caused by opium in its primary action to acute pain) is certainly not alien, not allopathic of the latter; there is a manifest relation of the medicinal symptom to the disease symptom, but it is the reverse of what should be; it is here intended that the annihilation of the disease symptom shall be effected by an opposite medicinal symptom, which is impossible. No doubt the antipathically chosen medicine touches precisely the same diseased point in the organism as the homoeopathic medicine chosen on account of the similar affection it produces; but the former covers the opposite symptom of the disease only as an opposite, and makes it unobservable for a short time only, so that in the first period of the action of the antagonistic palliative the vital force perceives nothing disagreeable from either if the two (neither from the disease symptom nor from the medicinal symptom), as they seem both to have mutually removed and dynamically neutralized one another as it were (for example, the stupefying power of opium does this to the pain). In the first minutes the vital force feels quite well, and perceives neither the stupefaction of the opium nor the pain of the disease. But as the antagonistic medicinal symptom cannot (as in the homoeopathic treatment) occupy the place of the morbid derangement present in the organism as a similar, stronger (artificial) disease, and cannot, therefore, like a homoeopathic medicine, affect the vital force with a similar artificial disease, so as to be able to step into the place of the original natural morbid derangement, the palliative medicine must, as a thing totally differing from, and the opposite of the disease derangement, leave the latter uneradicated; it renders it, as before said, by a semblance of dynamic neutralization,[1] at first unfelt by the vital force, but, like every medicinal disease, it is soon spontaneously extinguished, and not only leaves the disease behind, just as it was, but compels the vital force (as it must, like all palliatives, be given in large doses in order to effect the apparent removal) to produce an opposite condition (§§ 63,64) to this palliative medicine, the reverse of the medicinal action, consequently the analogue of the still present, undestroyed, natural morbid derangement, which is necessarily strengthened and increased[2] by this addition (reaction against the palliative) produced by the vital force. The disease symptom (this single part of the disease) consequently becomes worse after the term of the action of the palliative has expired; worse in proportion to the magnitude of the dose of the palliative. Accordingly (to keep to the same example) the larger the dose of opium given to allay the pain, so much the more does the pain increase beyond its original intensity as soon as the opium has exhausted its action.[3]

1. In the living human being no permanent neutralization of contrary or antagonistic sensations can take place, as happens with substances of opposite qualities in the chemical laboratory, where, for instance, sulphuric acid and potash unite to form a perfectly different substance, a neutral salt, which is now no longer either acid or alkali, and is not decomposed even by heat. Such amalgamations and thorough combinations to form something permanently neutral and indifferent do not, as has been said, ever take place with respect to dynamic impressions of an antagonistic nature in our sensific apparatus. Only a semblance of neutralization and mutual removal occurs in such cases at first, but the antagonistic sensations do not permanently remove one another. The tears of the mourner will be dried for but a short time by a laughable play; the jokes are, however, soon forgotten, and his tears then flow still more abundantly than before.

2. Plain as this proposition is, it has been misunderstood, and in opposition to it some have asserted "that the palliative in its secondary action, would then be similar to the disease present, must be capable of curing just as well as a homoeopathic medicine does by its primary action." But they did not reflect that the secondary action is not a product of the medicine, but invariably of the antagonistically acting vital force of the organism; that therefore this secondary action resulting

from the vital force on the employment of a palliative is a state similar to the symptoms of the disease which the palliative left uneradicated, and which the reaction of the vital force against the palliative consequently increased still more.

3. As when in a dark dungeon, where the prisoner could with difficulty recognize objects close to him, alcohol is suddenly lighted, everything is instantly illuminated in a most consolatory manner to the unhappy wretch; but when it is extinguished, the brighter the flame was previously the blacker is the night which now envelopes him, and renders everything about him much more difficult to be seen than before.

§ 69 SIXTH EDITION

In the antipathic (palliative) mode of treatment, however precisely the reverse of this takes place. The medicinal symptom which the physician opposes to the disease symptom (for example, the insensibility and stupefaction caused by opium in its primary action to acute pain) is certainly not alien, not allopathic of the latter; there is a manifest relation of the medicinal symptom to the disease symptom, but it is the reverse of what should be; it is here intended that the annihilation of the disease symptom shall be effected by an opposite medicinal symptom, which is nevertheless impossible. No doubt the antipathically chosen medicine touches precisely the same diseased point in the organism as the homoeopathic medicine chosen on account of the similar affection it produces; but the former covers the opposite symptom of the disease only as an opposite, and makes it unobservable to our life principle for a short time only, so that in the first period of the action of the antagonistic palliative the vital force perceives nothing disagreeable from either if the two (neither from the disease symptom nor from the medicinal symptom), as they seem both to have mutually removed and dynamically neutralized one another as it were (for example, the stupefying power of opium does this to the pain). In the first minutes the vital force feels quite well, and perceives neither the stupefaction of the opium nor the pain of the disease. But as the antagonistic medicinal symptom cannot (as in the homoeopathic treatment) occupy the place of the morbid derangement present in the organism in the sensation of the life principle as a similar, stronger (artificial) disease, and cannot, therefore, like a homoeopathic medicine, affect the vital force with a similar artificial disease, so as to be able to step into the place of the original natural morbid derangement, the palliative medicine must, as a thing totally differing from, and the opposite of the disease derangement, leave the latter uneradicated; it renders it, as before said, by a semblance of dynamic neutralization,1 at first unfelt by the vital force, but, like every medicinal disease, it is soon spontaneously extinguished, and not only leaves the disease behind, just as it was, but compels the vital force (as it must, like all palliatives, be given in large doses in order to effect the apparent removal) to produce an opposite condition (§§ 63,64) to this palliative medicine, the reverse of the medicinal action, consequently the analogue of the still present, undestroyed, natural morbid derangement, which is necessarily strengthened and increased2 by this addition (reaction against the palliative) produced by the vital force. The disease symptom (this single part of the disease) consequently becomes worse after the term of the action of the palliative has expired; worse in proportion to the magnitude of the dose of the

palliative. Accordingly (to keep to the same example) the larger the dose of opium given to allay the pain, so much the more does the pain increase beyond its original intensity as soon as the opium has exhausted its action.3

1. In the living human being no permanent neutralization of contrary or antagonistic sensations can take place, as happens with substances of opposite qualities in the chemical laboratory, where, for instance, sulphuric acid and potash unite to form a perfectly different substance, a neutral salt, which is now no longer either acid or alkali, and is not decomposed even by heat. Such amalgamations and thorough combinations to form something permanently neutral and indifferent do not, as has been said, ever take place with respect to synamic impressions of an antagonistic nature in our sensific apparatus. Only a semblance of neutralization and mutual removal occurs in such cases at first, but the antagonistic sensations do not permanently remove one another. The tears of the mourner will be dried for but a short time by a laughable play; the jokes are, however, soon forgotten, and his tears then flow still more abundantly than before.
2. Plain as this proposition is, it has been misunderstood, and in opposition to it some have asserted "that the palliative in its secondary action, would then be similar to the disease present, must be capable of curing just as well as a homoeopathic medicine does by its primary action." But they did not reflect that the secondary action is not a product of the medicine, but invariably of the antagonistically acting vital force of the organism; that therefore this secondary action resulting from the vital force on the employment of a palliative is a state similar to the symptoms of the disease which the palliative left uneradicated, and which the reaction of the vital force against the palliative consequently increased still more.
3. As when in a dark dungeon, where the prisoner could with difficulty recognize objects close to him, alcohol is suddenly lighted, everything is instantly illuminated in a most consolatory manner to the unhappy wretch; but when it is extinguished, the brighter the flame was previously the blacker is the night which now envelopes him, and renders everything about him much more difficult to be seen than before.

§ 70 FIFTH EDITION

From what has been already adduced we cannot fail to draw the following inferences:

That everything of a really morbid character and which ought to be cured that the physician can discover in diseases consists solely of the sufferings of the patient, and the sensible alterations in his health, in a word, solely of the totality of the symptoms, by means of which the disease demands the medicine requisite for its relief; while, on the other hand, every internal cause attributed to it, every occult quality or imaginary material morbific principle, is nothing but an idle dream;

That this derangement of the state of health, which we term disease, can only be converted into health by another revolution effected in the state of health by means of medicines, whose sole curative power, consequently, can only consist in altering man's state of health – that is to say, in a peculiar excitation of morbid symptoms, and is learned with most distinctness and purity by testing them on the healthy body;

That, according to all experience, a natural disease can never be cured by medicines that possess the power of producing in the healthy individual an alien morbid state (dissimilar morbid symptoms) differing from that of the disease to be cured (never, therefore, by an allopathic mode of treatment), and that even in nature no cure ever takes place in which an inherent disease is removed, annihilated and cured by the addition of another disease dissimilar to it, be the new one ever so strong;

That, moreover, all experience proves that, by means of medicines which have a tendency to produce in the healthy individual an artificial morbid symptom, antagonistic to the single symptom of disease sought to be cured, the cure of a long-standing affection will never be effected, but merely a very transientalleviation, always follows by its aggravation; and that, in a word, this antipathic and merely palliative treatment in long-standing diseases of a serious character is absolutely inefficacious;

That, however, the third and only other possible mode of treatment (the homoeopathic), in which there is employed for the totality of the symptoms of a natural disease a medicine capable of producing the most similar symptoms possible in the healthy individual, given in suitable dose, is the only efficacious remedial method whereby diseases, which are purely dynamic deranging irritations of the vital force, are overpowered, and being thus easily, perfectly and permanently extinguished, must necessarily cease to exist – and for this mode of procedure we have the example of unfettered Nature herself, when to an old disease there is added a new one similar to the first, whereby the new one is rapidly and forever annihilated and cured.

§ 70 SIXTH EDITION

From what has been already adduced we cannot fail to draw the following inferences:

That everything of a really morbid character and which ought to be cured that the physician can discover in diseases consists solely of the sufferings of the patient, and the sensible alterations in his health, in a word, solely of the totality of the symptoms, by means of which the disease demands the medicine requisite for its relief; while, on the other hand, every internal cause attributed to it, every occult quality or imaginary material morbific principle, is nothing but an idle dream;

That this derangement of the state of health, which we term disease, can only be converted into health by another revolution effected in the state of health by means of medicines, whose sole curative power, consequently, can only consist in altering man's state of health – that is to say, in a peculiar excitation of morbid symptoms, and is learned with most distinctness and purity by testing them on the healthy body;

That, according to all experience, a natural disease can never be cured by medicines that possess the power of producing in the healthy individual an alien morbid state (dissimilar morbid symptoms) differing from that of the disease to be cured (never, therefore, by an allopathic mode of treatment), and that even in nature no cure ever takes place in which an inherent disease is removed, annihilated and cured by the addition of another disease dissimilar to it, be the new one ever so strong;

That, moreover, all experience proves that, by means of medicines which have a tendency to produce in the healthy individual an artificial morbid symptom, antagonistic to the single symptom of disease sought to be cured, the cure of a long-standing affection will never be effected, but merely a very transientalleviation, always follows by its aggravation; and that, in a word, this antipathic and merely palliative treatment in long-standing diseases of a serious character is absolutely inefficacious;

That, however, the third and only other possible mode of treatment (the homoeopathic), in which there is employed for the totality of the symptoms of a natural disease a medicine capable of producing the most similar symptoms possible in the healthy individual, given in suitable dose, is the only efficacious remedial method whereby diseases, which are purely dynamic deranging irritations of the vital force, are overpowered, and being thus easily, perfectly and permanently extinguished, must necessarily cease to exist. This is brought about by means of the stronger similar deranging irritation of the homoeopathic medicine in the sensation of the life principle. – and for this mode of procedure we have the example of unfettered Nature herself, when to an old disease there is added a new one similar to the first, whereby the new one is rapidly and forever annihilated and cured.

§ 71

As it is now no longer a matter of doubt that the diseases of mankind consist merely of groups of certain symptoms, and may be annihilated and transformed into health by medicinal substances, but only by such as are capable of artificially producing similar morbid symptoms (and such is the process in all genuine cures), hence the operation of curing is comprised in the three following points:

I. How is the physician to ascertain what is necessary to be known in order to cure the disease?
II. How is he to gain a knowledge of the instruments adapted for the cure of the natural disease, the pathogenetic powers of the medicines?
III. What is the most suitable method of employing these artificial morbific agents (medicines) for the cure of natural disease?

§ 72

With respect to the first point, the following will serve as a general preliminary view. The disease to which man is liable are either rapid morbid processes of the abnormally deranged vital force, which have a tendency to finish their course more or less quickly, but always in a moderate time – these are termed acute diseases; – or they are diseases of such a character that, with small, often imperceptible beginnings, dynamically derange the living organism, each in its own peculiar manner, and cause it gradually to deviate from the healthy condition, in such a way that the automatic life energy, called vital force, whose office is to preserve the health, only opposes to them at the commencement and during their progress imperfect, unsuitable, useless resistance, but is unable of itself to extinguish them, but must helplessly suffer (them to spread and) itself to be ever more and more abnormally deranged, until at length the organism is destroyed; these are termed chronic diseases. They are caused by infection with a chronic miasm.

§ 73

As regards acute diseases, they are either of such a kind as attack human beings individually, the exciting cause being injurious influences to which they were particularly exposed. Excesses in food, or an insufficient supply of it, severe physical impression, chills, over heatings, dissipation, strains, etc., or physical irritations, mental emotions, and the like, are exciting causes of such acute febrile affections; in reality, however, they are generally only a transient explosion of latent psora, which spontaneously returns to its dormant state if the acute diseases were not of too violent a character and were soon quelled. Or they are of such a kind as attack several persons at the same time, here and there (sporadically), by means of meteoric or telluric influences and injurious agents, the susceptibility for being morbidly affected by which is possessed by only a few persons at one time. Allied to these are those diseases in which many persons are attacked with very similar sufferings from the same cause (epidemically); these diseases generally become infectious (contagious) when they prevail among thickly congregated masses of human beings. Thence arise fevers1, in each instance of a peculiar nature, and, because the cases of disease have an identical origin, they set up in all those they affect an identical morbid process, which when left to itself terminates in a moderate period of time in death or recovery. The calamities of war, inundations and famine are not infrequently their exciting causes and producers – sometimes they are peculiar acute miasms which recur in the same manner (hence known by some traditional name), which either attack persons but once in a lifetime, as the smallpox, measles, whooping-cough, the ancient, smooth, bright red scarlet fever2 of Sydenham, the mumps, etc., or such as recur frequently in pretty much the same manner, the plague of the Levant, the yellow fever of the sea-coast, the Asiatic cholera, etc.

1. The homoeopathic physician, who does not entertain the foregone conclusion devised by the ordinary school (who have fixed upon a few names of such fevers, besides which mighty nature dare not produce any others, so as to admit of their treating these disease according to some fixed method), does not acknowledge the names goal fever, bilious fever, typhus fever, putrid fever, nervous fever or mucous fever, but treats them each according to their several peculiarities.
2. Subsequently to the year 1801 a kind of pupura miliaris (roodvonk), which came from the West, was by physicians confounded with the scarlet fever, notwithstanding that they exhibited totally different symptoms, that the latter found its prophylatic and curative remedy in belladonna, the former in aconite, and that the former was generally merely sporadic, while the latter was invariable epidemic. Of late years it seems as if the two occasionally joined to form an eruptive fever of a peculiar kind, for which neither the one nor the other remedy, alone, will be found to be exactly homoeopathic.

§ 74 FIFTH EDITION

Among chronic diseases we must still, alas!, reckon those so commonly met with, artificially produced in allopathic treatment by the prolonged use of violent heroic medicines in large and increasing doses, by the abuse of calomel, corrosive sublimate, mercurial ointment, nitrate of silver, iodine and its ointments, opium, valerian, cinchona bark and quinine, foxglove, prussic acid, sulphur and sulphuric acid, perennial purgatives, venesections, leeches, issues, setons, etc., whereby the vital force is sometimes weakened to an unmerciful extent, sometimes, if it do not succumb, gradually abnormally deranged (by each substance in a peculiar manner) in such a way that, in order to maintain life against these inimical and destructive attacks, it must produce a revolution in the organism, and either deprive some part of its irritability and sensibility, or exalt these to an excessive degree, cause dilatation or contraction, relaxation or induration or even total destruction of certain parts, and develop faulty organic alterations here and there in the interior or the exterior1 (cripple the body internally or externally), in order to preserve the organism from complete destruction of the life by the ever-renewed, hostile assaults of such destructive forces.

1. If the patient succumbs, the practiser of such a treatment is in the habit of pointing out to the sorrowing relatives, at the post-mortem examination, these internal organic disfigurements, which are due to his pseudo-art, but which he artfully maintains to be the original incurable disease (see my book, Die Alloopathie, ein Wort deh Warnung an Kranke jeder Art, Leipzig, bei Baumgartner [translated in Lesser Writings]). Those deceitful records, the illustrated works on pathological anatomy, exhibit the products of such lamentable bungling.

§ 74 SIXTH EDITION

Among chronic diseases we must still, alas!, reckon those so commonly met with, artificially produced in allopathic treatment by the prolonged use of violent heroic medicines in large and increasing doses, by the abuse of calomel, corrosive sublimate, mercurial ointment, nitrate of silver, iodine and its ointments, opium, valerian, cinchona bark and quinine, foxglove, prussic acid, sulphur and sulphuric acid, perennial purgatives1, venesections, shedding streams of blood, leeches, issues, setons, etc., whereby the vital energy is sometimes weakened to an unmerciful extent, sometimes, if it do not succumb, gradually abnormally deranged (by each substance in a peculiar manner) in such a way that, in order to maintain life against these inimical and destructive attacks, it must produce a revolution in the organism, and either deprive some part of its irritability and sensibility, or exalt these to an excessive degree, cause dilatation or contraction, relaxation or induration or even total destruction of certain parts, and develop faulty organic alterations here and there in the interior or the exterior (cripple the body internally or externally), in order to preserve the organism from complete destruction of the life by the ever – renewed, hostile assaults of such destructive forces.3

1. The only possible case of plethora shows itself with the healthy woman, several days before her monthly period, with a feeling of a certain fullness of womb and breasts, but without inflammation.

2. Among all imaginable methods for the relief of sickness, no greater allopathic, irrational or inappropriate one can be thought of than this Brousseauic, debilitating treatment by means of venesection and hunger diet, which for many years has spread over a large part of the earth. No intelligent man can see in it anything medical, or medically helpful, whereas real medicines, even if chosen blindly and administered to a patient, may at times prove of benefit in a given case of sickness because they may accidentally have been homoeopathic to the case. But from venesection, healthy common sense can expect nothing more than certain lessening and shortening of life. It is a sorrowful and wholly groundless fallacy that most and indeed all diseases depend on local inflammation. Even for true local inflammation, the most certain and quickest cure is found in medicines capable of taking away dynamically the arterial irritation upon which the inflammation is based and this without the least loss of fluids and strength. Local venesections, even from the affected part, only tend to increase renewed inflammation of these parts. And precisely so it is generally inappropriate, aye, murderous to take away many pounds of blood from the veins in inflammatory fevers, when a few appropriate medicines would dispel this irritated arterial state, driving the hitherto quiet blood together with the disease in a few hours without the least loss of fluids and strength. Such great loss of blood is evidently irreplaceable for the remaining continuance of life, since the organs intended by the Creator for bloodmaking have thereby become so weakened that while they may manufacture blood in the same quantity but not again of the same good quality. And how impossible is it for this imagined plethora to have been produced in such remarkable rapidity and so to drain it off by frequent venesections when yet an hour before the pulse of this heated patient (before the fever and chill stage) was so quiet. No man, no sick person has ever too much blood or too much strength. On the contrary, every sick man lacks strength, otherwise his vital energy would have prevented the development of the disease. Thus it is irrational and cruel to add to this weakened patient, a greater, indeed the most serious source of debility that can be imagined. It is a murderous malpractice irrational and cruel based on a wholly groundless and absurd theory instead of taking away his disease which is ever dynamic and only to be removed by dynamic potencies.

§ 75

These inroads on human health effected by the allopathic non-healing art (more particularly in recent times) are of all chronic diseases the most deplorable, the most incurable; and I regret to add that it is apparently impossible to discover or to hit upon any remedies for their cure when they have reached any considerable height.

§ 76 FIFTH EDITION

Only for natural diseases has the beneficent Deity granted us, in Homoeopathy, the means of affording relief; but those devastations and maimings of the human organism exteriorly and interiorly, effected by years, frequently, of the unsparing exercise of a false art, with its hurtful

drugs and treatment, must be remedied by the vital force itself (appropriate aid being given for the eradication of any chronic miasm that may happen to be lurking in the background), if it has not already been too much weakened by such mischievous acts, and can devote several years to this huge operation undisturbed. A human healing art, for the restoration to the normal state of those innumerable abnormal conditions so often produced by the allopathic non-healing art, there is not and cannot be.

§ 76 SIXTH EDITION

Only for natural diseases has the beneficent Deity granted us, in Homoeopathy, the means of affording relief; but those devastations and maimings of the human organism exteriorly and interiorly, effected by years, frequently, of the unsparing exercise of a false art,1 with its hurtful drugs and treatment, must be remedied by the vital force itself (appropriate aid being given for the eradication of any chronic miasm that may happen to be lurking in the background), if it has not already been too much weakened by such mischievous acts, and can devote several years to this huge operation undisturbed. A human healing art, for the restoration to the normal state of those innumerable abnormal conditions so often produced by the allopathic non-healing art, there is not and cannot be.

1. If the patient succumbs, the practiser of such a treatment is in the habit of pointing out to the sorrowing relatives, at the post-mortem examination, these internal organic disfigurements, which are due to his pseudo-art, but which he artfully maintains to be the original incurable disease (see my book, Die Alloopathie, ein Wort deh Warnung an Kranke jeder Art, Leipzig, bei Baumgartner [translated in Lesser Writings]). Those deceitful records, the illustrated works on pathological anatomy, exhibit the products of such lamentable bungling. Deceased people from the country and those from the poor of cities who have died without such bungling with hurtful measures are not opened up through pathological anatomy as a rule. Such corruption and deformities would not be found in their corpses. From this fact can be judged the value of the evidence drawn from these beautiful illustrations as well as of the honesty of these authors and book makers.

§ 77

Those diseases are inappropriately named chronic, which persons incur who expose themselves continually to avoidable noxious influences, who are in the habit of indulging in injurious liquors or aliments, are addicted to dissipation of many kinds which undermine the health, who undergo prolonged abstinence from things that are necessary for the support of life, who reside in unhealthy localities, especially marshy districts, who are housed in cellars or other confined dwellings, who are deprived of exercise or of open air, who ruin their health by overexertion of body or mind, who live in a constant state of worry, etc. These states of ill-health, which persons bring upon themselves, disappear spontaneously, provided no chronic miasm lurks in the body, under an improved mode of living, and they cannot be called chronic diseases.

§ 78 FIFTH EDITION

The true natural chronic diseases are those that arise from a chronic miasm, which when left to themselves, and unchecked by the employment of those remedies that are specific for them, always go on increasing and growing worse, notwithstanding the best mental and corporeal regimen, and torment the patient to the end of his life with ever aggravated sufferings. These are the most numerous and greatest scourges of the human race; for the most robust constitution, the best regulated mode of living and the most vigorous energy of the vital force are insufficient for their eradication.

§ 78 SIXTH EDITION

The true natural chronic diseases are those that arise from a chronic miasm, which when left to themselves, and unchecked by the employment of those remedies that are specific for them, always go on increasing and growing worse, notwithstanding the best mental and corporeal regimen, and torment the patient to the end of his life with ever aggravated sufferings. These, excepting those produced by medical malpractice (§ 74), are the most numerous and greatest scourges of the human race; for the most robust constitution, the best regulated mode of living and the most vigorous energy of the vital force are insufficient for their eradication.[1]

1. During the flourishing years of youth and with the commencement of regular menstruation joined to a mode of life beneficial to soul, heart and body, they remain unrecognized for years. Those afflicted appeal in perfect health to their relatives and acquaintances and the disease that was received by infection or inheritance seems to have wholly disappeared. But in later years, after adverse events and conditions of life, they are sure to appear anew and develop the more rapidly and assume a more serious character in proportion as the vital principle has become disturbed by debilitating passions, worry and care, but especially when disordered by inappropriate medicinal treatment.

§ 79

Hitherto syphilis alone has been to some extent known as such a chronic miasmatic disease, which when uncured ceases only with the termination of life. Sycosis (the condylomatous disease), equally ineradicable by the vital force without proper medicinal treatment, was not recognized as a chronic miasmatic disease of a peculiar character, which it nevertheless undoubtedly is, and physicians imagined they had cured it when they had destroyed the growths upon the skin, but the persisting dyscrasia occasioned by it escaped their observation.

§ 80

Incalculably greater and more important than the two chronic miasms just named, however, is the chronic miasm of psora, which, while those two reveal their specific internal dyscrasia, the one by the venereal chancre, the other by the cauliflower-like growths, does also, after the completion of the internal infection of the whole organism, announce by a peculiar cutaneous eruption, sometimes consisting only of a few vesicles accompanied by intolerable voluptuous tickling itching (and a peculiar odor), the monstrous internal chronic miasm – the psora, the only real fundamental cause and producer of all the other numerous, I may say innumerable, forms of disease1, which, under the names of nervous debility, hysteria, hypochondriasis, mania, melancholia, imbecility, madness, epilepsy and convulsions of all sorts, softening of the bones (rachitis), scoliosis and cyphosis, caries, cancer, fungus nematodes, neoplasms, gout, haemorrhoids, jaundice, cyanosis, dropsy, amenorrhoea, haemorrhage from the stomach, nose, lungs, bladder and womb, of asthma and ulceration of the lungs, of impotence and barrenness, of megrim, deafness, cataract, amaurosis, urinary calculus, paralysis, defects of the senses and pains of thousands of kinds, etc., figure in systematic works on pathology as peculiar, independent diseases.

1. I spent twelve years in investigating the source of this incredibly large number of chronic affections, in ascertaining and collecting certain proofs of this great truth, which had remained unknown to all former or contemporary observers, and in discovering at the same time the principal (antipsoric) remedies, which collectively are nearly a match for this thousand-headed monster of disease in all its different developments and forms. I have published my observations on this subject in the book entitled The Chronic Diseases (4 vols., Dresden, Arnold. [2nd edit., Dusseldorf, Schaub.]) before I had obtained this knowledge I could only treat the whole number of chronic diseases as isolated, individual maladies, with those medicinal substances whose pure effects had been tested on healthy persons up to that period, so that every case of chronic disease was treated by my disciples according to the group of symptoms it presented, just like an idiopathic disease, and it was often so for cured that sick mankind rejoiced at the extensive remedial treasures already amassed by the new healing art. How much greater cause is there now for rejoicing that the desired goal has been so much more nearly attained, inasmuch as the recently discovered and far more specific homoeopathic remedies for chronic affections arising from psora (properly termed antipsoric remedies) and the special instructions for their preparation and employment have been published; and from among them the true physician can now select for his curative agents those whose medicinal symptoms correspond in the most similar (homoeopathic) manner to the chronic disease he has to cure; and thus, by the employment of (antipsoric) medicines more suitable for this miasm, he is enabled to render more essential service and almost invariably to effect a perfect cure.

§ 81

The fact that this extremely ancient infecting agent has gradually passed, in some hundreds of generations, through many millions of human organisms and has thus attained an incredible

development, renders it in some measure conceivable how it can now display such innumerable morbid forms in the great family of mankind, particularly when we consider what a number of circumstances1 contribute to the production of these great varieties of chronic diseases (secondary symptoms of psora), besides the indescribable diversity of men in respect of their congenital corporeal constitutions, so that it is no wonder if such a variety of injurious agencies, acting from within and from without and sometimes continually, on such a variety of organisms permeated with the psoric miasm, should produce an innumerable variety of defects, injuries, derangements and sufferings, which have hitherto been treated of in the old pathological works2, under a number of special names, as diseases of an independent character.

1. Some of these causes that exercise a modifying influence on the transformation of psora into chronic diseases manifestly depend sometimes on the climate and the peculiar physical character of the place of abode, sometimes on the very great varieties in the physical and mental training of youth, both of which may have been neglected, delayed or carried to excess, or on their abuse in the business or conditions of life, in the matter of diet and regimen, passions, manners, habits and customs of various kinds.

2. How many improper ambiguous names do not these works contain, under each of which are included excessively different morbid conditions, which often resemble each other in one single symptom only, as ague, jaundice, dropsy, consumption, leucorrhoea, haemorrhoids, rheumatism, apoplexy, convulsions, hysteria, hypochondriasis, melancholia, mania, quinsy, palsy, etc., which are represented as diseases of a fixed and unvarying character, and are treated, on account of their name, according to a determinate plan! How can the bestowal of such a name justify an identical medical treatment? And if the treatment is not always to be the same, why make use of an identical name which postulates an identity of treatment? "Nihil sane in artem medicam pestiferum magis unquam irrepsit malum, quam generalia quaedam medicinam," says Huxham, a man as clear-sighted as he was estimable on account of his conscientiousness (Op. phys. med., tom. I.). And in like manner Frittze laments (Annalen, I, p.80) "that essentially different diseases are designated by the same name." Even those epidemic diseases, which undoubtedly may be propagated in every separate epidemic by a peculiar contagious principle which remains unknown to us, are designated, in the old school of medicine by particular names, just as if they were well-known fixed diseases that invariably recurred under the same form, as hospital fever, goal fever, camp fever, putrid fever, bilious fever, nervous fever, mucous fever, although each epidemic of such roving fevers exhibits itself at every occurrence as another, a new disease, such as it has never before appeared in exactly the same form, differing very much, in every instance, in its course, as well as in many of its most striking symptoms and its whole appearance. Each is so for dissimilar to all previous epidemics, whatever names they may bear, that it would be dereliction of all logical accuracy in our ideas of things were we to give to these maladies, that differ so much among themselves, one of those names we meet with in pathological writings, and treat them all medicinally in conformity with this misused name. The candid Sydenham alone perceived this, when he (Obs. med., cap. ii, De morb, epid.) insists upon the necessity of not considering any epidemic disease as having occurred before and treating it in the same way as another, since all that occur successively, be they ever so numerous, differ from one another: "Nihil quicquam (opinor,) animum universae qua patet medicinae pomoeria perlustrantem,

> tanta admiratione percellet, quam discolor illa et sui plane dissimilis morborum Epidemicorum facies; non tam qua varias ejusdem anni tempestates, quam qua discrepantes divewrsorum ab invicem annorum constitutiones referunt, ab iisque dependent. Quae tam aperta praedictorum morborum diversitas tum propriis ac sibi peculiaribus symptomatis, tum etiam medendi ratione, quam hi ab illis disparem prorsus sibi vendicant, satis illucescit. Ex quibus constat morbus hosce, ut ut externa quadantenus specie, er symptomatis aliquot utrisque pariter super venientibus, convenire paulo incautioribus videantur, re tamen ipsa (si bene adverteris animum), alienae admondum esse indolis, et distare ut aera lupinis."

From all this it is clear that these useless and misused names of diseases ought to have no influence on the practice of the true physician, who knows that he has to judge of and to cure diseases, not according to the similarity of the name of a single one of their symptoms, but according to the totality of the signs of the individual state of each particular patient, whose affection it is his duty carefully to investigate, but never to give a hypothetical guess at it.

If, however, it is deemed necessary sometimes to make use of names of diseases, in order, when talking about a patient to ordinary persons, to render ourselves intelligible in few words, we ought only to employ them as collective names, and tell them, eg., the patient has a kind of St. Vitus's dance, a kind of dropsy, a kind of typhus, a kind of ague; but (in order to do away once and for all with the mistaken notions these names give rise to) we should never say he has the St. Vitus's dance, the typhus, the dropsy, the ague, as there are certainly no disease of these and similar names of fixed unvarying character.

§ 82

Although, by the discovery of that great source of chronic diseases, as also by the discovery of the specific homoeopathic remedies for the psora, medicine has advanced some steps nearer to a knowledge of the nature of the majority of diseases it has to cure, yet, for settling the indication in each case of chronic (psoric) disease he is called on to cure, the duty of a careful apprehension of its ascertainable symptoms and characteristics is as indispensable for the homoeopathic physician as it was before that discovery, as no real cure of this or of other diseases can take place without a strict particular treatment (individualization) of each case of disease – only that in this investigation some difference is to be made when the affection is an acute and rapidly developed disease, and when it is a chronic one; seeing that, in acute disease, the chief symptoms strike us and become evident to the senses more quickly, and hence much less time is requisite for tracing the picture of the disease and much fewer questions are required to be asked1, as almost everything is self-evident, than in a chronic disease which has been gradually progressing for several years, in which the symptoms are much more difficult to be ascertained.

1. Hence the following directions for investigating the symptoms are only partially applicable for acute diseases.

§ 83

This individualizing examination of a case of disease, for which I shall only give in this place general directions, of which the practitioner will bear in mind only what is applicable for each individual case, demands of the physician nothing but freedom from prejudice and sound senses, attention in observing and fidelity in tracing the picture of the disease.

§ 84

The patient details the history of his sufferings; those about him tell what they heard him complain of, how he has behaved and what they have noticed in him; the physician sees, hears, and remarks by his other senses what there is of an altered or unusual character about him. He writes down accurately all that the patient and his friends have told him in the very expressions used by them. Keeping silence himself he allows them to say all they have to say, and refrains from interrupting them1 unless they wander off to other matters. The physician advises them at the beginning of the examination to speak slowly, in order that he may take down in writing the important parts of what the speakers say.

1. Every interruption breaks the train of thought of the narrators, and all they would have said at first does not again occur to them in precisely the same manner after that.

§ 85

He begins a fresh line with every new circumstance mentioned by the patient or his friends, so that the symptoms shall be all ranged separately one below the other. He can thus add to any one, that may at first have been related in too vague a manner, but subsequently more explicitly explained.

§ 86

When the narrators have finished what they would say of their own accord, the physician then reverts to each particular symptom and elicits more precise information respecting it in the following manner; he reads over the symptoms as they were related to him one by one, and about each of them he inquires for further particulars, e.g., at what period did this symptom occur? Was it previous to taking the medicine he had hitherto been using? While taking the medicine? Or only some days after leaving off the medicine? What kind of pain, what sensation exactly, was it that occurred on this spot? Where was the precise spot? Did the pain occur in fits and by itself, at various times? Or was it continued, without intermission? How long did it last? At what time of the day or night, and in what position of the body was it worst, or ceased entirely? What was the exact nature of this or that event or circumstance mentioned – described in plain words?

§ 87

And thus the physician obtains more precise information respecting each particular detail, but without ever framing his questions so as to suggest the answer to the patient[1], so that he shall only have to answer yes or no; else he will be misled to answer in the affirmative or negative something untrue, half true, or not strictly correct, either from indolence or in order to please his interrogator, from which a false picture of the disease and an unsuitable mode of treatment must result.

1. For instance the physician should not ask, Was not this or that circumstance present? He should never be guilty of making such suggestions, which tend to seduce the patient into giving a false answer and a false account of his symptoms.

§ 88

If in these voluntary details nothing has been mentioned respecting several parts or functions of the body or his metal state, the physician asks what more can be told in regard to these parts and these functions, or the state of his disposition or mind[1], but in doing this he only makes use of general expressions, in order that his informants may be obliged to enter into special details concerning them.

1. For example what was the character of his stools? How does he pass his water? How is it with his day and night sleep? What is the state of his disposition, his humor, his memory? How about the thirst? What sort of taste has he in his mouth? What kinds of food and drink are most relished? What are most repugnant to him? Has each its full natural taste, or some other unusual taste? How does he feel after eating or drinking? Has he anything to tell about the head, the limbs or the abdomen?

§ 89

When the patient (for it is on him we have chiefly to rely for a description of his sensations, except in the case of feigned diseases) has by these details, given of his own accord and in answer to inquiries, furnished the requisite information and traced a tolerably perfect picture of the disease, the physician is at liberty and obliged (if he feels he has not yet gained all the information he needs) to ask more precise, more special questions.[1]

1. For example, how often are his bowels moved? What is the exact character of the stools? Did the whitish evacuation consist of mucus or faeces? Had he or had he not pains during the evacuation?

What was their exact character, and where were they seated? What did the patient vomit? Is the bad taste in the mouth putrid, or bitter, or sour, or what? before or after eating, or during the repast? At what period of the day was it worst? What is the taste of what is eructated? Does the urine only become turbid on standing, or is it turbid when first discharged? What is its color when first emitted? Of what color is the sediment? How does he behave during sleep? Does he whine, moan, talk or cry out in his sleep? Does he start during sleep? Does he snore during inspiration, or during expiration? Does he lie only on his back, or on which side? Does he cover himself well up, or can he not bear the clothes on him? Does he easily awake, or does he sleep too soundly? How often does this or that symptom occur? What is the cause that produces it each time it occurs? does it come on whilst sitting, lying, standing, or when in motion? only when fasting, or in the morning, or only in the evening, or only after a meal, or when does it usually appear? When did the rigor come on? was it merely a chilly sensation, or was he actually cold at the same time? if so, in what parts? or while feeling chilly, was he actually warm to the touch? was it merely a sensation of cold, without shivering? was he hot without redness of the face? what parts of him were hot to the touch? or did he complain of heat without being hot to the touch? How long did the chilliness last? how long the hot stage? When did the thirst come on – during the cold stage? during the heat? or previous to it? or subsequent to it? How great was the thirst, and what was the beverage desired? When did the sweat come on – at the beginning or the end of the heat? or how many hours after the heat? when asleep or when awake? How great was the sweat? was it warm or cold? on what parts? how did it smell? What does he complain of before or during the cold stage? what during the hot stage? what after it? what during or after the sweating stage?

(Added to the Sixth Edition)
In women, note the character of menstruation and other discharges, etc.

§ 90

When the physician has finished writing down these particulars, he then makes a note of what he himself observes in the patient1, and ascertains how much of that was peculiar to the patient in his healthy state.

1. For example, how the patient behaved during the visit – whether he was morose, quarrelsome, hasty, lachrymose, anxious, despairing or sad, or hopeful, calm etc. Whether he was in a drowsy state or in any way dull of comprehension; whether he spoke hoarsely, or in a low tone, or incoherently, or how other wise did he talk? what was the color of his face and eyes, and of his skin generally? what degree of liveliness and power was there in his expression and eyes? what was the state of his tongue, his breathing, the smell from his mouth, and his hearing? were his pupils dilated or contracted? how rapidly and to what extent did they alter in the dark and in the light? what was the character of the pulse? what was the condition of the abdomen? how moist or hot, how cold or dry to the touch, was the skin of this or that part or generally? whether he lay with head thrown back, with mouth half or wholly open, with the arms placed above the head, on his

back, or in what other position? what effort did he make to raise himself? and anything else in him that may strike the physician as being remarkable.

§ 91

The symptoms and feelings of the patient during a previous course of medicine do not furnish the pure picture of the disease; but on the other hand, those symptoms and ailments which he suffered from before the use of the medicines, or after they had been discontinued for several days, give the true fundamental idea of the original form of the disease, and these especially the physician must take note of. When the disease is of a chronic character, and the patient has been taking medicine up to the time he is seen, the physician may with advantage leave him some days quite without medicine, or in the meantime administer something of an unmedicinal nature and defer to a subsequent period the more precise scrutiny of the morbid symptoms, in order to be able to grasp in their purity the permanent uncontaminated symptoms of the old affection and to form a faithful picture of the disease.

§ 92

But if it be a disease of a rapid course, and if its serious character admit of no delay, the physician must content himself with observing the morbid condition, altered though it may be by medicines, if he cannot ascertain what symptoms were present before the employment of the medicines, – in order that he may at least form a just apprehension of the complete picture of the disease in its actual condition, that is to say, of the conjoint malady formed by the medicinal and original diseases, which from the use of inappropriate drugs is generally more serious and dangerous than was the original disease, and hence demands prompt and efficient aid; and by thus tracing out the complete picture of the disease he will be enabled to combat it with a suitable homoeopathic remedy, so that the patient shall not fall a sacrifice to the injurious drugs he was swallowed.

§ 93

If the disease has been brought on a short time or, in the case of a chronic affection, a considerable time previously, by some obvious cause, then the patient – or his friends when questioned privately – will mention it either spontaneously or when carefully interrogated.1

1. Any causes of a disgraceful character, which the patient or his friends do not like to confess, at least not voluntarily, the physician must endeavor to elicit by skilfully framing his questions, or by private information. To these belong poisoning or attempted suicide, onanism, indulgence in ordinary or unnatural debauchery, excess in wine, cordials, punch and other ardent beverages, or coffee, – over-indulgence in eating generally, or in some particular food of a hurtful character, – infection with venereal disease or itch, unfortunate love, jealousy, domestic infelicity, worry, grief

on account of some family misfortune, ill-usage, balked revenge, injured pride, embarrassment of a pecuniary nature, superstitious fear, – hunger, – or an imperfection in the private parts, a rupture, a prolapse, and so forth.

§ 94

While inquiring into the state of chronic disease, the particular circumstances of the patient with regard to his ordinary occupations, his usual mode of living and diet, his domestic situation, and so forth, must be well considered and scrutinized, to ascertain what there is in them that may tend to produce or to maintain disease, in order that by their removal the recovery may by prompted.1

1. In chronic diseases of females it is specially necessary to pay attention to pregnancy, sterility, sexual desire, accouchements, miscarriages, suckling, and the state of the menstrual discharge. With respect to the last-named more particularly, we should not neglect to ascertain if it recurs at too short intervals, or is delayed beyond the proper time, how many days it lasts, whether its flow is continuous or interrupted, what is its general quality, how dark is its color, whether there is leucorrhoea before its appearance or after its termination, but especially by what bodily or mental ailments, what sensations and pains, it is preceded, accompanied or followed; if there is leucorrhoea, what is its nature, what sensations attend its flow, in what quantity it is, and what are the conditions and occasions under which it occurs?

§ 95

In chronic disease the investigation of the signs of disease above mentioned, and of all others, must be pursued as carefully and circumstantially as possible, and the most minute peculiarities must be attended to, partly because in these diseases they are the most characteristic and least resemble those of acute diseases, and if a cure is to be affected they cannot be too accurately noted; partly because the patients become so used to their long sufferings that they pay little or no heed to the lesser accessory symptoms, which are often very pregnant with meaning (characteristic) – often very useful in determining the choice of the remedy – and regard them almost as a necessary part of their condition, almost as health, the real feeling of which they have well-nigh forgotten in the sometimes fifteen or twenty years of suffering, and they can scarcely bring themselves to believe that these accessory symptoms, these greater or less deviations from the healthy state, can have any connection with their principal malady.

§ 96

Besides this, patients themselves differ so much in their dispositions, that some, especially the so-called hypochondriacs and other persons of great sensitiveness and impatient of suffering,

portray their symptoms in too vivid colors and, in order to induce the physician to give them relief, describe their ailments in exaggerated expression.1

1. A pure fabrication of symptoms and sufferings will never be met with in hypochondriacs, even in the most impatient of them – a comparison of the sufferings they complain of at various times when the physician gives them nothing at all, or something quite unmedical, proves this plainly; – but we must deduct something from their exaggeration, at all events ascribe the strong character of their expressions to their expressions when talking of their ailments becomes of itself an important symptom in the list of features of which the portrait of the disease is composed. The case is different with insane persons and rascally feigners of disease.

§ 97

Other individuals of an opposite character, however, partly from indolence, partly from false modesty, partly from a kind of mildness of disposition or weakness of mind, refrain from mentioning a number of their symptoms, describe them in vague terms, or allege some of them to be of no consequence.

§ 98

Now, as certainly as we should listen particularly to the patient's description of his sufferings and sensations, and attach credence especially to his own expressions wherewith he endeavors to make us understand his ailments – because in the mouths of his friends and attendants they are usually altered and erroneously stated, – so certainly, on the other hand, in all diseases, but especially in the chronic ones, the investigation of the true, complete picture and its peculiarities demands especial circumspection, tact, knowledge of human nature, caution in conducting the inquiry and patience in an eminent degree.

§ 99

On the whole, the investigation of acute diseases, or of such as have existed but a short time, is much the easiest for the physician, because all the phenomena and deviations from the health that has been put recently lost are still fresh in the memory of the patient and his friends, still continue to be novel and striking. The physician certainly requires to know everything in such cases also; but he has much less to inquire into; they are for the most part spontaneously detailed to him.

§ 100

In investigating the totality of the symptoms of epidemic and sporadic diseases it is quite immaterial whether or not something similar has ever appeared in the world before under the same or any other name. The novelty or peculiarity of a disease of that kind makes no difference either in the mode of examining or of treating it, as the physician must any way regard to pure picture of every prevailing disease as if it were something new and unknown, and investigate it thoroughly for itself, if he desire to practice medicine in a real and radical manner, never substituting conjecture for actual observation, never taking for granted that the case of disease before him is already wholly or partially known, but always carefully examining it in all its phases; and this mode of procedure is all the more requisite in such cases, as a careful examination will show that every prevailing disease is in many respects a phenomenon of a unique character, differing vastly from all previous epidemics, to which certain names have been falsely applied – with the exception of those epidemics resulting from a contagious principle that always remains the same, such as smallpox, measles, etc.

§ 101

It may easily happen that in the first case of an epidemic disease that presents itself to the physician's notice he does not at once obtain a knowledge of its complete picture, as it is only by a close observation of several cases of every such collective disease that he can become conversant with the totality of its signs and symptoms. The carefully observing physician can, however, from the examination of even the first and second patients, often arrive so nearly at a knowledge of the true state as to have in his mind a characteristic portrait of it, and even to succeed in finding a suitable, homoeopathically adapted remedy for it.

§ 102

In the course of writing down the symptoms of several cases of this kind the sketch of the disease picture becomes ever more and more complete, not more spun out and verbose, but more significant (more characteristic), and including more of the peculiarities of this collective disease; on the one hand, the general symptoms (e.g., loss of appetite, sleeplessness, etc.) become precisely defined as to their peculiarities; and on the other, the more marked and special symptoms which are peculiar to but few diseases and of rarer occurrence, at least in the same combination, become prominent and constitute what is characteristic of this malady.1 All those affected with the disease prevailing at a given time have certainly contracted it from one and the same source and hence are suffering from the same disease; but the whole extent of such an epidemic disease and the totality of its symptoms (the knowledge whereof, which is essential for enabling us to choose the most suitable homoeopathic remedy for this array of symptoms, is obtained by a complete survey of the morbid picture) cannot be learned from one single patient, but is only to be perfectly deduced (abstracted) and ascertained from the sufferings of several patients of different constitutions.

1. The physician who has already, in the first cases, been able to choose a remedy approximating to the homoeopathic specific, will, from the subsequence cases, be enabled either to verify the suitableness of the medicine chosen, or to discover a more appropriate, the most appropriate homoeopathic remedy.

§ 103

In the same manner as has here been taught relative to the epidemic disease, which are generally of an acute character, the miasmatic chronic maladies, which, as I have shown, always remain the same in their essential nature, especially the psora, must be investigated, as to the whole sphere of their symptoms, in a much more minute manner than has ever been done before, for in them also one patient only exhibits a portion of their symptoms, a second, a third, and so on, present some other symptoms, which also are but a (dissevered, as it were), portion of the totality of the symptoms which constitute the entire extent of this malady, so that the whole array of the symptoms belonging to such a miasmatic, chronic disease, and especially to the psora, can only be ascertained from the observation of very many single patients affected with such a chronic disease, and without a complete survey and collective picture of these symptoms the medicines capable of curing the whole malady homoeopathically (to wit, the antipsorics) cannot be discovered; and these medicines are, at the same time, the true remedies of the several patients suffering from such chronic affections.

§ 104

When the totality of the symptoms that specially mark and distinguish the case of disease or, in other words, when the picture of the disease, whatever be its kind, is once accurately sketched,1 the most difficult part of the task is accomplished. The physician has then the picture of the disease, especially if it be a chronic one, always before him to guide him in his treatment; he can investigate it in all its parts and can pick out the characteristic symptoms, in order to oppose to these, that is to say, to the whole malady itself, a very similar artificial morbific force, in the shape of a homoeopathically chosen medicinal substance, selected from the lists of symptoms of all the medicines whose pure effects have been ascertained. And when, during the treatment, he wishes to ascertain what has been the effect of the medicine, and what change has taken place in the patient's state, at this fresh examination of the patient he only needs to strike out of the list of the symptoms noted down at the first visit those that have become ameliorated, to mark what still remain, and add any new symptoms that may have supervened.

1. The old school physician gave himself very little trouble in this matter in his mode of treatment. He would not listen to any minute detail of all the circumstances of his case by the patient; indeed,

he frequently cut him short in his relation of his sufferings, in order that he might not be delayed in the rapid writing of his prescription, composed of a variety of ingredients unknown to him in their true effects. No allopathic physician, as has been said, sought to learn all the circumstances of the patient's case, and still less did he make a note in writing of them. On seeing the patient again several days afterwards he recollected nothing concerning the few details he had heard at the first visit (having in the meantime seen so many other patients laboring under different affections); he had allowed everything to go in at one ear and out at the other. At subsequent visits he only asked a few general questions, went through the ceremony of feeling the pulse at the wrist, looked at the tongue, and at the same moment wrote another prescription, on equally irrational principles, or ordered the first one to be continued (in considerable quantities several times a day), and, with a graceful bow, he hurried off to the fiftieth or sixtieth patient he had to visit, in this thoughtless way, in the course of that forenoon. The profession which of all others requires actually the most reflection, a conscientious, careful examination of the state of each individual patient and a special treatment founded thereon, was conducted in this manner by persons who called themselves physicians, rational practitioners. The result, as might naturally be expected, was almost invariably bad; and yet patients had to go to them for advise, partly because there were none better to be had, partly for fashion's sake.

§ 105

The second point of the business of a true physician related to acquiring a knowledge of the instruments intended for the cure of the natural diseases, investigating the pathogenetic power of the medicines, in order, when called on to cure, to be able to select from among them one, from the list of whose symptoms an artificial disease may be constructed, as similar as possible to the totality of the principal symptoms of the natural disease sought to be cured.

§ 106

The whole pathogenetic effect of the several medicines must be known; that is to say, all the morbid symptoms and alterations in the health that each of them is specially capable of developing in the healthy individual must first have been observed as far as possible, before we can hope to be able to find among them, and to select, suitable homoeopathic remedies for most of the natural disease.

§ 107

If, in order to ascertain this, medicines be given to sick persons only, even though they be administered singly and alone, then little or nothing precise is seen of their true effects, as

those peculiar alterations of the health to be expected from the medicine are mixed up with the symptoms of the disease and can seldom be distinctly observed.

§ 108

There is, therefore, no other possible way in which the peculiar effects of medicines on the health of individuals can be accurately ascertained – there is no sure, no more natural way of accomplishing this object, than to administer the several medicines experimentally, in moderate doses, to healthy persons, in order to ascertain what changes, symptoms and signs of their influence each individually produces on the health of the body and of the mind; that is to say, what disease elements they are able and tend to produce1, since, as has been demonstrated (§§ 24-27), all the curative power of medicines lies in this power they possess of changing the state of man's health, and is revealed by observation of the latter.

1. Not one single physician, as far as I know, during the previous two thousand five hundred years, thought of this so natural, so absolutely necessary and only genuine mode of testing medicines for their pure and peculiar effects in deranging the health of man, in order to learn what morbid state each medicine is capable of curing, except the great and immoral Albrecht von Haller. He alone, besides myself, saw the necessity of this (vide the Preface to the Pharmacopoeia Helvet, Basil, 1771, fol., p.12); Nempe primum in corpore sano medela tentanda est, sine peregrina ulla miscela; odoreque et sapore ejus exploratis, exigua illiu dosis ingerenda et ad ommes, quae inde contingunt, affectiones, quis pulsus, qui calor, quae respiratia, quaenam excretiones, attendum. Inde ad ductum phaenomenorum, in sano obviorum, transeas ad experimenta in corpore aegroro," etc. But no one, not a single physician, attended to or followed up this invaluable hint.

§ 109

I was the first that opened up this path, which I have pursued with a perseverance that could only arise and be kept up by a perfect conviction of the great truth, fraught with such blessings to humanity, that it is only by the homoeopathic employment of medicines1 that the certain cure of human maladies is possible.2

1. It is impossible that there can be another true, best method of curing dynamic diseases (i.e., all diseases not strictly surgical) besides homoeopathy, just as it is impossible to draw more than one straight line betwixt two given points. He who imagines that there are other modes of curing diseases besides it could not have appreciated homoeopathy fundamentally nor practised it with sufficient care, nor could he ever have seen or read cases of properly performed homoeopathic cures; nor, on the other hand, could he have discerned the baselessness of all allopathic modes of treating diseases and their bad or even dreadful effects, if, with such lax indifference, he places the only true healing art on an equality with those hurtful methods of treatment, or alleges the

latter to be auxiliaries to homoeopathy which it could not do without! My true, conscientious followers, the pure homoeopathists, with their successful, almost never-failing treatment, might teach these persons better.

2. The first fruits of these labors, as perfect as they could be at that time, I recorded in the Fragmenta de viribus medicamentorum positivis, sive in sano corpore humano observatis, pts. I, ii, Lipsiae, 8, 1805, ap. J. A. Barth; the more mature fruits in the Reine Arzneimittellebre, I Th., dritte Ausg.; II Th., dritte Ausg., 1833; III Th., zweite Ausg., 1825; IV Th., zw. Ausg., 1827 (English translation, Materia Medica Pura, vols I and ii); and in the second, third, and fourth parts of Die chronischen Krankheiten, 1828, 1830, Dresden bei Arnold (2nd edit., with a fifth part, Dusseldorf bei Schaub, 1835, 1839).

§ 110

I saw, moreover, that the morbid lesions which previous authors had observed to result from medicinal substances when taken into the stomach of healthy persons, either in large doses given by mistake or in order to produce death in themselves or others, or under other circumstances, accorded very much with my own observations when experimenting with the same substances on myself and other healthy individuals. These authors give details of what occurred as histories of poisoning and as proofs of the pernicious effects of these powerful substances, chiefly in order to warn others from their use; partly also for the sake of exalting their own skill, when, under the use of the remedies they employed to combat these dangerous accidents, health gradually returned; but partly also, when the persons so affected died under their treatment, in order to seek their own justification in the dangerous character of these substances, which they then termed poisons. None of these observers ever dreamed that the symptoms they recorded merely as proofs of the noxious and poisonous character of these substances were sure revelations of the power of these drugs to extinguish curatively similar symptoms occurring in natural disease, that these their pathogenetic phenomena were intimations of their homoeopathic curative action, and that the only possible way to ascertain their medicinal powers is to observe those changes of health medicines are capable of producing in the healthy organism; for the pure, peculiar powers of medicines available for the cure of disease are to be learned neither by any ingenious a priori speculations, nor by the smell, taste or appearance of the drugs, nor by their chemical analysis, nor yet by the employment of several of them at one time in a mixture (prescription) in diseases; it was never suspected that these histories of medicinal diseases would one day furnish the first rudiments of the true, pure materia medica, which from the earliest times until now has consisted solely of false conjectures and fictions of the imagination – that is to say, did not exist at all.1

1. See what I have said on this subject in the "Examination of the Sources of the Ordinary Materia Medica," prefixed to the third part of my Reine Arzneimittellebre (translated in the Materia Medica Pura, vol. ii).

§ 111

The agreement of my observations on the pure effects of medicines with these older ones – although they were recorded without reference to any therapeutic object, – and the very concordance of these accounts with others of the same kind by different authors must easily convince us that medicinal substances act in the morbid changes they produce in the healthy human body according to fixed, eternal laws of nature, and by virtue of these are enabled to produce certain, reliable disease symptoms each according to its own peculiar character.

§ 112

In those older prescriptions of the often dangerous effects of medicines ingested in excessively large doses we notice certain states that were produced, not at the commencement, but towards the termination of these sad events, and which were of an exactly opposite nature to those that first appeared. These symptoms, the very reverse of the primary action (§ 63) or proper action of the medicines on the vital force are the reaction of the vital force of the organism, its secondary action (§§ 62-67), of which, however, there is seldom or hardly ever the least trace from experiments with moderate doses on healthy bodies, and from small doses none whatever. In the homoeopathic curative operation the living organism reacts from these only so much as is requisite to raise the health again to the normal healthy state (§ 67).

§ 113

The only exceptions to this are the narcotic medicines. As they, in their primary action, take away sometimes the sensibility and sensation, sometimes the irritability, it frequently happens that in their secondary action, even from moderate experimental doses on healthy bodies, an increased sensibility (and a greater irritability) is observable.

§ 114

With the exception of these narcotic substances, in experiments with moderate doses of medicine on healthy bodies, we observe only their primary action, i.e., those symptoms wherewith the medicine deranges the health of the human being and develops in him a morbid state of longer or shorter duration.

§ 115

Among these symptoms, there occur in the case of some medicines not a few which are partially, or under certain conditions, directly opposite to other symptoms that have previously or subsequently appeared, but which are not therefore to be regarded as actual secondary action or the mere reaction of the vital force, but which only represent the alternating state of the various paroxysms of the primary action; they are termed alternating actions.

§ 116

Some symptoms are produced by the medicines more frequently – that is to say, in many individuals, others more rarely or in few persons, some only in very few healthy bodies.

§ 117

To the latter category belong the so-called idiosyncrasies, by which are meant peculiar corporeal constitutions which, although otherwise healthy, possess a disposition to be brought into a more or less morbid state by certain things which seem to produce no impression and no change in many other individuals.1 But this inability to make an impression on every one is only apparent. For as two things are required for the production of these as well as all other morbid alterations in the health of man – to wit., the inherent power of the influencing substance, and the capability of the vital force that animates the organism to be influenced by it – the obvious derangements of health in the so-called idiosyncrasies cannot be laid to the account of these peculiar constitutions alone, but they must also be ascribed to these things that produce them, in which must lie the power of making the same impressions on all human bodies, yet in such a manner that but a small number of healthy constitutions have a tendency to allow themselves to be brought into such an obvious morbid condition by them. That these agents do actually make this impression on every healthy body is shown by this, that when employed as remedies they render effectual homoeopathic service2 to all sick persons for morbid symptoms similar to those they seem to be only capable of producing in so-called idiosyncratic individuals.

1. Some few persons are apt to faint from the smell of roses and to fall into many other morbid, and sometimes dangerous states from partaking of mussels, crabs or the roe of the barbel, from touching the leaves of some kinds of sumach, etc.
2. Thus the Princess Maria Porphyroghnita restored her brother, the Emperor Alexius, who suffered from faintings, by sprinkling him with rose water in the presence of his aunt Eudoxia (Hist. byz. Alexias, lib. xv, p. 503, ed. Posser); and Horstius (Oper., iii, p.59) saw great benefit from rose vinegar in cases of syncope.

§ 118

Every medicine exhibits peculiar actions on the human frame, which are not produced in exactly the same manner by any other medicinal substance of a different kind.1

1. This fact was also perceived by the estimable A. v. Haller, who says (Preface to his Hist. stirp. helv.): "Latet immensa virium diversitas in iis ipsis plantis, quarum facies externas dudum novimus, animas quasi et quodcunque caelestius habent, nondum perspeximus."

§ 119

As certainly as every species of plant differs in its external form, mode of life and growth, in its taste and smell from every other species and genus of plant, as certainly as every mineral and salt differs from all others, in its external as well as its internal physical and chemical properties (which alone should have sufficed to prevent any confounding of one with another), so certainly do they all differ and diverge among themselves in their pathogenetic – consequently also in their therapeutic – effects.1 Each of these substances produces alterations in the health of human beings in a peculiar, different, yet determinate manner, so as to preclude the possibility of confounding one with another.2

1. Anyone who has a thorough knowledge of, and can appreciate the remarkable difference of, effects on the health of man of every single substance from those of every other, will readily perceive that among them there can be, in a medical point of view, no equivalent remedies whatever, no surrogates. Only those who do not know the pure, positive effects of the different medicines can be so foolish as to try to persuade us that one can serve in the stead of the other, and can in the same disease prove just as serviceable as the other. Thus do ignorant children confound the most essential different things, because they scarcely know their external appearances, far less their real value, their true importance and their very dissimilar inherent properties.
2. If this be pure truth, as it undoubtedly is, then no physician who would not be regarded as devoid of reason, and who would not act contrary to the dictates of his conscience, the sole arbiter of real worth, can employ in the treatment of diseases any medicinal substance but one with whose real significance he is thoroughly and perfectly conversant, i.e., whose positive action on the health of healthy individuals he has so accurately tested that he knows for certain that it is capable of producing a very similar morbid state, more similar than any other medicine with which he is perfectly acquainted, to that presented by the case of disease he intends to cure by means of it; for, as has been shown above, neither man, nor mighty Nature herself, can effect a perfect, rapid and permanent cure otherwise than with a homoeopathic remedy. Henceforth no true physician can abstain from making such experiment, in order to obtain this most necessary and only knowledge of the medicines that are essential to cure, this knowledge which has hitherto been neglected by the physicians in all ages. In all former ages – posterity will scarcely believe it – physicians have hitherto contented themselves with blindly prescribing for diseases medicines whose value was unknown, and which had never been tested relative to their highly important, very various, pure dynamic action on the health of man; and, moreover, they mingled several of these unknown medicines that differed so vastly among each other in one formula, and left it to chance to determine what effects should thereby be produced on the patient. This is just as if a madman should force his way into the workshop of an artisan, seize upon handfuls of very different tools, with the uses of all of which he is quite unacquainted, in order, as he imagines, to work at the

objects of art he sees around him. I need hardly remark that these would be destroyed, I may say utterly ruined, by his senseless operations.

§ 120

Therefore medicines, on which depend man's life and death, disease and health, must be thoroughly and most carefully distinguished from one another, and for this purpose tested by careful, pure experiments on the healthy body for the purpose of ascertaining their powers and real effects, in order to obtain an accurate knowledge of them, and to enable us to avoid any mistake in their employment in diseases, for it is only by correct selection of them that the greatest of all earthly blessings, the health of the body and of the mind, can be rapidly and permanently restored.

§ 121

In proving medicines to ascertain their effects on the healthy body, it must be borne in mind that the strong, heroic substances, as they are termed, are liable even in small doses to produce changes in the health even of robust persons. Those of milder power must be given for these experiments in more considerable quantities; in order to observe the action of the very weakest, however, the subjects of experiment should be persons free from disease, and who are delicate, irritable and sensitive.

§ 122

In these experiments – on which depends the exactitude of the whole medical art, and the weal of all future generations of mankind – no other medicines should be employed except such as are perfectly well known, and of whose purity, genuineness and energy we are thoroughly assured.

§ 123

Each of these medicines must be taken in a perfectly simple, unadulterated form; the indigenous plants in the form of freshly expressed juice, mixed with a little alcohol to prevent it spoiling; exotic vegetable substances, however, in the form of powder, or tincture prepared with alcohol when they were in the fresh state and afterwards mingled with a certain proportion of water; salts and gums, however, should be dissolved in water just before being taken. If the plant can only be procured in its dry state, and if its powers are naturally weak, in that case there may be used for the experiment an infusion of it, made by cutting the herb into small pieces and pouring boiling water on it, so as to extract its medicinal parts; immediately after its preparation it must be swallowed while still warm, as all expressed vegetable juices and all aqueous infusions of herbs, without the addition of spirit, pass rapidly into fermentation and decomposition, whereby all their medicinal properties are lost.

§ 124

For these experiments every medicinal substance must be employed quite alone and perfectly pure, without the admixture of any foreign substance, and without taking anything else of a medicinal nature the same day, nor yet on the subsequent days, nor during all the time we wish to observe the effects of the medicine.

§ 125

During all the time the experiment lasts the diet must be strictly regulated; it should be as much as possible destitute of spices, of a purely nutritious and simple character, green vegetables,1 roots and all salads and herb soups (which, even when most carefully prepared, possess some disturbing medicinal qualities) should be avoided. The drinks are to be those usually partaken of, as little stimulating as possible.2

1. Young green peas, green French beans ('boiled potatoes' in the Sixth Edition) and in all cases carrots are allowable, as the least medicinal vegetables.
2. The subject of experiment must either be not in the habit of taking pure wine, brandy, coffee or tea, or he must have totally abstained for a considerable time previously from the use of these injurious beverages, some of which are stimulating, others medicinal.

§ 126 FIFTH EDITION

The person who is proving the medicine must during the whole time of the experiment avoid all over-exertion of mind and body, all sorts of dissipation and disturbing passions; he should have no urgent business to distract his attention; he must devote himself to careful self-observation and not be disturbed while so engaged; his body must be in what is for him a good state of health, and he must possess a sufficient amount of intelligence to be able to express and describe his sensations in accurate terms.

§ 126 SIXTH EDITION

The person who is proving the medicine must be pre-eminently trustworthy and conscientious and during the whole time of the experiment avoid all over-exertion of mind and body, all sorts of dissipation and disturbing passions; he should have no urgent business to distract his attention;

he must devote himself to careful self-observation and not be disturbed while so engaged; his body must be in what is for him a good state of health, and he must possess a sufficient amount of intelligence to be able to express and describe his sensations in accurate terms.

§ 127

The medicines must be tested on both males and females, in order also to reveal the alterations of the health they produce in the sexual sphere.

§ 128 FIFTH EDITION

The most recent observations have shown that medicinal substances, when taken in their crude state by the experimenter for the purpose of testing their peculiar effects, do not exhibit nearly the full amount of the powers that lie hidden in them which they do when they are taken for the same object in high dilutions potentized by proper trituration and succussion, by which simple operations the powers which in their crude state lay hidden, and, as it were, dormant, are developed and roused into activity to an incredible extent. In this manner we now find it best to investigate the medicinal powers even of such substances as are deemed weak, and the plan we adopt is to give to the experimenter, on an empty stomach, daily from four to six very small globules of the thirtieth potentized dilution of such a substance, moistened with a little water, and let him continue this for several days.

§ 128 SIXTH EDITION

The most recent observations have shown that medicinal substances, when taken in their crude state by the experimenter for the purpose of testing their peculiar effects, do not exhibit nearly the full amount of the powers that lie hidden in them which they do when they are taken for the same object in high dilutions potentized by proper trituration and succussion, by which simple operations the powers which in their crude state lay hidden, and, as it were, dormant, are developed and roused into activity to an incredible extent. In this manner we now find it best to investigate the medicinal powers even of such substances as are deemed weak, and the plan we adopt is to give to the experimenter, on an empty stomach, daily from four to six very small globules of the thirtieth potency of such a substance, moistened with a little water or dissolved in more or less water and thoroughly mixed, and let him continue this for several days.

§ 129

If the effects that result from such a dose are but slight, a few more globules may be taken daily, until they become more distinct and stronger and the alterations of the health more conspicuous;

for all persons are not effected by a medicine in an equally great degree; on the contrary, there is a vast variety in this respect, so that sometimes an apparently weak individual may by scarcely at all affected by moderate doses of a medicine known to be of a powerful character, while he is strongly enough acted on by others of a much weaker kind. And, on the other hand, there are very robust persons who experience very considerable morbid symptoms from an apparently mild medicine, and only slighter symptoms from stronger drugs. Now, as this cannot be known beforehand, it is advisable to commence in every instance with a small dose of the drug and, where suitable and requisite, to increase the dose more and more from day to day.

§ 130

If, at the very commencement, the first dose administered shall have been sufficiently strong, this advantage is gained, that the experimenter learns the order of succession of the symptoms and can note down accurately the period at which each occurs, which is very useful in leading to a knowledge of the genius of the medicine, for then the order of the primary actions, as also that of the alternating actions, is observed in the most unambiguous manner. A very moderate dose, even, often suffices for the experiment, provided only the experimenter is endowed with sufficiently delicate sensitiveness, and is very attentive to his sensations. The duration of the action of a drug can only be ascertained by a comparison of several experiments.

§ 131

If, however, in order to ascertain anything at all, the same medicine must be given to the same person to test for several successive days in ever increasing doses, we thereby learn, no doubt, the various morbid states this medicine is capable of producing in a general manner, but we do not ascertain their order of succession; and the subsequent dose often removes, curatively, some one or other of the symptoms caused by the previous dose, or develops in its stead an opposite state; such symptoms should be enclosed in brackets, to mark their ambiguity, until subsequent purer experiments show whether they are the reaction of the organism and secondary action or an alternating action of this medicine.

§ 132

But when the object is, without reference to the sequential order of the phenomena and the duration of the action of the drug, only to ascertain the symptoms themselves, especially those of a weak medicinal substance, in that case the preferable course to pursue is to give it for several successive days, increasing the dose every day. In this manner the action of an unknown medicine, even of the mildest nature, will be revealed, especially if tested on sensitive persons.

§ 133

On experiencing any particular sensation from the medicine, it is useful, indeed necessary, in order to determine the exact character of the symptom, to assume various positions while it lasts, and to observe whether, by moving the part affected, by walking in the room or the open air, by standing, sitting or lying the symptom is increased, diminished or removed, and whether it returns on again assuming the position in which it was first observed, – whether it is altered by eating or drinking, or by any other condition, or by speaking, coughing, sneezing or any other action of the body, and at the same time to note at what time of the day or night it usually occurs in the most marked manner, whereby what is peculiar to and characteristic of each symptom will become apparent.

§ 134

All external influences, and more especially medicines, possess the property of producing in the health of the living organism a particular kind of alteration peculiar to themselves; but all the symptoms peculiar to a medicine do not appear in one person, nor all at once, nor in the same experiment, but some occur in one person chiefly at one time, others again during a second or third trail; in another person some other symptoms appear, but in such a manner that probably some of the phenomena are observed in the fourth, eighth or tenth person which had already appeared in the second, sixth or ninth person, and so forth; moreover, they may not recur at the same hour.

§ 135

The whole of the elements of disease a medicine is capable of producing can only be brought to anything like completeness by numerous observations on suitable persons of both sexes and of various constitutions. We can only be assured that a medicine has been thoroughly proved in regard to the morbid states it can produce – that is to say, in regard to its pure powers of altering the health of man – when subsequent experimenters can notice little of a novel character from its action, and almost always only the same symptoms as had been already observed by others.

§ 136

Although, as has been said, a medicine, on being proved on healthy subjects, cannot develop in one person all the alterations of health it is capable of causing, but can only do this when given to many different individuals, varying in their corporeal and mental constitution, yet the tendency to excite all these symptoms in every human being exists in it (§ 117), according to an eternal and immutable law of nature, by virtue of which all its effects, even those that are but rarely developed in the healthy person, are brought into operation in the case of every individual if administered to him when he is in a morbid state presenting similar symptoms; it then, even in the smallest dose, being homoeopathically selected, silently produces in the patient an artificial state closely resembling the natural disease, which rapidly and permanently (homoeopathically) frees and cures him of his original malady.

§ 137

The more moderate, within certain limits, the doses of the medicine used for such experiments are – provided we endeavor to facilitate the observation by the selection of a person who is a lover of truth, temperate in all respects, of delicate feelings, and who can direct the most minute attention to his sensation – so much the more distinctly are the primary effects developed, and only these, which are most worth knowing, occur without any admixture of secondary effects or reactions of the vital force. When, however, excessively large doses are used there occur at the same time not only a number of secondary effects among the symptoms, but the primary effects developed, and only these, which are most worth knowing, occur without any admixture of secondary effects or reactions of the vital force. When, however, excessively large doses are used there occur at the same time not only a number of secondary effects among the symptoms, but the primary effects also come on in such hurried confusion and with such impetuosity that nothing can be accurately observed; let alone the danger attending them, which no one who has any regard for his fellow-creatures, and who looks on the meanest of mankind as his brother, will deem an indifferent manner.

§ 138

All the sufferings, accidents and changes of the health of the experimenter during the action of a medicine (provided the above condition [§§ 124-127] essential to a good and pure experiment are complied with) are solely derived from this medicine, and must be regarded and registered as belonging peculiarly to this medicine, as symptoms of this medicine, even though the experimenter had observed, a considerable time previously, the spontaneous occurrence of similar phenomena in himself. The reappearance of these during the trial of the medicine only shows that this individual is, by virtue of his peculiar constitution, particularly disposed to have such symptoms excited in him. In this case they are the effect of the medicine; the symptoms do not arise spontaneously while the medicine that has been taken is exercising an influence over the health of the whole system, but are produced by the medicine.

§ 139

When the physician does not make the trial of the medicine on himself, but gives it to another person, the latter must note down distinctly the sensations, sufferings, accidents and changes of health he experiences at the time of their occurrence, mentioning the time after the ingestion of the drug when each symptom arose and, if it lasts long, the period of its duration. The physician looks over the report in the presence of the experimenter immediately after the experiment is concluded, or if the trial lasts several days he does this every day, in order, while everything is still fresh in his memory, to question him about the exact nature of every one of these circumstances, and to write down the more precise details so elicited, or to make such alterations as the experimenter may suggest.1

1. He who makes known to the medical world the results of such experiments becomes thereby responsible for the trustworthiness of the person experimented on and his statements, and justly so, as the weal of suffering humanity is here at stake.

§ 140

If the person cannot write, the physician must be informed by him every day of what has occurred to him, and how it took place. What is noted down as authentic information on this point, however, must be chiefly the voluntary narration of the person who makes the experiment, nothing conjectural and as little as possible derived from answers to leading questions should be admitted; everything must be ascertained with the same caution as I have counselled above (§§ 84-99) for the investigation of the phenomena and for tracing the picture of natural diseases.

§ 141

But the best provings of the pure effects of simple medicines in altering the human health, and of the artificial diseases and symptoms they are capable of developing in the healthy individual, are those which the healthy, unprejudiced and sensitive physician institutes on himself with all the caution and care here enjoined. He knows with the greatest certainty the things he has experienced in his own person.1

1. Those trials made by the physician on himself have for him other and inestimable advantages. In the first place, the great truth that the medicinal virtue of all drugs, whereon depends their curative power, lies in the changes of health he has himself undergone from the medicines he has proved, and the morbid states he has himself experienced from them, becomes for him an incontrovertible fact. Again by such noteworthy observations on himself he will be brought to understand his own sensations, his mode of thinking and his disposition (the foundation of all true wisdom "), and he will be also trained to be, what every physician ought to be, a good observer. All our observations on others are not nearly so interesting as those made on ourselves. The observer of others must always dread lest the experimenter did not feel exactly what he said, or lest he did not describe his sensations with the most appropriate expressions. He must always remain in doubt whether he has not been deceived, at least to some extent. These obstacles to the knowledge of the truth, which can never be thoroughly surmounted in our investigations

of the artificial morbid symptoms that occur in others from the ingestion of medicines, cease entirely when we make the trials on ourselves. He who makes these trials on himself knows for certain what he has felt, and each trial is a new inducement for him to investigate the powers of other medicines. He thus becomes more and more practised in the art of observing, of such importance to the physician, by continuing to observe himself, the one on whom he can most rely and who will never deceive him; and this he will do all the more zealously as these experiments on himself promise to give him a reliable knowledge of the true value and significance of the instruments of cure that are still to a great degree unknown to our art. Let it not be imagined that such slight indispositions caused by taking medicines for the purpose of proving them can be in the main injurious to the health. Experience shows on the contrary, that the organism of the prover becomes, by these frequent attacks on his health, all the more expert in repelling all external influences inimical to his frame and all artificial and natural morbific noxious agents, and becomes more hardened to resist everything of an injurious character, by means of these moderate experiments on his own person with medicines. His health becomes more unalterable; he becomes more robust, as all experience shows.

§ 142

But how some symptoms[1] of the simple medicine employed for a curative purpose can be distinguished amongst the symptoms of the original malady, even in diseases, especially in those of a chronic character that usually remain unaltered, is a subject appertaining to the higher art of judgement, and must be left exclusively to masters in observation.

1. Symptoms which, during the whole course of the disease, might have been observed only a long time previously, or never before, consequently new ones, belonging to the medicine.

§ 143

If we have thus tested on the healthy individual a considerable number of simple medicines and carefully and faithfully registered all the disease elements and symptoms they are capable of developing as artificial disease-producers, then only have we a true materia medica – a collection of real, pure, reliable[1] modes of action of simple medicinal substances, a volume of the book of nature, wherein is recorded a considerable array of the peculiar changes of the health and symptoms ascertained to belong to each of the powerful medicines, as they were revealed to the attention of the observer, in which the likeness of the (homoeopathic) disease elements of many natural diseases to be hereafter cured by them are present, which, in a word, contain artificial morbid states, that furnish for the similar natural morbid states the only true, homoeopathic, that is to say, specific, therapeutic instruments for effecting their certain and permanent cure.

1. Latterly it has been the habit to entrust the proving of medicines to unknown persons at a distance, who were paid for their work, and the formation so obtained was printed. But by so doing, the

work which is of all others the most important, which is to form the basis of the only true healing art, and which demands the greatest moral certainty and trustworthiness seems to me, I regret to say, to become doubtful and uncertain in its results and to lose all value.

§ 144

From such a materia medica everything that is conjectural, all that is mere assertion or imaginary should be strictly excluded; everything should be the pure language of nature carefully and honestly interrogated.

§ 145 FIFTH EDITION

Of a truth, it is only by a very considerable store of medicines accurately known in respect of these their pure modes of action in altering the health of man, that we can be placed in a position to discover a homoeopathic remedy, a suitable artificial (curative) morbific analogue for each of the infinitely numerous morbid states in nature, for every malady in the world.1 In the meantime, even now – thanks to the truthful character of the symptoms, and to the abundance of disease elements which every one of the powerful medicinal substances has already shown in its action on the healthy body – but few disease remain, for which a tolerably suitable homoeopathic remedy may not be met with among those now proved as to their pure action,2 which, without much disturbance, restores health in a gentle, sure and permanent manner - infinitely more surely and safely than can be effected by all the general and special therapeutics of the old allopathic medical art with its unknown composite remedies, which do but alter and aggravate but cannot cure chronic diseases, and rather retard than promote recovery from acute diseases.

1. At first, I was the only person who made the provings of the pure powders of medicines the most important of his occupations. Since then I have been assisted in this by some young men, who instituted experiments on themselves, and whose observations I have critically revised. Following these some genuine work of this kind was done by a few others. But what shall we not be able to effect in the way of curing in the whole extent of the infinitely large domain of disease, when numbers of accurate and trustworthy observers shall have rendered their services in enriching this, the only true materia medica, by careful experiments on themselves! The healing art will then come near the mathematical sciences in certainty.
2. See the second note to §109.

§ 145 SIXTH EDITION

Of a truth, it is only by a very considerable store of medicines accurately known in respect of these their pure modes of action in altering the health of man, that we can be placed in a position to discover a homoeopathic remedy, a suitable artificial (curative) morbific analogue for each of the infinitely numerous morbid states in nature, for every malady in the world.1 In the meantime, even now – thanks to the truthful character of the symptoms, and to the abundance of disease elements which every one of the powerful medicinal substances has already shown in its action on the healthy body – but few disease remain, for which a tolerably suitable homoeopathic remedy may not be met with among those now proved as to their pure action,2 which, without much disturbance, restores health in a gentle, sure and permanent manner - infinitely more surely and safely than can be effected by all the general and special therapeutics of the old allopathic medical art with its unknown composite remedies, which do but alter and aggravate but cannot cure chronic diseases, and rather retard than promote recovery from acute diseases and frequently endanger life.

1. At first, about forty years ago, I was the only person who made the provings of the pure powders of medicines the most important of his occupations. Since then I have been assisted in this by some young men, who instituted experiments on themselves, and whose observations I have critically revised. Following these some genuine work of this kind was done by a few others. But what shall we not be able to effect in the way of curing in the whole extent of the infinitely large domain of disease, when numbers of accurate and trustworthy observers shall have rendered their services in enriching this, the only true materia medica, by careful experiments on themselves! The healing art will then come near the mathematical sciences in certainty.
2. See the second note to §109.

§ 146

The third point of the business of a true physician relates to the judicious employment of the artificial morbific agents (medicines) that have been proved on healthy individuals to ascertain their pure action in order to effect the homoeopathic cure of natural diseases.

§ 147

Whichever of these medicines that have been investigated as to their power of altering man's health we find to contain in the symptoms observed from its use the greatest similarity to the totality of the symptoms of a given natural disease, this medicine will and must be the most suitable, the most certain homoeopathic remedy for the disease; in it is found the specific remedy of this case of disease.

§ 148 FIFTH EDITION

A medicine selected in this manner, which has the power and the tendency to produce symptoms the most similar possible to the disease to be cured, consequently a similar artificial disease, given in a suitable dose, affects, in its dynamic action on the morbidly deranged vital force of the individual, those very parts and points in the organism now suffering from the natural disease, and produces in them its own artificial disease, which, on account of its great similarity and preponderjng strength, occupies precisely the seat hitherto occupied by the natural morbid derangement, so that the instinctive, automatic vital force is from that time forward no longer affected by the natural disease but solely by the stronger, similar medicinal disease; which in its turn, on account of the small dose of the remedy, being, like every moderate medicinal disease, overcome by the increased energy of the vital force, soon spontaneously disappears, leaving the body free from all disease, that is to say, healthy and permanently cured.

§ 148 SIXTH EDITION

The natural disease is never to be considered as a noxious material situated somewhere within the interior or exterior of man (§ 11-13) but as one produced by an inimical spirit-like (conceptual) agency which, like a kind of infection (note to § 11) disturbs in its instinctive existence of the spirit-like (conceptual) principle of life within the organism torturing it as an evil spirit and compelling it to produce certain ailments and disorders in the regular course of its life. These are known as symptoms (disease). If, now, the influence of this inimical agency that not only caused but strives to continue this disorder, be taken away as is done when the physician administers an artificial potency, capable of altering the life principle in the most similar manner (a homoeopathic medicine) which exceeds in energy even in the smallest dose the similar natural disease (§§ 33, 279), then the influence of the original noxious morbid agent on the life principle is lost during the action of this stronger similar artificial disease. Thence the evil no longer exists for the life principle – it is destroyed. If, as has been said, the selected homoeopathic remedy is administered properly, then the acute natural disease which is to be overruled if recently developed, will disappear imperceptibly in a few hours.

An older, more chronic disease will yield somewhat later together with all traces of discomfort, by the use of several doses of the same more highly potentized remedy or after careful selection1 of one or another more similar homoeopathic medicine. Health, recovery, follow in imperceptible, often rapid transitions. The life principle is freed again and capable of resuming the life of the organism in health as before and strength returns.

1. But this laborious, sometimes very laborious, search for and selection of the homoeopathic remedy most suitable in every respect to each morbid state, is an operation which, notwithstanding all the admirable books for facilitating it, still demands the study of the original sources themselves, and at the same time a great amount of circumspection and serious deliberation, which have their best rewards in the consciousness of having faithfully discharged our duty. How could his laborious, care-demanding task, by which alone the best way of curing diseases is rendered possible, please the gentlemen of the new mongrel sect, who assume the honorable name of homoeopathists, and even seem to employ medicines in form and appearance homoeopathic, but determined upon by them anyhow (quidquid in buccam venit), and who, when the unsuitable remedy does not immediately give relief,

in place of laying the blame on their unpardonable ignorance and laxity in performing the most and important and serious of all human affairs, ascribe it to homoeopathy, which they accuse of great imperfection (if the truth be told, its imperfection consists in this, that the most suitable homoeopathic remedy for each morbid condition does not spontaneously fly into their mouths like roasted pigeons, without any trouble on their own part). They know, however, from frequent practice, how to make up for the inefficiency of the scarcely half homoeopathic remedy by the employment of allopathic means, that come much more handy to them, among which one or more dozens of leeches applied to the affected part, or little harmless venesections to the extent of eight ounces, and so forth, play an important part; and should the patient, in spite of all this, recover, they extol their venesections, leeches, etc., alleging that, had it not been for these, the patient would not have been pulled through, and they give us to understand, in no doubtful language, that these operations, derived without much exercise of genius from the pernicious routine of the old school, in reality contributed the best share towards the cure. But if the patient die under the treatment, as not unfrequently happens, they seek to console the friends by saying that "they themselves were witnesses that everything conceivable had been done for the lamented deceased". Who would do this frivolous and pernicious tribe the honour to call them, after the name of the very laborious but salutary art, homoeopathic physicians? May the just recompense await them, that, when taken ill, they may be treated in the same manner!

§ 149 FIFTH EDITION

When the suitable homoeopathic remedy has been thus selected and rightly employed, the acute disease we wish to cure, even though it be of a grave character and attended by many sufferings subsides insensibly, in a few hours if it be of recent date, in a few days if it be of a somewhat longer standing, along with all traces of indisposition, and nothing or almost nothing more of the artificial medicinal disease is perceived; there occurs, by rapid, imperceptible transitions, noting but restored health, recovery. Disease of long standing (and especially such as are of a complicated character) require for their cure a proportionately longer time. More especially do the chronic medicinal dyscrasia so often produced by allopathic bungling, along with the natural disease left uncured by it, require a much longer time for their recovery; often, indeed, are they incurable, in consequence of the shameful robbery of the patient's strength and juices, the principal feat performed by allopathy in its so-called methods of treatment.

§ 149 SIXTH EDITION

Diseases of long standing (and especially such as are of a complicated character) require for their cure a proportionately longer time. More especially do the chronic medicinal dyscrasia so often produced by allopathic bungling along with the natural disease left uncured by it, require a much longer time for their recovery; often, indeed, are they incurable, in consequence of the shameful robbery of the patient's strength and juices (venesections, purgatives, etc.), on account of long continued use of large doses of violently acting remedies given on the basis of empty, false theories for alleged usefulness in cases of disease appearing similar, also in prescribing unsuitable mineral baths, etc., the principal feat performed by allopathy in its so-called methods of treatment.

§ 150

If a patient complain of one or more trivial symptoms, that have been only observed a short time previously, the physician should not regard this as a fully developed disease but requires serious medical aid. A slight alteration in the diet and regimen will usually suffice to dispel such an indisposition.

§ 151

But if the patient complain of a few violent sufferings, the physician will usually find, on investigation, several other symptoms besides, although of a slighter character, which furnish a complete picture of the disease.

§ 152

The worse of the acute disease is, of so much the more numerous and striking symptoms is it generally composed, but with so much the more certainly may a suitable remedy for it be found, if there be a sufficient number of medicines known, with respect to their positive action, to choose from. Among the lists of symptoms of many medicines it will not be difficult to find one from whose separate disease elements an antitype of curative artificial disease, very like the totality of the symptoms of the natural disease, may be constructed, and such a medicine is the desired remedy.

§ 153 FIFTH EDITION

In this search for a homoeopathic specific remedy, that is to say, in this comparison of the collective symptoms of the natural disease with the list of symptoms of known medicines, in order to find among these an artificial morbific agent corresponding by similarity to the disease to be cured, the more striking, singular, uncommon and peculiar (characteristic) signs and symptoms1 of the case of disease are chiefly and most solely to be kept in view; for it is more particularly these that very similar ones in the list of symptoms of the selected medicine must correspond to, in order to constitute it the most suitable for effecting the cure. The more general and undefined symptoms: loss of appetite, headache, debility, restless sleep, discomfort, and so forth, demand but little attention when of that vague and indefinite character, if they cannot be more accurately described, as symptoms of such a general nature are observed in almost every disease and from almost every drug.

1. Dr. von Bonninghausen, who has already distinguished himself by his labours in connection with the new system of medicine, has lately increased our obligation to him by the publication of his important little book setting forth the characteristic symptoms, more particularly of the antipsoric medicines, entitled Uebersicht der Hauptwirkungs-Sphure der antips. Arz., Munster, bei Coppenrath, 1883, and the appendix thereto (containing the antisyphilitic and the antisycotic medicines) at the end of the second edition of his Systematisch-alphabetisches Repertorium der antipsorischen Arzneien, bei Coppenrath in Munster.

§ 153 SIXTH EDITION

In this search for a homoeopathic specific remedy, that is to say, in this comparison of the collective symptoms of the natural disease with the list of symptoms of known medicines, in order to find among these an artificial morbific agent corresponding by similarity to the disease to be cured, the more striking, singular, uncommon and peculiar (characteristic) signs and symptoms1 of the case of disease are chiefly and most solely to be kept in view; for it is more particularly these that very similar ones in the list of symptoms of the selected medicine must correspond to, in order to constitute it the most suitable for effecting the cure. The more general and undefined symptoms: loss of appetite, headache, debility, restless sleep, discomfort, and so forth, demand but little attention when of that vague and indefinite character, if they cannot be more accurately described, as symptoms of such a general nature are observed in almost every disease and from almost every drug.

1. Dr. von Bonninghausen, by the publication of the characteristic symptoms of homoeopathic medicines and his repertory has rendered a great service to Homoeopathy as well as Dr. J. H. G. Jahr in his handbook of principal symptoms.

§ 154

If the antitype constructed from the list of symptoms of the most suitable medicine contain those peculiar, uncommon, singular and distinguishing (characteristic) symptoms, which are to be met with in the disease to be cured in the greatest number and in the greatest similarity, this medicine is the most appropriate homoeopathic specific remedy for this morbid state; the disease, if it be not one of very long standing, will generally be removed and extinguished by the first dose of it, without any considerable disturbance.

§ 155 FIFTH EDITION

I say without any considerable disturbance. For in the employment of this most appropriate homoeopathic remedy it is only the symptoms of the medicine that correspond to the symptoms of the disease that are called into play, the former occupying the place of the latter (weaker) in the organism, and thereby annihilating them by overpowering them; but the other symptoms of the homoeopathic medicine, which are often very numerous, being in no way applicable to the case of disease in question, are not called into play at all. The patient, growing hourly better, feels almost nothing of them at all, because the excessively minute dose requisite for homoeopathic use is much too weak to produce the other symptoms of the medicine that are not homoeopathic to the case, in those parts of the body that are free from disease, and consequently can allow only the homoeopathic symptoms to act on the parts of the organism that are already most irritated and excited by the similar symptoms of the disease, thus changing the morbid affection of the vital force into a similar but stronger medicinal disease, whereby the original malady is extinguished.

§ 155 SIXTH EDITION

I say without any considerable disturbance. For in the employment of this most appropriate homoeopathic remedy it is only the symptoms of the medicine that correspond to the symptoms of the disease that are called into play, the former occupying the place of the latter (weaker) in the organism, i.e., in the sensation of the life principle, and thereby annihilating them by overpowering them; but the other symptoms of the homoeopathic medicine, which are often very numerous, being in no way applicable to the case of disease in question, are not called into play at all. The patient, growing hourly better, feels almost nothing of them at all, because the excessively minute dose requisite for homoeopathic use is much too weak to produce the other symptoms of the medicine that are not homoeopathic to the case, in those parts of the body that are free from disease, and consequently can allow only the homoeopathic symptoms to act on the parts of the organism that are already most irritated and excited by the similar symptoms of the disease, in order that the sick life principle may react only to a similar but stronger medicinal disease, whereby the original malady is extinguished.

§ 156

There is, however, almost no homoeopathic medicine, be it ever so suitably chosen, that, especially if it should be given in an insufficiently minute dose, will not produce, in very irritable and sensitive patients, at least one trifling, unusual disturbance, some slight new symptom while its action lasts; for it is next to impossible that medicine and disease should cover one another symptomatically as exactly as two triangles with equal sides and equal angles. But this (in ordinary circumstances) unimportant difference will be easily done away with by the potential activity (energy) of the living organism, and is not perceptible by patients not excessively delicate; the restoration goes forward, notwithstanding, to the goal of perfect recovery, if it be not prevented by the action of heterogeneous medicinal influences upon the patient, by errors of regimen or by excitement of the passions.

§ 157 FIFTH EDITION

But though it is certain that a homoeopathically selected remedy does, by reason of its appropriateness and the minuteness of the dose, gently remove and annihilate the acute disease analogous to it, without manifesting its other unhomoeopathic symptoms, that is to say, without the production of new, serious disturbances, yet it usually, immediately after ingestion – for the first hour, or for a few hours – causes a kind of slight aggravation (where the dose has been somewhat too large, however, for a considerable number of hours), which has so much resemblance to the original disease that it seems to the patient to be an aggravation of his own disease. But it is, in reality, nothing more than an extremely similar medicinal disease, somewhat exceeding in strength the original affection.

§ 157 SIXTH EDITION

But though it is certain that a homoeopathically selected remedy does, by reason of its appropriateness and the minuteness of the dose, gently remove and annihilate the acute disease analogous to it, without manifesting its other unhomoeopathic symptoms, that is to say, without the production of new, serious disturbances, yet it usually, immediately after ingestion – for the first hour, or for a few hours – causes a kind of slight aggravation when the dose has not been sufficiently small and (where the dose has been somewhat too large, however, for a considerable number of hours), which has so much resemblance to the original disease that it seems to the patient to be an aggravation of his own disease. But it is, in reality, nothing more than an extremely similar medicinal disease, somewhat exceeding in strength the original affection.

§ 158

This slight homoeopathic aggravation during the first hours – a very good prognostic that the acute disease will most probably yield to the first dose – is quite as it ought to be, as the medicinal disease must naturally be somewhat stronger than the malady to be cured if it is to overpower and extinguish the latter, just as a natural disease can remove and annihilate another one similar to it only when it is stronger than the latter (§§ 43 – 48).

§ 159 FIFTH EDITION

The smaller the dose of the homoeopathic remedy is, so much the slighter and shorter is the apparent increase of the disease during the first hours.

§ 159 SIXTH EDITION

The smaller the dose of the homoeopathic remedy is in the treatment of acute diseases so much the slighter and shorter is the apparent increase of the disease during the first hours.

§ 160

But as the dose of a homoeopathic remedy can scarcely ever be made so small that it shall not be able to relieve, overpower, indeed completely cure and annihilate the uncomplicated natural disease of not long standing that is analogous to it (§ 249, note), we can understand why a does of an appropriate homoeopathic medicine, not the very smallest possible, does always, during the first hour after its ingestion, produce a perceptible homoeopathic aggravation of this kind.1

1. This exaltation of the medicinal symptoms over those disease symptoms analogous to them, which looks like an aggravation, has been observed by other physicians also, when by accident they employed a homoeopathic remedy. When a patient suffering from itch complains of an increase of the eruption after sulphur, his physician who knows not the cause of this, consoles him with the assurance that the itch must first come out properly before it can be cured; he knows not, however, that this is a sulphur eruption, that assumes the appearance of an increase of the itch.

"The facial eruption which the viola tricolor cured was aggravated by it at the commencement of its action," Leroy tells us (Heilk, fur Mutter, p.406), but he knew not that the apparent aggravation was owing to the somewhat too large dose of the remedy, which in this instance was to a certain extent homoeopathic. Lysons says (Med. Transact., vol ii, London, 1772), "The bark of the elm cures most certainly those skin diseases which it increases at the beginning of its action." Had he not given the bark in the monstrous doses usual in the allopathic system, but in the quite small doses requisite when the medicine shows similarity of symptoms, that is to say, when it is used homoeopathically, he would have effected a cure without, or almost without, seeing this apparent increase of the disease (homoeopathic aggravation).

§ 161 SIXTH EDITION

When I here limit the so-called homoeopathic aggravation, or rather the primary action of the homoeopathic medicine that seems to increase somewhat the symptoms of the original disease, to the first or few hours, this is certainly true with respect to diseases of a more acute character and of recent origin, but where medicines of long action have to combat a malady of, considerable or of very long standing, where no such apparent increase of the original disease ought to appear during treatment and it does not so appear if the accurately chosen medicine was given in proper small, gradually higher doses, each somewhat modified with renewed dynamization (§ 247). Such increase of the original symptoms of a chronic disease can appear only at the end of treatment when the cure is almost or quite finished.

§ 162

Sometimes happens, owing to the moderate number of medicines yet known with respect to their true, pure action, that but a portion of the symptoms of the disease under treatment are to be met with in the list of symptoms of the most appropriate medicine, consequently this imperfect medicinal morbific agent must be employed for lack of a more perfect one.

§ 163

In this case we cannot indeed expect from this medicine a complete, untroubled cure; for during its use some symptoms appear which were not previously observable in the disease, accessory symptoms of the not perfectly appropriate remedy. This does by no means prevent a considerable part of the disease (the symptoms of the disease that resemble those of the medicine) from being eradicated by this medicine, thereby establishing a fair commencement of the cure, but still this does not take place without those accessory symptoms, which are, however, always moderate when the dose of the medicine is sufficiently minute.

§ 164

The small number of homoeopathic symptoms present in the best selected medicine is no obstacle to the cure in cases where these few medicinal symptoms are chiefly of an uncommon kind and such as are peculiarly distinctive (characteristic) of the disease; the cure takes place under such circumstances without any particular disturbance.

§ 165

If, however, among the symptoms of the remedy selected, there be none that accurately resemble the distinctive (characteristic), peculiar, uncommon symptoms of the case of disease, and if the remedy correspond to the disease only in the general, vaguely described, indefinite states (nausea, debility, headache, and so forth), and if there be among the known medicines none more homoeopathically appropriate, in that case the physician cannot promise himself any immediate favorable result from the employment of this unhomoeopathic medicine.

§ 166

Such a case is, however, very rare, owing to the increased number of medicines whose pure effects are now known, and the bad effects resulting from it, when they do occur, are diminished whenever a subsequent medicine, of more accurate resemblance, can be selected.

§ 167

Thus if there occur, during the use of this imperfectly homoeopathic remedy first employed, accessory symptoms of some moment, then, in the case of acute diseases, we do not allow this first dose to exhaust its action, nor leave the patient to the full duration of the action of the remedy, but we investigate afresh the morbid state in its now altered condition, and add the remainder of the original symptoms to those newly developed in tracing a new picture of the disease.

§ 168

We shall then be able much more readily to discover, among the known medicines, an analogue to the morbid state before us, a single dose of which, if it do not entirely destroy the disease, will advance it considerably on the way to be cured. And thus we go on, if even this medicine be not quite sufficient to effect the restoration of health, examining again and again the morbid state that still remains, and selecting a homoeopathic medicine as suitable as possible for it, until our object, namely, putting the patient in the possession of perfect health, is accomplished.

§ 169 FIFTH EDITION

If, on the first examination of a disease and the first selection of a medicine, we should find that the totality of the symptoms of the disease would not be effectually covered by the disease elements of a single medicine – owing to the insufficient number of known medicines, – but that two medicines contend for the preference in point of appropriateness, one of which is more homoeopathically suitable for one part, the other for another part of the symptoms of the disease, it is not advisable, after the employment of the more suitable of the two medicines, to administer the other without fresh examination, for the medicine that seemed to be the next best would not, under the change of circumstances that has in the meantime taken place, be suitable for the rest of the symptoms that then remain; in which case, consequently, a more appropriate homoeopathic remedy must be selected in place of the second medicine for the set of symptoms as they appear on a new inspection.

§ 169 SIXTH EDITION

If, on the first examination of a disease and the first selection of a medicine, we should find that the totality of the symptoms of the disease would not be effectually covered by the disease elements of a single medicine – owing to the insufficient number of known medicines, – but that two medicines contend for the preference in point of appropriateness, one of which is more homoeopathically suitable for one part, the other for another part of the symptoms of the disease, it is not advisable, after the employment of the more suitable of the two medicines, to administer the other without fresh examination, and much less to give both together (§ 272, note) for the medicine that seemed to be the next best would not, under the change of circumstances that has in the meantime taken place, be suitable for the rest of the symptoms that then remain; in which case, consequently, a more appropriate homoeopathic remedy must be selected in place of the second medicine for the set of symptoms as they appear on a new inspection.

§ 170

Hence in this as in every case where a change of the morbid state has occurred, the remaining set of symptoms now present must be inquired into, and (without paying any attention to the medicine which at first appeared to be the next in point of suitableness) another homoeopathic medicine, as appropriate as possible to the new state now before us, must be selected. If it should so happen, as is not often the case, that the medicine which at first appeared to be the next best seems still to be well adapted for the morbid state that remains, so much the more will it merit our confidence, and deserve to be employed in preference to another.

§ 171 FIFTH EDITION

In non-venereal chronic disease, those, therefore, that arise from psora, we often require, in order to effect a cure, to give several antipsoric remedies in succession, every successive one being homoeopathically chosen in consonance with the group of symptoms remaining after the expiry of the action of the previous remedy (which may have been employed in a single dose or in several successive doses).

§ 171 SIXTH EDITION

In non-venereal chronic disease, those, therefore, that arise from psora, we often require, in order to effect a cure, to give several antipsoric remedies in succession, every successive one being homoeopathically chosen in consonance with the group of symptoms remaining after completion of the action of the previous remedy.

§ 172

A similar difficulty in the way of the cure occurs from the symptoms of the disease being too few – a circumstances that deserves our careful attention, for by its removal almost all the difficulties that can lie in the way of this most perfect of all possible modes of treatment (except that its apparatus of known homoeopathic medicines is still incomplete) are removed.

§ 173

The only diseases that seem to have but few symptoms, and on that account to be less amenable to cure, are those which may be termed one-sided, because they display only one or two principal symptoms which obscure almost all the others. They belong chiefly to the class of chronic diseases.

§ 174

Their principal symptom may be either an internal complaint (e.g. a headache of many years' duration, a diarrhoea of long standing, an ancient cardialgia, etc.), or it may be an affection more of an external kind. Diseases of the latter character are generally distinguished by the name of local maladies.

§ 175

In one-sided diseases of the first kind it is often to be attributed to the medical observer's want of discernment that he does not fully discover the symptoms actually present which would enable him to complete the sketch of the portrait of the disease.

§ 176

There are, however, still a few diseases, which, after the most careful initial examination (§§ 84-98), present but one or two severe, violent symptoms, while all the others are but indistinctly perceptible.

§ 177

In order to meet most successfully such a case as this, which is of very rare occurrence, we are in the first place to select, guided by these few symptoms, the medicine which in our judgment is the most homoeopathically indicated.

§ 178

It will, no doubt, sometimes happen that this medicine, selected in strict observance of the homoeopathic law, furnishes the similar artificial disease suited for the annihilation of the malady present; and this is much more likely to happen when these few morbid symptoms are very striking, decided, uncommon and peculiarly distinctive (characteristic).

§ 179

More frequently, however, the medicine first chosen in such a case will be only partially, that is to say, not exactly suitable, as there was no considerable number of symptoms to guide to an accurate selection.

§ 180

In this case the medicine, which has been chosen as well as was possible, but which, for the reason above stated, is only imperfectly homoeopathic, will, in its action upon the disease that is only partially analogous to it – just as in the case mentioned above (§ 162, et seq.) where the limited number of homoeopathic remedies renders the selection imperfect – produce accessory symptoms, and several phenomena from its own array of symptoms are mixed up with the patient's state of health, which are, however, at the same time, symptoms of the disease itself, although they may have been hitherto never or very rarely perceived; some symptoms which the patient had never previously experienced appear, or others he had only felt indistinctly become more pronounced.

§ 181

Let is not be objected that the accessory phenomena and new symptoms of this disease that now appear should be laid to the account of the medicament just employed. They owe their origin to it1 certainly, but they are always only symptoms of such a nature as this disease was itself capable of producing in this organism, and which were summoned forth and induced to make their appearance by the medicine given, owing to its power to cause similar symptoms. In a word, we have to regard the whole collection of symptoms now perceptible as belonging to the disease itself, as the actual existing condition, and to direct our further treatment accordingly.

1. When they were not caused by an important error in regimen, a violent emotion, or a tumultuous revolution in the organism, such as the occurrence or cessation of the menses, conception, childbirth, and so forth.

§ 182

Thus the imperfect selection of the medicament, which was in this case almost inevitable owing to the too limited number of the symptoms present, serves to complete the display of the symptoms of the disease, and in this way facilitates the discovery of a second, more accurately suitable, homoeopathic medicine.

§ 183

Whenever, therefore, the dose of the first medicine ceases to have a beneficial effect (if the newly developed symptoms do not, by reason of their gravity, demand more speedy aid – which, however, from the minuteness of the dose of homoeopathic medicine, and in very chronic diseases, is excessively rare), a new examination of the disease must be instituted, the status morbi as it now is must be noted down, and a second homoeopathic remedy selected in accordance with it, which shall exactly suit the present state, and one which shall be all the more appropriate can then be found, as the group of symptoms has become larger and more complete.1

1. In cases where the patient (which, however, happens excessively seldom in chronic, but not infrequently in acute, diseases) feels very ill, although his symptoms are very indistinct, so that this state may be attributed more to the benumbed state of the nerves, which does not permit the patient's pains and sufferings to be distinctly perceived, this torpor of the internal sensibility is removed by opium, and in its secondary action the symptoms of the disease become distinctly apparent.

§ 184 FIFTH EDITION

In like manner, after each new dose of medicine has exhausted its action, the state of the disease that still remains is to be noted anew with respect to its remaining symptoms, and another homoeopathic remedy sought for, as suitable as possible for the group of symptoms now observed, and so on until the recovery is complete.

§ 184 SIXTH EDITION

In like manner, after each new dose of medicine has exhausted its action, when it is no longer suitable and helpful, the state of the disease that still remains is to be noted anew with respect to its remaining symptoms, and another homoeopathic remedy sought for, as suitable as possible for the group of symptoms now observed, and so on until the recovery is complete.

§ 185

Among the one-sided disease an important place is occupied by the so-called local maladies, by which term is signified those changes and ailments that appear on the external parts of the body. Till now the idea prevalent in the schools was that these parts were alone morbidly affected, and that the rest of the body did not participate in the disease – a theoretical, absurd doctrine, which has led to the most disastrous medical treatment.

§ 186 FIFTH EDITION

Those so-called local maladies which have been produced a short time previously, solely by an external lesion, still appear at first sight to deserve the name of local disease. But then the lesion must be very trivial, and in that case it would be of no great moment. For in the case of injuries accruing to the body from without, if they be at all severe, the whole living organism sympathizes; there occur fever, etc. The treatment of such diseases is relegated to surgery; but this is right only in so far as the affected parts require mechanical aid, whereby the external obstacles to the cure, which can only be expected to take place by the agency of the vital force, may be removed by mechanical means, e.g., by the reduction of dislocations, by bandages to bring together the lips of wounds, by the extraction of foreign bodies that have penetrated into the living parts, by making an opening into a cavity of the body in order to remove an irritating substance or to procure the evacuation of effusions or collections of fluids, by bringing into apposition the broken extremities of a fractured bone and retaining them in exact contact by an appropriate bandage, etc. But when in such injuries the whole living organism requires, as it always does, active dynamic aid to put it in a position to accomplish the work of healing, e.g. when the violent fever resulting from extensive contusions, lacerated muscles, tendons and blood-vessels requires to be removed by medicine given internally, or when the external pain of scalded or burnt parts needs to be homoeopathically subdued, then the services of the dynamic physician and his helpful homoeopathy come into requisition.

§ 186 SIXTH EDITION

Those so-called local maladies which have been produced a short time previously, solely by an external lesion, still appear at first sight to deserve the name of local disease. But then the lesion must be very trivial, and in that case it would be of no great moment. For in the case of injuries accruing to the body from without, if they be at all severe, the whole living organism sympathizes; there occur fever, etc. The treatment of such diseases is relegated to surgery; but this is right only in so far as the affected parts require mechanical aid, whereby the external obstacles to the cure, which can only be expected to take place by the agency of the vital force, may be removed by mechanical means, e.g., by the reduction of dislocations, by needles and bandages to bring together the lips of wounds, by mechanical pressure to still the flow of blood from open arteries, by the extraction of foreign bodies that have penetrated into the living parts, by making an opening into a cavity of the body in order to remove an irritating substance or to procure the evacuation of effusions or collections of fluids, by bringing into apposition the broken extremities of a fractured bone and retaining them in exact contact by an appropriate bandage, etc. But when in such injuries the whole living organism requires, as it always does, active dynamic aid to put it in a position to accomplish the work of healing, e.g. when the violent fever resulting from extensive contusions, lacerated muscles, tendons and blood-vessels requires to be removed by medicine given internally, or when the external pain of scalded or burnt parts needs to be homoeopathically subdued, then the services of the dynamic physician and his helpful homoeopathy come into requisition.

§ 187

But those affections, alterations and ailments appearing on the external parts, that do not arise from any external injury or that have only some slight external wound for their immediate exciting cause, are produced in quite another manner; their source lies in some internal malady. To consider them as mere local affections, and at the same time to treat them only, or almost only, as it were surgically, with topical applications – as the old school have done from the remotest ages – is as absurd as it is pernicious in its results.

§ 188

These affections were considered to be merely topical, and were therefore called local diseases, as if they were maladies exclusively limited to those parts wherein the organism took little or no part, or affections of these particular visible parts of which the rest of the living organism, so to speak, knew nothing.1

1. One of the many great and pernicious blunders of the old school.

§ 189

And yet very little reflection will suffice to convince us that no external malady (not occasioned by some important injury from without) can arise, persist or even grow worse without some internal cause, without the co-operation of the whole organism, which must consequently be in a diseased state. It could not make its appearance at all without the consent of the whole of the rest of the health, and without the participation of the rest of the living whole (of the vital force that pervades all the other sensitive and irritable parts of the organism); indeed, it is impossible to conceive its production without the instrumentality of the whole (deranged) life; so intimately are all parts of the organism connected together to form an indivisible whole in sensation and functions. No eruption on the lips, no whitlow can occur without previous and simultaneous internal ill-health.

§ 190

All true medical treatment of a disease on the external parts of the body that has occurred from little or no injury from without must, therefore, be directed against the whole, must effect the annihilation and cure of the general malady by means of internal remedies, if it is wished that the treatment should be judicious, sure, efficacious and radical.

§ 191

This is confirmed in the most unambiguous manner by experience, which shows in all cases that every powerful internal medicine immediately after its ingestion causes important changes in the general health of such a patient, and particularly in the affected external parts (which the ordinary medical school regards as quite isolated), even in a so-called local disease of the most external parts of the body, and the change it produces is most salutary, being the restoration to health of the entire body, along with the disappearance of the external affection (without the aid of any external remedy), provided the internal remedy directed towards the whole state was suitable chosen in a homoeopathic sense.

§ 192

This is best effected when, in the investigation of the case of disease, along with the exact character of the local affection, all the changes, sufferings and symptoms observable in the patient's health, and which may have been previously noticed when no medicines had been used, are taken in conjunction to form a complete picture of the disease before searching among the medicines, whose peculiar pathogenetic effects are known, for a remedy corresponding to the totality of the symptoms, so that the selection may be truly homoeopathic.

§ 193

By means of this medicine, employed only internally (and, if the disease be but of recent origin, often by the very first dose of it), the general morbid state of the body is removed along with the local affection, and the latter is cured at the same time as the former, proving that the local affection depended solely on a disease of the rest of the body, and should only be regarded as an inseparable part of the whole, as one of the most considerable and striking symptoms of the whole disease.

§ 194

It is not useful, either in acute local diseases of recent origin or in local affections that have already existed a long time, to rub in or apply externally to the spot an external remedy, even though it be the specific and, when used internally, salutary by reason of its homoeopathicity, even although it should be at the same time administered internally; for the acute topical affections (e.g., inflammations of the individual parts, erysipelas, etc.), which have not been caused by external injury of proportionate violence, but by dynamic or internal causes, yield most surely to internal remedies homoeopathically adapted to the perceptible state of the health present in the exterior and interior, selected from the general store of proved medicines,1 and generally without any other aid; but if these diseases do not yield to them completely, and if there still remain in the affected spot and in the whole state, notwithstanding good regimen, a relic of disease which the vital force is not competent to restore to the normal state, then the acute disease was (as not infrequently happens) a product of psora which had hitherto remained latent in the interior, but has now burst forth and is on the point of developing into a palpable chronic disease.

1. As, for instance, aconite, rhus, belladonna, mercury, etc.

§ 195

In order to effect a radical cure in such cases, which are by no means rare, after the acute state has pretty well subsided, an appropriate antipsoric treatment (as is taught in my work on Chronic Diseases) must then be directed against the symptoms that still remain and the morbid state of health to which the patient was previously subject. In chronic local maladies that are not obviously venereal, the antipsoric internal treatment is, moreover, alone requisite.

§ 196

It might, indeed, seen as though the cure of such diseases would be hastened by employing the medicinal substance which is known to be truly homoeopathic to the totality of the symptoms, not only internally, but also externally, because the action of a medicine applied to the seat of the local affection might effect a more rapid change in it.

§ 197 FIFTH EDITION

This treatment, however, is quite inadmissible, not only for the local symptoms arising from the miasm of psora, but also and especially for those originating in the miasm of syphilis or sycosis, for the simultaneous local application, along with the internal employment, of the remedy in diseases whose chief symptom is a constant local affection, has this great disadvantage, that, by such a topical application, this chief symptom (local affection)1 will usually be annihilated sooner than the internal disease, and we shall now be deceived by the semblance of a perfect cure; or at least it will be difficult, and in some cases impossible, to determine, from the premature disappearance of the local symptom, if the general disease is destroyed by the simultaneous employment of the internal medicine.

1. Recent itch eruption, chancre, condylomata.

§ 197 SIXTH EDITION

This treatment, however, is quite inadmissible, not only for the local symptoms arising from the miasm of psora, but also and especially for those originating in the miasm of syphilis or sycosis, for the simultaneous local application, along with the internal employment, of the remedy in diseases whose chief symptom is a constant local affection, has this great disadvantage, that, by such a topical application, this chief symptom (local affection)1 will usually be annihilated sooner than the internal disease, and we shall now be deceived by the semblance of a perfect cure; or at least it will be difficult, and in some cases impossible, to determine, from the premature disappearance of the local symptom, if the general disease is destroyed by the simultaneous employment of the internal medicine.

1. Recent itch eruption, chancre, condylomata, as I have indicated in my book of Chronic Diseases.

§ 198

The mere topical employment of medicines, that are powerful for cure when given internally, to the local symptoms of chronic miasmatic diseases is for the same reason quite inadmissible; for if the local affection of the chronic disease be only removed locally and in a one-sided manner, the internal treatment indispensable for the complete restoration of the health remains in dubious obscurity; the chief symptom (the local affection) is gone, and there remain only the other, less distinguishable symptoms, which are less constant and less persistent than the local affection, and frequently not sufficiently peculiar and too slightly characteristic to display after that, a picture of the disease in clear and peculiar outlines.

§ 199

If the remedy perfectly homoeopathic to the disease had not yet been discovered1 at the time when the local symptoms were destroyed by a corrosive or desiccative external remedy or by the knife, then the case becomes much more difficult on account of the too indefinite (uncharacteristic) and inconstant appearance of the remaining symptoms; for what might have contributed most to determine the selection of the most suitable remedy, and its internal employment until the disease should have been completely annihilated, namely, the external principal symptom, has been removed from our observation.

1. As was the case before my time with the remedies for the condylomatous disease (and the antipsoric medicines).

§ 200 FIFTH EDITION

Had it still been present to guide the internal treatment, the homoeopathic remedy for the whole disease might have been discovered, and had that been found, the persistence of the local affection during its internal employment would have shown that the cure was not yet completed; but were it cured on its seat, this would be a convincing proof that the disease was completely eradicated, and the desired recovery from the entire disease was fully accomplished – an inestimable, indispensable advantage.

§ 200 SIXTH EDITION

Had it still been present to guide the internal treatment, the homoeopathic remedy for the whole disease might have been discovered, and had that been found, the persistence of the local affection during its internal employment would have shown that the cure was not yet completed; but were it cured on its seat, this would be a convincing proof that the disease was completely eradicated, and the desired recovery from the entire disease was fully accomplished – an inestimable, indispensable advantage to reach a perfect cure.

§ 201 FIFTH EDITION

It is evident that man's vital force, when encumbered with a chronic disease which it is unable to overcome by its own powers, adopts the plan of developing a local malady on some external part, solely for this object, that by making and keeping in a diseased state this part which is not indispensable to human life, it may thereby silence the internal disease, which otherwise threatens to destroy the vital organs (and to deprive the patient of life), and that it may thereby, so to speak, transfer the internal disease to the vicarious local affection and, as it were, draw it thither. The presence of the local affection thus silences, for a time, the internal disease, though without being able either to cure it or to diminish it materially.1 The local affection, however, is never anything else than a part of the general disease, but a part of it increased all in one direction by the organic vital force, and transferred to a less dangerous (external) part of the body, in order to allay the internal ailment. But (as has been said) by this local symptom that silences the internal disease, so far from anything being gained by the vital force towards diminishing or curing the whole malady, the internal disease, on the contrary, continues, in spite of it, gradually to increase and Nature is constrained to enlarge and aggravate the local symptom always more and more, in order that it may still suffice as a substitute for the increased internal disease and may still keep it under. Old ulcers on the legs get worse as long as the internal psora is uncured, the chancre enlarges as long as the internal syphilis remains uncured, just as the general internal disease continues to increase as time goes on.

1. The issues of the old-school do something similar; as artificial ulcers on external parts, they silence some internal chronic diseases, but only for a short time, without being able to cure them; but, on the other hand, they weaken and destroy the general health much more than is done by most of the metastases effected by the instinctive vital force.

§ 201 SIXTH EDITION

It is evident that man's vital force, when encumbered with a chronic disease which it is unable to overcome by its own powers instinctively, adopts the plan of developing a local malady on some external part, solely for this object, that by making and keeping in a diseased state this part which is not indispensable to human life, it may thereby silence the internal disease, which otherwise threatens to destroy the vital organs (and to deprive the patient of life), and that it may thereby, so to speak, transfer the internal disease to the vicarious local affection and, as it were, draw it thither. The presence of the local affection thus silences, for a time, the internal disease, though without being able either to cure it or to diminish it materially.1 The local affection, however, is never anything else than a part of the general disease, but a part of it increased all in one direction by the organic vital force, and transferred to a less dangerous (external) part of the body, in order to allay the internal ailment. But (as has been said) by this local symptom that silences the internal disease, so far from anything being gained by the vital force towards diminishing or curing the whole malady, the internal disease, on the contrary, continues, in spite of it, gradually to increase and Nature is constrained to enlarge and aggravate the local symptom always more and more, in order that it may still suffice as a substitute for the increased internal disease and may still keep it under. Old ulcers on the legs get worse as long as the internal psora is uncured, the chancre enlarges as long as the internal syphilis remains uncured, the fig warts increased and grow while the sycosis is not cured whereby the latter is rendered more and more difficult to cure, just as the general internal disease continues to increase as time goes on.

1. The issues of the old-school do something similar; as artificial ulcers on external parts, they silence some internal chronic diseases, but only for a short time, as long as they cause a painful

irritation to which the sick organism is not used, without being able to cure them; but, on the other hand, they weaken and destroy the general health much more than is done by most of the metastases effected by the instinctive vital force.

§ 202

If the old-school physician should now destroy the local symptom by the topical application of external remedies, under the belief that he thereby cures the whole disease, Nature makes up for its loss by rousing the internal malady and the other symptoms that previously existed in a latent state side by side with the local affection; that is to say, she increases the internal disease. When this occurs it is usual to say, though incorrectly that the local affection has been driven back into the system or upon the nerves by the external remedies.

§ 203

Every external treatment of such local symptoms, the object of which is to remove them from the surface of the body, while the internal miasmatic disease is left uncured, as, for instance, driving off the skin the psoric eruption by all sorts of ointments, burning away the chancre by caustics and destroying the condylomata on their seat by the knife, the ligature or the actual cautery; this pernicious external mode of treatment, hitherto so universally practised, has been the most prolific source of all the innumerable named or unnamed chronic maladies under which mankind groans; it is one of the most criminal procedures the medical world can be guilty of, and yet it has hitherto been the one generally adopted, and taught from the professional chairs as the only one.1

1. For any medicines that might at the same time be given internally served but to aggravate the malady, as these remedies possessed no specific power of curing the whole disease, but assailed the organism, weakened it and inflicted on it, in addition, other chronic medicinal diseases.

§ 204 FIFTH EDITION

If we deduct all chronic affections, ailments and diseases that depend on a persistent unhealthy mode of living, (§ 77) as also those innumerable medicinal maladies (v. § 74) caused by the irrational, persistent, harassing and pernicious treatment of diseases often only of trivial character by physicians of the old school, all the remainder, without exception, result from the development of these three chronic miasms, internal syphilis, internal sycosis, but chiefly and in infinitely greater proportion, internal psora, each of which was already in possession of the whole organism, and had penetrated it in all directions before the appearance of the primary, vicarious local symptom of each of them (in the case of psora the scabious eruption, in syphilis the chancre or the bubo, and in sycosis the condylomata) that prevented their outburst; and these chronic miasmatic diseases, if deprived of their local symptom, are inevitably destined by mighty Nature sooner or later to become developed and to burst forth, and thereby propagate all the nameless misery, the incredible number of chronic diseases which have plagued mankind for hundreds and thousands of years, none of which would so frequently have come into existence had physicians striven in a rational manner to cure radically and to extinguish in the organism these three miasms by the internal homoeopathic medicines suited for each of them, without employing topical remedies for their external symptoms. (See note to § 282).

§ 204 SIXTH EDITION

If we deduct all chronic affections, ailments and diseases that depend on a persistent unhealthy mode of living, (§ 77) as also those innumerable medicinal maladies (v. § 74) caused by the irrational, persistent, harassing and pernicious treatment of diseases often only of trivial character by physicians of the old school, most the remainder of chronic diseases result from the development of these three chronic miasms, internal syphilis, internal sycosis, but chiefly and in infinitely greater proportion, internal psora, each of which was already in possession of the whole organism, and had penetrated it in all directions before the appearance of the primary, vicarious local symptom of each of them (in the case of psora the scabious eruption, in syphilis the chancre or the bubo, and in sycosis the condylomata) that prevented their outburst; and these chronic miasmatic diseases, if deprived of their local symptom, are inevitably destined by mighty Nature sooner or later to become developed and to burst forth, and thereby propagate all the nameless misery, the incredible number of chronic diseases which have plagued mankind for hundreds and thousands of years, none of which would so frequently have come into existence had physicians striven in a rational manner to cure radically and to extinguish in the organism these three miasms by the internal homoeopathic medicines suited for each of them, without employing topical remedies for their external symptoms. (See note to § 282).

§ 205 FIFTH EDITION

The homoeopathic physician never treats one of these primary symptoms of chronic miasms, nor yet one of their secondary affections that result from their further development, by local remedies (neither by those external agents that act dynamically,1 nor yet by those that act mechanically), but he cures, in cases where the one or the other appears, only the great miasm on which they depend, whereupon its primary, as also its secondary symptoms disappear spontaneously; but as this was not the mode pursued by the old-school practitioners who preceded him in the treatment of the case, the homoeopathic physician generally, alas!, finds that the primary symptoms2 have already been destroyed by them by means of external remedies, and that he has now to do more with the secondary ones, i.e., the affections resulting from the breaking forth and development of these inherent miasms, but especially with the chronic disease evolved from internal psora, the internal treatment of which, as far as a single physician can elucidate it by many years of reflection, observation and experience, I have endeavored to point out in my work on Chronic Diseases, to which I must refer the reader.

1. I cannot therefore advise, for instance, the local extirpation of the so-called cancer of the lips and face by means of the arsenical remedy of Frere Cosme, not only because it is excessively painful and often fails, but more for this reason, because, if this dynamic remedy should indeed succeed in freeing the affected part of the body from the malignant ulcer locally, the basic malady is thereby not diminished in the slightest, the preserving vital force is therefore necessitated to transfer the field of operation of the great internal malady to some more important part (as it does in every case of metastasis), and the consequence is blindness, deafness, insanity, suffocative asthma, dropsy, apoplexy, etc. But this ambiguous local liberation of the part from the malignant ulcer by the topical arsenical remedy only succeeds, after all, in those cases where the ulcer has not yet attained any great size, and when the vital force is still very energetic; but it is just in such a state of things that the complete internal cure of the whole original disease is also still practicable.

    The result is the same without previous cure of the inner miasm when cancer of the face or breast is removed by the knife alone and when encysted tumors are enucleated; something worse ensues, or at any rate death is hastened. This has been the case times without number, but the old school still goes blindly on in the same way in every new case, with the same disastrous results.
2. Itch eruption, chancre (bubo), condylomata.

§ 205 SIXTH EDITION

The homoeopathic physician never treats one of these primary symptoms of chronic miasms, nor yet one of their secondary affections that result from their further development, by local remedies (neither by those external agents that act dynamically,1 nor yet by those that act mechanically), but he cures, in cases where the one or the other appears, only the great miasm on which they depend, whereupon its primary, as also its secondary symptoms disappear spontaneously; but as this was not the mode pursued by the old-school practitioners who preceded him in the treatment of the case, the homoeopathic physician generally, alas!, finds that the primary symptoms2 have already been destroyed by them by means of external remedies, and that he has now to do more with the secondary ones, i.e., the affections resulting from the breaking forth and development of these inherent miasms, but especially with the chronic disease evolved from internal psora, the internal treatment of which, as far as a single physician can elucidate it by many years of reflection, observation and experience, I have endeavored to point out in my work on Chronic Diseases, to which I must refer the reader.

1. I cannot therefore advise, for instance, the local extirpation of the so-called cancer of the lips and face (the product of highly developed psora, not infrequently in conjunction with syphilis) by means of the arsenical remedy of Frere Cosme, not only because it is excessively painful and often fails, but more for this reason, because, if this dynamic remedy should indeed succeed in freeing the affected part of the body from the malignant ulcer locally, the basic malady is thereby not

diminished in the slightest, the preserving vital force is therefore necessitated to transfer the field of operation of the great internal malady to some more important part (as it does in every case of metastasis), and the consequence is blindness, deafness, insanity, suffocative asthma, dropsy, apoplexy, etc. But this ambiguous local liberation of the part from the malignant ulcer by the topical arsenical remedy only succeeds, after all, in those cases where the ulcer has not yet attained any great size, and when the vital force is still very energetic; but it is just in such a state of things that the complete internal cure of the whole original disease is also still practicable.

The result is the same without previous cure of the inner miasm when cancer of the face or breast is removed by the knife alone and when encysted tumors are enucleated; something worse ensues, or at any rate death is hastened. This has been the case times without number, but the old school still goes blindly on in the same way in every new case, with the same disastrous results.

2. Itch eruption, chancre (bubo), condylomata.

§ 206 FIFTH EDITION

Before commencing the treatment of a chronic disease, it is necessary to make the most careful investigation1 as to whether the patient has had a venereal infection (or an infection with condylomatous gonorrhoea); for then the treatment must be directed towards this alone, when only the signs of syphilis (or of the rarer condylomatous disease) are present, but this disease is very seldom met with alone nowadays. If such infection have previously occurred, this must also be borne in mind in the treatment of those cases in which psora is present, because in them the latter is complicated with the former, as is always the case when the symptoms are not those of pure syphilis; for when the physician thinks he has a case of old venereal disease before him, he has always, or almost always, to treat a syphilitic affection accompanied mostly by (complicated with) psora, for the internal itch dyscrasia (the psora) is far the most frequent (most certain) fundamental cause of chronic diseases, either united (complicated) with syphilis (or with sycosis), if the latter infections have avowedly occurred; or, as is much more frequently the case, psora is the sole fundamental cause of all other chronic maladies, whatever names they may bear, which are, moreover, so often bungled, increased and disfigured to a monstrous extent by allopathic unskillfulness.

1. In investigations of this nature we must not allow ourselves to be deceived by the assertions of the patients of their friends, who frequently assign as the cause of chronic, even of the severest and most inveterate diseases, either a cold caught (a thorough wetting, drinking cold water after being heated) many years ago, or a former fright, a sprain, a vexation (sometimes even a bewitchment), etc. These causes are much too insignificant to develop a chronic disease in a healthy body, to keep it up for years, and to aggravate it year by year, as is the case with all chronic diseases from developed psora. Causes of a much more important character than those remembered noxious influences must lie at the root of the initiation and progress of a serious, obstinate disease of long standing; the assigned causes could only rouse into activity the latent chronic miasm.

§ 206 SIXTH EDITION

Before commencing the treatment of a chronic disease, it is necessary to make the most careful investigation1 as to whether the patient has had a venereal infection (or an infection with condylomatous gonorrhoea); for then the treatment must be directed towards this alone, when only the signs of syphilis (or of the rarer condylomatous disease) are present, but this disease is very seldom met with alone nowadays. If such infection have previously occurred, this must also be borne in mind in the treatment of those cases in which psora is present, because in them the latter is complicated with the former, as is always the case when the symptoms are not those of pure syphilis; for when the physician thinks he has a case of old venereal disease before him, he has always, or almost always, to treat a syphilitic affection accompanied mostly by (complicated with) psora, for the internal itch dyscrasia (the psora) is far the most frequent fundamental cause of chronic diseases. At times, both miasms may be complicated also with sycosis in chronically diseased organisms, or, as is much more frequently the case, psora is the sole fundamental cause of all other chronic maladies, whatever names they may bear, which are, moreover, so often bungled, increased and disfigured to a monstrous extent by allopathic unskillfulness.

1. In investigations of this nature we must not allow ourselves to be deceived by the assertions of the patients of their friends, who frequently assign as the cause of chronic, even of the severest and most inveterate diseases, either a cold caught (a thorough wetting, drinking cold water after being heated) many years ago, or a former fright, a sprain, a vexation (sometimes even a bewitchment), etc. These causes are much too insignificant to develop a chronic disease in a healthy body, to keep it up for years, and to aggravate it year by year, as is the case with all chronic diseases from developed psora. Causes of a much more important character than those remembered noxious influences must lie at the root of the initiation and progress of a serious, obstinate disease of long standing; the assigned causes could only rouse into activity the latent chronic miasm.

§ 207

When the above information has been gained, it still remains for the homoeopathic physician to ascertain what kinds of allopathic treatment had up to that date been adopted for the chronic disease, what perturbing medicines had been chiefly and most frequently employed, also what mineral baths had been used and what effects these had produced, in order to understand in some measure the degeneration of the disease from its original state, and, where possible, to correct in part these pernicious artificial operations, or to enable him to avoid the employment of medicines that have already been improperly used.

§ 208

The age of the patient, his mode of living and diet, his occupation, his domestic position, his social relation and so forth, must next be taken into consideration, in order to ascertain whether these things have tended to increase his malady, or in how far they may favor or hinder the treatment. In like manner the state of his disposition and mind must be attended to, to learn whether that presents any obstacles to the treatment, or requires to be directed encouraged or modified.

§ 209

After this is done, the physician should endeavor in repeated conversations with the patient to trace the picture of his disease as completely as possible, according to the directions given above, in order to be able to elucidate the most striking and peculiar (characteristic) symptoms, in accordance with which he selects the first antipsoric or other remedy having the greatest symptomatic resemblance, for the commencement of the treatment, and so forth.

§ 210

Of psoric origin are almost all those diseases that I have above termed one-sided, which appear to be more difficult to cure in consequence of this one-sidedness, all their other morbid symptoms disappearing, as it were, before the single, great, prominent symptom. Of this character are what are termed mental diseases. They do not, however, constitute a class of disease the condition of the disposition and mind is always altered;1 and in all cases of disease we are called on to cure the state of the patient's disposition is to be particularly noted, along with the totality of the symptoms, if we would trace an accurate picture of the disease, in order to be able therefrom to treat it homoeopathically with success.

1. How often, for instance, do we not meet with a mild, soft disposition in patients who have for years been afflicted with the most painful diseases, so that the physician feels constrained to esteem and compassionate the sufferer! But if he subdue the disease and restore the patient to health – as is frequently done in homoeopathic practice – he is often astonished and horrified at the frightful alteration in his disposition. He often witnesses the occurrence of ingratitude, cruelty, refined malice and propensities most disgraceful and degrading to humanity, which were precisely the qualities possessed by the patient before he grew ill.

Those who were patient when well often become obstinate, violent, hasty, or even intolerant and capricious, or impatient or disponding when ill; those formerly chaste and modest often frequently become lascivious and shameless. A clear-headed person not infrequently becomes obtuse of intellect, while one ordinarily weak-minded becomes more prudent and thoughtful; and a man slow to make up his mind sometimes acquires great presence of mind and quickness of resolve, etc.

§ 211

This holds good to such an extent, that the state of the disposition of the patient often chiefly determines the selection of the homoeopathic remedy, as being a decidedly characteristic symptom which can least of all remain concealed from the accurately observing physician.

§ 212

The Creator of therapeutic agents has also had particular regard to this main feature of all diseases, the altered state of the disposition and mind, for there is no powerful medicinal substance in the world which does not very notably alter the state of the disposition and mind in the healthy individual who tests it, and every medicine does so in a different manner.

§ 213

We shall, therefore, never be able to cure conformably to nature – that is to say, homoeopathically – if we do not, in every case of disease, even in such as are acute, observe, along with the other symptoms, those relating to the changes in the state of the mind and disposition, and if we do not select, for the patient's relief, from among the medicines a disease-force which, in addition to the similarity of its other symptoms to those of the disease, is also capable of producing a similar state of the disposition and mind.1

1. Thus aconite will seldom or never effect a rapid or permanent cure in a patient of a quiet, calm, equable disposition; and just as little will nux vomica be serviceable where the disposition is mild and phlegmatic, pulsatilla where it is happy, gay and obstinate, or ignatia where it is imperturbable and disposed neither to be frightened nor vexed.

§ 214

The instructions I have to give relative to the cure of mental diseases may be confined to a very few remarks, as they are to be cured in the same way as all other diseases, namely, by a remedy which shows, by the symptoms it causes in the body and mind of a healthy individual, a power of producing a morbid state as similar as possible to the case of disease before us, and in no other way can they be cured.

§ 215

Almost all the so-called mental and emotional diseases are nothing more than corporeal diseases in which the symptom of derangement of the mind and disposition peculiar to each of them is increased, while the corporeal symptoms decline (more or less rapidly), till it a length attains the most striking one-sidedness, almost as though it were a local disease in the invisible subtle organ of the mind or disposition.

§ 216

The cases are not rare in which a so-called corporeal disease that threatens to be fatal – a suppuration of the lungs, or the deterioration of some other important viscus, or some other disease of acute character, e.g., in childbed, etc. – becomes transformed into insanity, into a kind of melancholia or into mania by a rapid increase of the psychical symptoms that were previously present, whereupon the corporeal symptoms lose all their danger; these latter improve almost to perfect health, or rather they decrease to such a degree that their obscured presence can only be detected by the observation of a physician gifted with perseverance and penetration. In this manner they become transformed into a one-sided and, as it were, a local disease, in which the symptom of the mental disturbance, which was at first but slight, increases so as to be the chief symptom, and in a great measure occupies the place of the other (corporeal) symptoms, whose intensity it subdues in a palliative manner, so that, in short, the affections of the grosser corporeal organs become, as it were, transferred and conducted to the almost spiritual, mental and emotional organs, which the anatomist has never yet and never will reach with his scalpel.

§ 217

In these diseases we must be very careful to make ourselves acquainted with the whole of the phenomena, both those belonging to the corporeal symptoms, and also, and indeed particularly, those appertaining to the accurate apprehension of the precise character of the chief symptom, of the peculiar and always predominating state of the mind and disposition, in order to discover, for the purpose of extinguishing the entire disease, among the remedies whose pure effects are known, a homoeopathic medicinal pathogenetic force – that is to say, a remedy which in its list of symptoms displays, with the greatest possible similarity, not only the corporeal morbid symptoms present in the case of disease before us, but also especially this mental and emotional state.

§ 218

To this collection of symptoms belongs in the first place to accurate description of all the phenomena of the previous so-called corporeal disease, before it degenerated into a one-sided increase of the physical symptom, and became a disease of the mind and disposition. This may be learned from the report of the patient's friends.

§ 219

A comparison of these previous symptoms of the corporeal disease with the traces of them that still remain, though they have become less perceptible (but which even now sometimes become prominent, when a lucid interval and a transient alleviation of the psychical disease occurs), will serve to prove them to be still present, though obscured.

§ 220

By adding to this the state of the mind and disposition accurately observed by the patient's friends and by the physician himself, we have thus constructed the complete picture of the disease, for which in order to effect the homoeopathic cure of the disease, a medicine capable of producing strikingly similar symptoms, and especially an analogous disorder of the mind, must be sought for among the antipsoric remedies, if the physical disease have already lasted some time.

§ 221

If, however, insanity or mania (caused by fright, vexation, the abuse of spirituous liquors, etc.) have suddenly broken out as an acute disease in the patient's ordinary calm state, although it almost always arises from internal psora, like a flame bursting forth from it, yet when it occurs in this acute manner it should not be immediately treated with antipsoric, but in the first place with remedies indicated for it out of the order class of proved medicaments (e.g., aconite, belladonna, stramonium, hyoscyamus, mercury, etc.) in highly potentized, minute, homoeopathic doses, in order to subdue it so far that the psora shall for the time revert to its former latent state, wherein the patient appears as if quite well.

§ 222

But such a patient, who has recovered from an acute mental or emotional disease by the use of these non-antipsoric medicines, should never be regarded as cured; on the contrary, no time should be lost in attempting to free him completely,1 by means of a prolonged antipsoric treatment, from the chronic miasm of the psora, which, it is true, has now become once more latent but is quite ready to break out anew; if this be done, there is no fear of another similar attack, if he attend faithfully to the diet and regimen prescribed for him.

1. It very rarely happens that a mental or emotional disease of long standing ceases spontaneously (for the internal dyscrasia transfers itself again to the grosser corporeal organs); such are the few cases met with now and then, where a former inmate of a madhouse has been dismissed apparently recovered. Hitherto, moreover, all madhouses have continued to be chokefull, so that

the multitude of other insane persons who seek for admission into such institutions could scarcely find room in them unless some of the insane in the house died. Not one is ever really and permanently cured in them! A convincing proof, among many others, of the complete nullity of the non-healing art hitherto practised, which has been ridiculously honored by allopathic ostentation with the title of rational medicine. How often, on the other hand, has not the true healing art, genuine pure homoeopathy, been able to restore such unfortunate beings to the possession of their mental and corporeal health, and so give them back again to their delighted friends and to the world!

§ 223

But if the antipsoric treatment be omitted, then we may almost assuredly expect, from a much slighter cause than brought on the first attack of the insanity, the speedy occurrence of a new and more lasting the severe fit, during which the psora usually develops itself completely, and passes into either a periodic or continued mental derangement, which is then more difficult to be cured by antipsorics.

§ 224

If the mental disease be not quite developed, and if it be still somewhat doubtful whether it really arose from a corporeal affection, or did not rather result from faults of education, bad practices, corrupt morals, neglect of the mind, superstition or ignorance; the mode of deciding this point will be, that if it proceed from one or other of the latter causes it will diminish and be improved by sensible friendly exhortations, consolatory arguments, serious representations and sensible advice, whereas a real moral or mental malady, depending on bodily disease, would be speedily aggravated by such a course, the melancholic would become still more dejected, querulous, inconsolable and reserved, the spiteful maniac would thereby become still more exasperated, and the chattering fool would become manifestly more foolish.1

1. It would seem as though the mind, in these cases, felt with uneasiness and grief the truth of these rational representations and acted upon the body as it wished to restore the lost harmony, but that the body, by means of its disease, reacted upon the organs of the mind and disposition and put them in still greater disorder by a fresh transference of its sufferings on to them.

§ 225

There are, however, as has just been stated, certainly a few emotional diseases which have not merely been developed into that form out of corporeal diseases, but which, in an inverse manner, the body being but slightly indisposed, originate and are kept up by emotional causes, such as continued anxiety, worry, vexation, wrongs and the frequent occurrence of great fear and fright. This kind of emotional diseases in time destroys the corporeal health, often to a great degree.

§ 226

It is only such emotional diseases as these, which were first engendered and subsequently kept up by the mind itself, that, while they are yet recent and before they have made very great inroads on the corporeal state, may, by means of psychical remedies, such as a display of confidence, friendly exhortations, sensible advice, and often by a well-disguised deception, be rapidly changed into a healthy state of the mind (and with appropriate diet and regimen, seemingly into a healthy state of the body also.)

§ 227

But the fundamental cause in these cases also is a psoric miasm, which was only not yet quite near its full development, and for security's sake, the seemingly cured patient should be subjected to a radical, antipsoric treatment, in order that he may not again, as might easily occur, fall into a similar state of mental disease.

§ 228

In mental and emotional diseases resulting from corporeal maladies, which can only be cured by homoeopathic antipsoric medicine conjoined with carefully regulated mode of life, an appropriate psychical behavior towards the patient on the part of those about him and of the physician must be scrupulously observed, by way of an auxiliary mental regimen. To furious mania we must oppose clam intrepidity and cool, firm resolution – to doleful, querulous lamentation, a mute display of commiseration in looks and gestures – to senseless chattering, a silence not wholly inattentive – to disgusting and abominable conduct and to conversation of a similar character, total inattention. We must merely endeavor to prevent the destruction and injury of surrounding objects, without reproaching the patient for his acts, and everything must be arranged in such a way that the necessity for any corporeal punishments and tortures1 whatever may be avoided. This is so much the more easily effected, because in the administration of the medicine – the only circumstance in which the employment of coercion could be justified – in the homoeopathic system the small doses of the appropriate medicine never offend the taste, and may consequently be given to the patient without his knowledge in his drink, so that all compulsion is unnecessary.

1. It is impossible to marvel at the hard-heartedness and indiscretion of the medical men in many establishments for patients of this kind, who, without attempting to discover the true and only efficacious mode of curing such disease, which is by homoeopathic medicinal (antipsoric) means,

content themselves with torturing these most pitiable of all human beings with the most violent blows and other painful torments. By this unconscientious and revolting procedure they debase themselves beneath the level of the turnkeys in a house of correction, for the latter inflict such chastisement as the duty devolving on their office, and on criminals only, whilst the former appear, from a humiliating consciousness of their uselessness as physicians, only to vent their spite at the supposed incurability of mental diseases in harshness towards the pitiable, innocent sufferers, for they are too ignorant to be of any use and too indolent to adopt a judicious mode of treatment.

§ 229

On the other hand, contradiction, eager explanations, rude corrections and invectives, as also weak, timorous yielding, are quite out of place with such patients; they are equally pernicious modes of treating mental and emotional maladies. But such patients are most of all exasperated and their complaint aggravated by contumely, fraud, and deceptions that they can detect. The physician and keeper must always pretend to believe them to be possessed of reason.

All kinds of external disturbing influences on their senses and disposition should be if possible removed; there are no amusements for their clouded spirit, no salutary distractions, no means of instruction, no soothing effects from conversation, books or other things for the soul that pines or frets in the chains of the diseased body, no invigoration for it, but the care; it is only when the bodily health is changed for the better that tranquillity and comfort again beam upon their mind.1

1. Foot-note in Sixth Edition only.

The treatment of the violent insane manic and melancholic can take place only in an institution specially arranged for their treatment but not within the family circle of the patient.

§ 230

If the antipsoric remedies selected for each particular case of mental or emotional disease (there are incredibly numerous varieties of them) be quite homoeopathically suited for the faithfully traced picture of the morbid state, which, if there be a sufficient number of this kind of medicines known in respect of their pure effects, is ascertained by an indefatigable search for the most appropriate homoeopathic remedy all the more easily, as the emotional and mental state, constituting the principal symptom of such a patient, is so unmistakably perceptible, – then the most striking improvement in no very long time, which could not be brought about by physicking the patient to death with the largest oft – repeated doses of all other unsuitable (allopathic) medicines. Indeed, I can confidently assert, from great experience, that the vast superiority of the homoeopathic system over all other conceivable methods of the treatment is nowhere displayed in a more triumphant light than in mental and emotional diseases of long standing, which originally sprang from corporeal maladies or were developed simultaneously with them.

§ 231

The intermittent disease deserve a special consideration, as well those that recur at certain periods – like the great number of intermittent fevers, and the apparently non-febrile affections that recur at intervals like intermittent fevers – as also those in which certain morbid states alternate at uncertain intervals with morbid states of a different kind.

§ 232

These latter, alternating diseases, are also very numerous,1 but all belong to the class of chronic diseases; they are generally a manifestation of developed psora alone, sometimes, but seldom, complicated with a syphilitic miasm, and therefore in the former case may be cured by antipsoric medicines; in the latter, however, in alternation with antisyphilitics as taught in my work on the Chronic Diseases.

1. Two or three states may alternate with one another. Thus, for instance, in the case of double alternating diseases, certain pains may occur persistently in the legs, etc., immediately on the disappearance of a kind of ophthalmia, which latter again appears as soon as the pain in the limbs has gone off for the time – convulsions and spasms may alternate immediately with any other affection of the body or some part of it – in a case of threefold alternating states in a common indisposition, periods of apparent increase of health and unusual exaltation of the corporeal and mental powers (extravagant gaiety, extraordinary activity of the body, excess of comfortable feeling, inordinate appetite, etc.) may occur, after which, and quite unexpectedly, gloomy, melancholy humor, intolerable hypochondriacal derangement of the disposition, with disorder of several of the vital operations, the digestion, sleep, etc., appear, which again, and just as suddenly, give place to the habitual moderate ill-health; and so also several and very various alternating states. When the new state makes its appearance, there is often no perceptible trace of the former one. In other cases only slight traces of the former alternating state remain when the new one occurs; few of the symptoms of the first state remain on the appearance and during the continuance of the second. Sometimes the morbid alternating states are quite of opposite natures, as for instance, melancholy periodically alternating with gay insanity or frenzy.

§ 233

The typical intermittent disease are those where a morbid state of unvarying character returns at a tolerably fixed period, while the patient is apparently in good health, and takes its departure at an equally fixed period; this is observed in those apparently non-febrile morbid states that come and go in a periodical manner (at certain times), as well as in those of a febrile character, to wit, the numerous varieties of intermittent fevers.

§ 234

Those apparently non-febrile, typical, periodically recurring morbid states just alluded to observed in one single patient at a time (they do not usually appear sporadically or epidemically) always belong to the chronic diseases, mostly to those that are purely psoric, are but seldom complicated with syphilis, and are successfully treated by the same means; yet it is sometimes necessary to employ as an intermediate remedy a small dose of a potentized solution of cinchona bark, in order to extinguish completely their intermittent type.

§ 235

With regard to the intermittent fevers,1 that prevail sporadically or epidemically (not those endemically located in marshy districts), we often find every paroxysm likewise composed of two opposite alternating states (cold, heat – heat, cold), more frequently still of three (cold, heat, sweat). Therefore the remedy selected for them from the general class of proved (common, not antipsoric) medicines must either (and remedies of this sort are the surest) be able likewise to produce in the healthy body two (or all three) similar alternating states, or else must correspond by similarity of symptoms, in the most homoeopathic manner possible, to the strongest, best marked, and most peculiar alternating state (either to the cold stage, or to the hot stage, or to the sweating state, each with its accessory symptoms, according as the one or other alternating state is the strongest and most peculiar); but the symptoms of the patient's health during the intervals when he is free from fever must be the chief guide to the most appropriate homoeopathic remedy.2

1. The pathology hitherto in vogue, which is still in the stage of irrational infancy, recognizes but one single intermittent fever, which it likewise termed ague, and admits of no varieties but such as are constituted by the different intervals at which the paroxysms recur, quotidian, tertian, quartan etc. But there are much more important differences among them than what are marked by the periods of their recurrence; there are innumerable varieties of these fevers, some of which cannot even be denominated ague, as their fits consist solely of heat; others, again, are characterised by cold alone, with or without subsequent perspiration; yet others which exhibit general coldness of the surface, with a sensation on the patient's part, or whilst the body feels externally hot, the patient feels cold; others, again, in which one paroxysm consists entirely of a rigor or simple chilliness followed by an interval of health, while the next consists of heat alone, followed or not by perspiration; others, again, in which the heat comes first and the cold stage not till that is gone; others, again, wherein after a cold or hot stage apyrexia ensues, and then perspiration comes on like a second fit, often many hours subsequently; others, again, in which no perspiration at all comes on, and yet others in which the whole attack consists of perspiration alone, without any cold or hot stage, or in which the perspiration is only present during the heat; and there are innumerable other

differences, especially in regard to the accessory symptoms, such as headache of a peculiar kind, bad taste of the mouth, nausea, vomiting, diarrhoea, want of or excessive thirst, peculiar pains in the body or limbs, disturbed sleep, deliria, alterations of temper, spasms, etc., before, during or after the sweating stage, and countless other varieties. All these are manifestly intermittent fevers of very different kinds, each of which, as might naturally be supposed, requires a special (homoeopathic) treatment. It must be confessed that they can almost all be suppressed (as is often done) by enormous doses of bark and of its pharmaceutical preparation, the sulphate of quinine; that is to say, their periodical recurrence (their typus) may be extinguished by it, but the patients who suffered from intermittent fevers for which cinchona bark is not suitable, as is the case with all those epidemic intermittent fevers that traverse whole countries and even mountainous districts, are not restored to health by the extinction of the typus; on the contrary, they now remain ill in another manner, and worse, often much worse, than before; they are affected by peculiar, chronic bark dyscrasias, and can scarcely be restored to health even by a prolonged treatment by the true system of medicine – and yet that is what is called curing, forsooth!

2. Dr. von Bonninghausen, who has rendered more services to our beneficent system of medicine than any other of my disciples, has best elucidated this subject, which demands so much care, and has facilitated the choice of the efficient remedy for the various epidemics of fever, in his work entitled Versuch einer homoopathischen Therapie der Wechselfieber, 1833, Muster bi Regensberg.

§ 236

The most appropriate and efficacious time for administering the medicine in these cases is immediately or very soon after the termination of the paroxysm, as soon as the patient has in some degree recovered from its effects; it has then time to effect all the changes in the organism requisite for the restoration of health, without any great disturbance or violent commotion; whereas the action of a medicine, be it ever so specifically appropriate, if given immediately before the paroxysm, coincides with the natural recurrence of the disease and causes such a reaction in the organism, such a violent contention, that an attack of that nature produces at the very least a great loss of strength, if it do not endanger life.1 But if the medicine be given immediately after the termination of the fit, that is to say, at the period when the apyretic interval has commenced and a long time before there are any preparations for the next paroxysm, then the vital force of the organism is in the best possible condition to allow itself to be quietly altered by the remedy, and thus restored to the healthy state.

1. This is observed in the fatal cases, by no means rare, in which a moderate dose of opium given during the cold stage quickly deprived the patients of life.

§ 237

But if the stage of apyrexia be very short, as happens in some very bad fevers, or if it be disturbed by some of the after sufferings of the previous paroxysm, the dose of the homoeopathic

medicine should be administered when the perspiration begins to abate, or the other subsequent phenomena of the expiring paroxysm begin to diminish.

§ 238 FIFTH EDITION

It is only when the suitable medicine has with a single dose destroyed several fits and manifest health and ensued, but after some time indications of a new paroxysm appear, only then can and must the same medicine be given again, provided always the totality of the symptoms is still the same. This recurrence of the same fever after an interval of health is, however, only possible when the noxious influence that first excited the intermittent fever still continues to act upon the convalescent, as happens in marshy districts; in which case a permanent cure is often only possible by the removal of this exciting cause (as, for instance, a residence in a mountainous country if the case was one of marsh intermittent fever).

§ 238 SIXTH EDITION

Not infrequently, the suitable medicine has with a single dose destroyed several attacks and brought about the return of health, but in the majority of cases, another dose must be administered after such attack. Better still, however, when the character of the symptoms has not changed, doses of the same medicine given according to the newer discovery of repetition of doses (see note to § 270), may be given without difficulty in dynamizing each successive dose with 10-12 succussions of the vial containing the medicinal substance. Nevertheless, there are at times cases, though seldom, where the intermittent fever returns after several days' well being. This return of the same fever after a healthy interval is only possible when the noxious principle that first caused the fever, is still acting upon the convalescent, as is the case in marshy regions. Here a permanent restoration can often take place only by getting away from this causative factor, as is possible by seeking a mountainous retreat, if the cause was a marshy fever.

§ 239

As almost every medicine causes in its pure action a special, peculiar fever and even a kind of intermittent fever with its alternating states, differing from all other fevers that are caused by other medicines, homoeopathic remedies may be found in the extensive domain of medicines for all the numerous varieties of natural intermittent fevers and, for a great many of such fevers, even in the moderate collection of medicines already proved on the healthy individual.

§ 240

But if the remedy found to be the homoeopathic specific for a prevalent epidemic of intermittent fever do not effect a perfect cure in some one or other patient, if it be not the influence of a marshy district that prevents the cure, it must always be the psoric miasm in the background, in which case antipsoric medicines must be employed until complete relief is obtained.

§ 241

Epidemics of intermittent fever, in situations where none are endemic, are of the nature of chronic diseases, composed of single acute paroxysms; each single epidemic is of a peculiar, uniform character common to all the individuals attacked, and when this character is found in the totality of the symptoms common to all, it guides us to the discovery of the homoeopathic (specific) remedy suitable for all the cases, which is almost universally serviceable in those patients who enjoyed tolerable health before the occurrence of the epidemic, that is to say, who were not chronic sufferers from developed psora.

§ 242

If, however, in such an epidemic intermittent fever the first paroxysms have been left uncured, or if the patients have been weakened by improper allopathic treatment; then the inherent psora that exists, alas! in so many persons, although in a latent state, becomes developed, takes on the type of the intermittent fever, and to all appearance continues to play the part of the epidemic intermittent fever, so that the medicine, which would have been useful in the first paroxysms (rarely an antipsoric), is now no longer suitable and cannot be of any service. We have now to do with a psoric intermittent fever only, and this will generally be subdued by minute and rarely repeated doses of sulphur or hepar sulphuris in a high potency.

§ 243

In those often very pernicious intermittent fevers which attack a single person, not residing in a marshy district, we must also at first, as in the case of acute diseases generally, which they resemble in respect to their psoric origin, employ for some days, to render what service it may, a homoeopathic remedy selected for the special case from the other class of proved (not antipsoric) medicines; but if, notwithstanding this procedure, the recovery is deferred, we know that we have psora on the point of its development, and that in this case antipsoric medicines alone can effect a radical cure.

§ 244 FIFTH EDITION

The intermittent fevers endemic in marshy districts and tracts of country frequently exposed to inundations, give a great deal of work to physicians of the old school, and yet a healthy man may in his youth become habituated even to marshy districts and remain in good health, provided he preserves a faultless regimen and his system is not lowered by want, fatigue or pernicious passions. The intermittent fevers endemic there would at the most only attack him on his first arrival; but one or two very small doses of a highly potentized solution of cinchona bark would, conjointly with the well-regulated mode of living just alluded to, speedily free him from the disease. But persons who, while taking sufficient corporeal exercise and pursuing a healthy system of intellectual occupations and bodily regimen, cannot be cured of marsh intermittent fever by one or a few of such small doses of cinchona – in such persons psora, striving to develop itself, always lies at the root of their malady, and their intermittent fever cannot be cured in the marshy district without antipsoric treatment.1 It sometimes happens that when these patients exchange, without delay, the marshy district for one that is dry and mountainous, recovery apparently ensues (the fever leaves them) if they be not yet deeply sunk in disease, that is to say, if the psora was not completely developed in them and can consequently return to its latent state; but they will never regain perfect health without antipsoric treatment.

1. Large, oft-repeated doses of cinchona bark, as also concentrated cinchona remedies, such as the sulphate of quinine, have certainly the power of freeing such patients from the periodical fits of the marsh ague; but those thus deceived into the belief that they are cured remain diseased in another way.

§ 244 SIXTH EDITION

The intermittent fevers endemic in marshy districts and tracts of country frequently exposed to inundations, give a great deal of work to physicians of the old school, and yet a healthy man may in his youth become habituated even to marshy districts and remain in good health, provided he preserves a faultless regimen and his system is not lowered by want, fatigue or pernicious passions. The intermittent fevers endemic there would at the most only attack him on his first arrival; but one or two very small doses of a highly potentized solution of cinchona bark would, conjointly with the well-regulated mode of living just alluded to, speedily free him from the disease. But persons who, while taking sufficient corporeal exercise and pursuing a healthy system of intellectual occupations and bodily regimen, cannot be cured of marsh intermittent fever by one or a few of such small doses of cinchona – in such persons psora, striving to develop itself, always lies at the root of their malady, and their intermittent fever cannot be cured in the marshy district without antipsoric treatment.1 It sometimes happens that when these patients exchange, without delay, the marshy district for one that is dry and mountainous, recovery apparently ensues (the fever leaves them) if they be not yet deeply sunk in disease, that is to say, if the psora was not completely developed in them and can consequently return to its latent state; but they will never regain perfect health without antipsoric treatment.

1. Large, oft-repeated doses of cinchona bark, as also concentrated cinchona remedies, such as the sulphate of quinine, have certainly the power of freeing such patients from the periodical fits of the marsh ague; but those thus deceived into the belief that they are cured remain diseased in another way, frequently with an incurable Quinin intoxication (see §276 note.)

§ 245 FIFTH EDITION

Having thus seen what attention should, in the homoeopathic treatment, be paid to the chief varieties of diseases and to the peculiar circumstances connected with them, we now pass on to what we have to say respecting the remedies and the mode of employing them, together with the diet and regimen to be observed during their use.

§ 245 SIXTH EDITION

Having thus seen what attention should, in the homoeopathic treatment, be paid to the chief varieties of diseases and to the peculiar circumstances connected with them, we now pass on to what we have to say respecting the remedies and the mode of employing them, together with the diet and regimen to be observed during their use.

Every perceptibly progressive and strikingly increasing amelioration in a transient (acute) or persistent (chronic) disease, is a condition which, as long as it lasts, completely precludes every repetition of the administration of any medicine whatsoever, because all the good the medicine taken continues to effect is new hastening towards its completion. Every new dose of any medicine whatsoever, even of the one last administered, that has hitherto shown itself to be salutary, would in this case disturb the work of amelioration.

§ 246 FIFTH EDITION

On the other hand, the slowly progressive amelioration consequent on a very minute dose, whose selection has been accurately homoeopathic, when it has met with no hindrance to the duration of its action, sometimes accomplishes all the good the remedy in question is capable from its nature of performing in a given case, in periods of forty, fifty or a hundred days. This is, however, but rarely the case; and besides, it must be a matter of great importance to the physician as well as to the patient that were it possible, this period should be diminished to one-half, one-quarter, and even still less, so that a much more rapid cure might be obtained. And this may be very happily affected, as recent and oft-repeated observations have shown, under three conditions: firstly, if the medicine selected with the utmost care was perfectly homoeopathic; secondly, if it was given in the minutest dose, so as to produce the least possible excitation of the vital force,

and yet sufficient to effect the necessary change in it; and thirdly, if this minutest yet powerful dose of the best selected medicine be repeated at suitable intervals,1 which experience shall have pronounced to be the best adapted for accelerating the cure to the utmost extent, yet without the vital force, which it is sought to influence to the production of a similar medicinal disease, being able to feel itself excited and roused to adverse reactions.

1. In the former editions of the Organon I have advised that a single dose of a well-selected homoeopathic medicine should always be allowed first fully to expend its action before a new medicine is given or the same one repeated – a doctrine which was the result of the positive experience that neither by a larger dose of the remedy, which may have been well chosen (as has been again recently proposed, but which would be very like a retrograde movement), nor, what amounts to the same thing, by several doses of it given in quick succession, can the greatest possible good be effected in the treatment of diseases, more especially of chronic ones; and the reason of this is, that by such a procedure the vital force dose not quietly adapt itself to the transition from the natural disease to the similar medicinal disease, but is usually so violently excited and disturbed by a larger dose, or by smaller doses of even a homoeopathically chosen remedy given rapidly one after the other, that in most cases its reaction will be anything but salutary and will do more harm than good. As long as no more efficacious mode of proceeding than that then taught by me was discovered, the safe philanthropic maxim of sin non juvat, modo ne noceat, rendered it imperative for the homoeopathic practitioner, for whom the weal of his fellow-creatures was the highest object, to allow, as a general rule in diseases, but a single dose at a time, and that the very smallest, of the carefully selected remedy to act upon the patient and, moreover, to exhaust its action. The very smallest, I repeat, for it holds good and will continue to hold good as a homoeopathic therapeutic maxim not to be refuted by any experience in the world, that the best doses of the properly selected remedy is always the very smallest on in one of the high potencies (X), as well for chronic as for acute as for acute diseases – a truth that is the inestimable property of pure homoeopathy and which as long as allopathy and the new mongrel sect, whose treatment is a mixture of allopathic and homoeopathic processes is not much better continues to gnaw like a cancer at the life of sick human beings, and to ruin them by large and ever larger doses of drugs, will keep pure homoeopathy separated from these spurious arts as by an impassable gulf.

On the other hand, however, practice shows us that though a single one of these small doses may suffice to accomplish almost all that it was possible for this medicine to do under the circumstances, in some, and especially in slight cases of disease, particularly in those of young children and very delicate and excitable adults, yet that in many, indeed in most cases, not only of very chronic diseases that have already made great progress and have frequently been aggravated by a previous employment of inappropriate medicines, but also of serious acute diseases, one such smallest dose of medicine in our highly potentized dynamization is evidently insufficient to effect all the curative action that might be expected from that medicine, for it may unquestionably be requisite to administer several of them, in order that the vital force may be pathogenetically altered by them to such a degree and its salutary reaction stimulated to such a height, as to enable it to completely extinguish, by its reaction, the whole of that portion of the original disease that it lay in the power of the well-selected homoeopathic remedy to eradicate; the best chosen medicine in such a small dose, given but once, might certainly be of some service, but would not be nearly sufficient.

But the careful homoeopathic physician would not venture soon to repeat the same dose of the same remedy again, as from such a practice he has frequently experienced no advantage, but most frequently, on close observation, decided disadvantage. He generally witnessed aggravation, from even the smallest dose of the most suitable remedy, which he has given one day, when he repeated the next day and the next.

Now, in cases where he was convinced of the correctness of his choice of the homoeopathic medicine, in order to obtain more benefit for the patient than he was able to get hitherto from prescribing a single small dose, the idea often naturally struck him to increase the dose, since, for the reason given above, one single dose only should be given; an, for instance, in place of giving a single very minute globule moistened with the medicine in the highest dynamization, to administer six, seven or eight of them at once, and even a half or a whole drop. But the result was almost always less favourable than it should have been; it was often actually unfavourable, often even very bad – an injury that, in a patient so treated, is difficult to repair.

The difficulty in this case is not solved by giving, instead, lower dynamizations of the remedy in a large dose.

Thus, increasing the strength of the single doses of the homoeopathic medicine with the view of effecting the degree of pathogenic excitation of the vital force necessary to produce satisfactory salutary reaction, fails altogether, as experience teaches, to accomplish the desired object. This vital force is thereby too violent and too suddenly assailed and excited to allow it time to exercise a gradual equable, salutary reaction, to adapt itself to the modification effected in it; hence it strives to repel, as if it were an enemy, the medicine attacking it in excessive force, by means of vomiting, diarrhoea, fever, perspiration, and so forth, and thus in a great measure it diverts and renders nugatory the aim of the incautious physician – little or no good towards curing the disease will be thereby accomplished; on the contrary, the patient will be thereby perceptibly weakened and, for a long time, the administration of even the smallest dose of the same remedy must not be thought of if we would not wish it to injure the patient.

But it happens, moreover, that a number of the smallest doses given for the same object in quick succession accumulate in the organism into a kind of excessively large dose, with (a few cases excepted) similar bad results; in this case the vital force, not being able to recover itself betwixt every dose, though it be but small, becomes oppressed and overwhelmed, and thus being incapable of reacting in a salutary manner, it is necessitated passively to allow involuntary the continuance of the over-strong medicinal disease that has thus been forced upon it, just in the same manner as we may every day observe from the allopathic abuse of large cumulative doses of one and the same medicine, to the lasting injury of the patient.

Now, therefore, in order, whilst avoiding the erroneous method I have here pointed out, to attain the desired object more certainly than hitherto, and to administer the medicine selected in such a manner that it must exercise all its efficacy without injury to the patient, that it may effect all the good it is capable of performing in a given case of disease, I have lately adopted a particular method.

I perceived that, in order to discover this true middle path, we must be guided as well by the nature of the different medicinal substances, as also by the corporeal constitution of the patient and the magnitude of the disease, so that – to give an example from the use of sulphur in chronic (psoric) diseases – the smallest dose of it (tinct, sulph. X?) can seldom be repeated with advantage, seen in the most robust patients and in fully developed psora, oftener than every seven days, a period of time which must be proportionally lengthened when we have to treat weaker and more excitable patients of this kind; in such cases we would do well to give such a dose only every nine, twelve, or fourteen days, and continue to repeat the medicine until it ceases to be of service. We thus find (to abide by the instance of sulphur) that in sporic diseases seldom fewer than four, often however, six, eight and even ten doses (tinct. sulph. X?) are required to be successively administered at these intervals for the complete annihilation of the whole portion of the chronic disease that is eradicated by sulphur – provided always there had been no previous allopathic abuse of sulphur in the case. Thus even a (primary) scabious eruption of recent origin, though it may have spread all over the body, may be perfectly cured, in persons who are not too weakly, by a dose of tinct sulph. X? given every seven days, in the course of from ten to twelve weeks (accordingly with ten or twelve such globules), so that it will seldom be necessary to aid the cure with a few doses of carb. veg. X? (also given at the rate of one dose per week) without the slightest external treatment besides frequent changes of linen and good regimen.

When for other serious chronic diseases also we may consider it requisite, as far as we can calculate, to give eight, nine or ten doses of tinct. sulph. (at X?) it is yet more expedient in such cases, instead of giving them in uninterrupted succession, to interpose after every, or every second or third dose, a dose of another medicine, which in this case is next in point of homoeopathic suitableness to sulphur (usually hep. sulph.) and to allow this likewise to act for eight, nine, twelve or fourteen days before again commencing a course of three doses of sulphur.

But it not infrequently happens that the vital force refuses to permit several doses of sulphur, even though they may be essential for the cure of the chronic malady and are given at the intervals mentioned above, to act quietly on itself; this refusal it reveals by some, though moderate, sulphur symptoms, which it allows to appear in the patient during the treatment. In such cases it is sometimes advisable to administer a small dose of nux vom. X?, allowing it to act for eight or ten days, in order to dispose the system again to allow succeeding doses of the sulphur to act quietly and effectually upon it. In those cases for which it is adapted, puls. X? is preferable.

But the vital force shows the greatest resistance to the salutary action upon itself of the strongly indicated sulphur, and even exhibits manifest aggravation of the chronic disease, though the sulphur be given in the very smallest dose, though only a globule of the size of a mustard seed moistened with tinct. sulph X? be smelt, if the sulphur have formerly (it may be years since) been improperly given allopathically in large doses. This is one lamentable circumstance that renders the best medical treatment of chronic disease almost impossible among the many that the ordinary bungling treatment of chronic diseases by the old school would leave us nothing to do but to deplore, were there not some mode of getting over the difficulty.

In such cases we have only to let the patient smell a single time strongly at a globule the size of a mustard seed moistened with mercur metall. X, and allow this olfaction to act for about nine days, in order to make the vital force again disposed to permit the sulphur (at least the olfaction of tinct. sulph. X?) to exercise a beneficial influence on itself – a discovery for which we are indepted to Dr. Griesselich, of Carlsruhe.

§ 246 SIXTH EDITION

Every perceptibly progressive and strikingly increasing amelioration during treatment is a condition which, as long as it lasts, completely precludes every repetition of the administration of any medicine whatsoever, because all the good the medicine taken continues to effect is now hastening towards its completion. This is not infrequently the cause in acute diseases, but in more chronic diseases, on the other hand, a single dose of an appropriately selected homoeopathic remedy will at times complete even with but slowly progressive improvement and give the help which such a remedy in such a case can accomplish naturally within 40, 50, 60, 100 days. This is, however, but rarely the case; and besides, it must be a matter of great importance to the physician as well as to the patient that were it possible, this period should be diminished to one-half, one-quarter, and even still less, so that a much more rapid cure might be obtained. And this may be very happily affected, as recent and oft-repeated observations have taught me under the following conditions: firstly, if the medicine selected with the utmost care was perfectly homoeopathic; secondly, if it is highly potentized, dissolved in water and given in proper small dose that experience has taught as the most suitable in definite intervals for the quickest accomplishment of the cure but with the precaution, that the degree of every dose deviate somewhat from the preceding and following in order that the vital principle which is to be altered to a similar medicinal disease be not aroused to untoward reactions and revolt as is always the case1 with unmodified and especially rapidly repeated doses.

1. What I said in the fifth edition of the organon, in a long note to this paragraph in order to prevent these undesirable reactions of the vital energy, was all the experience I then had justified. But during the last four or five years, however, all these difficulties are wholly solved by my new altered but perfected method. The same carefully selected medicine may now be given daily and for months, if necessary in this way, namely, after the lower degree of potency has been used for one or two weeks in the treatment of chronic disease, advance is made in the same way to higher degrees, (beginning according to the new dynamization method, taught herewith with the use of the lowest degrees).

§ 247 FIFTH EDITION

Under these conditions, the smallest doses of the best selected homoeopathic medicine may be repeated with the best, often with incredible results, at intervals of fourteen, twelve, ten, eight, seven days, and, where rapidity is requisite, in chronic diseases resembling cases of acute disease, at still shorter intervals, but in acute diseases at very much shorter periods – every twenty – four, twelve, eight, four hours, in the very acutest every hour, up to as often as every five minutes, – in ever case in proportion to the more or less rapid course of the diseases and of the action of the medicine employed, as is more distinctly explained in the last note.

§ 247 SIXTH EDITION

It is impractical to repeat the same unchanged dose of a remedy once, not to mention its frequent repetition (and at short intervals in order not to delay the cure). The vital principle does not accept such unchanged doses without resistance, that is, without other symptoms of the medicine to manifest themselves than those similar to the disease to be cured, because the former dose has already accomplished the expected change in the vital principle and a second dynamically wholly similar, unchanged dose of the same medicine no longer finds, therefore, the same conditions of the vital force. The patient may indeed be made sick in another way by receiving other such unchanged doses, even sicker than he was, for now only those symptoms of the given remedy remain active which were not homoeopathic to the original disease, hence no step towards cure can follow, only a true aggravation of the condition of the patient. But if the succeeding dose is changed slightly every time, namely potentized somewhat higher (§§ 269-270) then the vital principle may be altered without difficulty by the same medicine (the sensation of natural disease diminishing) and thus the cure brought nearer.1

1. We ought not even with the best chosen homoeopathic medicine, for instance one pellet of the same potency that was beneficial at first, to let the patient have a second or third dose, taken dry. In the same way, if the medicine was dissolved in water and the first dose proved beneficial, a second or third and even smaller dose from the bottle standing undisturbed, even in intervals of a few days, would prove no longer beneficial, even though the original preparation had been potentized with ten succussions or as I suggested later with but two succussions in order to obviate this disadvantage and this according to above reasons. But through modification of every dose in its dynamiztion degree, as I herewith teach, there exists no offence, even if the doses be repeated more frequently, even if the medicine be ever so highly potentized with ever so many succussions. It almost seems as if the best selected homoeopathic remedy could best extract the morbid disorder from the vital force and in chronic disease to extinguish the same only if applied in several different forms.

§ 248 FIFTH EDITION

The dose of the same medicine may be repeated several times according to circumstances, but only so long as until either recovery ensues, or the same remedy ceases to do good and the rest of the disease, presenting a different group of symptoms, demands a different homoeopathic remedy.

§ 248 SIXTH EDITION

For this purpose, we potentize anew the medicinal solution1 (with perhaps 8, 10, 12 succussions) from which we give the patient one or (increasingly) several teaspoonful doses, in long lasting diseases daily or every second day, in acute diseases every two to six hours and in very urgent cases every hour or oftener. Thus in chronic diseases, every correctly chosen homoeopathic medicine, even those whose action is of long duration, may be repeated daily for months with ever increasing success. If the solution is used up (in seven to fifteen days) it is necessary to add to the next solution of the same medicine if still indicated one or (though rarely) several pellets of a higher potency with which we continue so long as the patient experiences continued improvement without encountering one or another complaint that he never had before in his life. For if this happens, if the balance of the disease appears in a group of altered symptoms then another, one more homoeopathically related medicine must be chosen in place of the last and administered in the same repeated doses, mindful, however, of modifying the solution of every dose with thorough vigorous succussions, thus changing its degree of potency and increasing it somewhat. On the other hand, should there appear during almost daily repetition of the well indicated homoeopathic remedy, towards the end of the treatment of a chronic disease, so-called (§ 161) homoeopathic aggravations by which the balance of the morbid symptoms seem to again increase somewhat (the medicinal disease, similar to the original, now alone persistently manifests itself). The doses in that case must then be reduced still further and repeated in longer intervals and possibly stopped several days, in order to see if the convalescence need no further medicinal aid. The apparent symptoms (Schein – Symptome) caused by the excess of the homoeopathic medicine will soon disappear and leave undisturbed health in its wake. If only a small vial say a dram of dilute alcohol is used in the treatment, in which is contained and dissolved through succussion one globule of the medicine which is to be used by olfaction every two, three or four days, this also must be thoroughly succussed eight to ten times before each olfaction.

1. Made in 40, 30, 20, 15 or 8 tablespoons of water with the addition of some alcohol or a piece of charcoal in order to preserve it. If charcoal is used, it is suspended by means of a thread in the vial and is taken out when the vial is succussed. The solution of the medicinal globule (and it is rarely necessary to use more than one globule) of a thoroughly potentized medicine in a large quantity of water can be obviated by making a solution in only 7-8 tablespoons of water and after thorough succussion of the vial take from it one tablespoon and put it in a glass of water (containing about 7 to 8 spoonfuls), this stirred thoroughly and then given a dose to the patient. If he is unusually excited and sensitive, a teaspoon of this solution may be put in a second glass of water, thoroughly stirred and teaspoonful doses or more be given. There are patients of so great sensitiveness that a third or fourth glass, similarly prepared, may be necessary. Each such prepared glass must be made fresh daily. the globule of the high potency is best crushed in a few grains of sugar of milk which the patient can put in the vial and be dissolved in the requisite quantity of water.

§ 249

Every medicine prescribed for a case of disease which, in the course of its action, produces new and troublesome symptoms not appertaining to the disease to be cured, is not capable of effecting real improvement,1 and cannot be considered as homoeopathically selected; it must, therefore, either, if the aggravation be considerable, be first partially neutralized as soon as possible by an antidote before giving the next remedy chosen more accurately according to similarity of action; or if the troublesome symptoms be not very violent, the next remedy must be given immediately, in order to take the place of the improperly selected one.2

1. As all experience shows that the dose of the specially suited homoeopathic medicine can scarcely be prepared too small to effect perceptible amelioration in the disease for which it is appropriate (§§ 275-278), we should act injudiciously and hurtfully were we when no improvement, or some, though it be even slight, aggravation ensues, to repeat or even increase the dose of the same medicine, as is done in the old system, under the delusion that it was not efficacious on account of its small quantity (its too small dose). Every aggravation by the production of new symptoms – when nothing untoward has occurred in the mental or physical regimen – invariably proves unsuitableness on the part of the medicine formerly given in the case of disease before us, but never indicates that the dose has been too weak.
2. The well informed and conscientiously careful physician will never be in a position to require an antidote in his practice if he will begin, as he should, to give the selected medicine in the smallest possible dose. Like minute doses of a better chosen remedy will re-establish order throughout.

§ 250

When, to the observant practitioner who accurately investigates the state of the disease, it is evident, in urgent cases after the lapse of only six, eight or twelve hours, that he has made a bad selection in the medicine last given, in that the patient's state is growing perceptibly, however slightly, worse from hour to hour, by the occurrence of new symptoms and sufferings, it is not only allowable for him, but it is his duty to remedy his mistake, by the selection and administration of a homoeopathic medicine not merely tolerably suitable, but the most appropriate possible for the existing state of the disease (§ 167).

§ 251

There are some medicines (e.g., ignatia, also bryonia and rhus, and sometimes belladonna) whose power of altering man's health consists chiefly in alternating actions – a kind of primary-action symptoms that are in part opposed to each other. Should the practitioner find, on prescribing one of these, selected on strict homoeopathic principles, that no improvement follows, he will in most cases soon effect his object by giving (in acute diseases, even within a few hours) a fresh and equally small dose of the same medicine.1

1. As I have more particularly described in the introduction to "Ignatia" (in the first volume of the Materia Medica Pura).

§ 252

But should we find, during the employment of the other medicines in chronic (psoric) diseases, that the best selected homoeopathic (antipsoric) medicine in the suitable (minutest) dose does not effect an improvement, this is a sure sign that the cause that keeps up the disease still persists, and that there is some circumstances in the mode of life of the patient or in the situation in which he is placed, that must be removed in order that a permanent cure may ensue.

§ 253

Among the signs that, in all diseases, especially in such as are of an acute nature, inform us of a slight commencement of amelioration or aggravation that is not perceptible to every one, the state of mind and the whole demeanor of the patient are the most certain and instructive. In the case of ever so slight an improvement we observe a greater degree of comfort, increased calmness and freedom of the mind, higher spirits – a kind of return of the natural state. In the case of ever so small a commencement of aggravation we have, on the contrary, the exact opposite of this: a constrained helpless, pitiable state of the disposition, of the mind, of the whole demeanor, and of all gestures, postures and actions, which may be easily perceived on close observation, but cannot be described in words.1

1. The signs of improvement in the disposition and mind, however, may be expected only soon after the medicine has been taken when the dose has been sufficiently minute (i.e., as small as possible), an unnecessary large dose of even the most suitable homoeopathic medicine acts too violently, and at first produces too great and too lasting a disturbance of the mind and disposition to allow us soon to perceive the improvement in them. I must here observe that this so essential rule is chiefly transgressed by presumptuous tryos in homoeopathy, and by physicians who are converted to homoeopathy from the ranks of the old school. From old prejudices these persons abhor the smallest doses of the lowest dilutions of medicine in such cases, and hence they fail to experience the great advantages and blessings of that mode of proceeding which a thousandfold experience has shown to be the most salutary; they cannot effect all that homoeopathy is capable of doing, and hence they have no claim to be considered its adherents.

§ 254

The other new or increased symptoms or, on the contrary, the diminution of the original ones without any addition of new ones, will soon dispel all doubts from the mind of the attentively observing and investigating practitioner with regard to the aggravation or amelioration; though there are among patients persons who are either incapable of giving an account of this amelioration or aggravation, or are unwilling to confess it.

§ 255 FIFTH EDITION

But even with such individuals we may convince ourselves on this point by going with them through all the symptoms enumerated in our notes of the disease one by one, and finding that they complain of no new unusual symptoms in addition to these, and that none of the old symptoms are worse. If this be the case, and if an improvement in the disposition and mind have already been observed, the medicine must have effected positive diminution of the disease, or, if sufficient time have not yet elapsed for this, it will soon effect it. Now, supposing the remedy is perfectly appropriate, if the improvement delay too long in making its appearance, this depends either on some error of conduct on the part of the patient, or on the homoeopathic aggravation produced by medicine lasting too long (§ 157), consequently on the dose not being small enough.

§ 255 SIXTH EDITION

But even with such individuals we may convince ourselves on this point by going with them through all the symptoms enumerated in our notes of the disease one by one, and finding that they complain of no new unusual symptoms in addition to these, and that none of the old symptoms are worse. If this be the case, and if an improvement in the disposition and mind have already been observed, the medicine must have effected positive diminution of the disease, or, if sufficient time have not yet elapsed for this, it will soon effect it. Now, supposing the remedy is perfectly appropriate, if the improvement delay too long in making its appearance, this depends either on some error of conduct on the part of the patient, or on other interfering circumstances.

§ 256 FIFTH EDITION

On the other hand, if the patient mention the occurrence of some fresh accidents and symptoms of importance – signs that the medicine chosen has not been strictly homoeopathic – even though he should good-naturedly assure us that he feels better, we must not believe this assurance, but regard his state as aggravated as it will soon be perfectly apparent it is.

§ 256 SIXTH EDITION

On the other hand, if the patient mention the occurrence of some fresh accidents and symptoms of importance – signs that the medicine chosen has not been strictly homoeopathic – even though he should good-naturedly assure us that he feels better, as is not infrequently the case in phthisical patients with lung abscess, we must not believe this assurance, but regard his state as aggravated as it will soon be perfectly apparent it is.

§ 257

The true physician will take care to avoid making favorite remedies of medicines, the employment of which he has, by chance, perhaps found often useful, and which he has had opportunities of using with good effect. If he do so, some remedies or rarer use, which would have been more homoeopathically suitable, consequently more serviceable, will often be neglected.

§ 258

The true practitioner, moreover, will not in his practice with mistrustful weakness neglect the employment of those remedies that he may now and then have employed with bad effects, owing to an erroneous selection (from his own fault, therefore), or avoid them for other (false) reasons, as that they were unhomoeopathic for the case of disease before him; he must bear in mind the truth, that of medicinal agents that one alone invariably deserves the preference in every case of disease which correspond most accurately by similarity to the totality of the characteristic symptoms, and that no paltry prejudices should interfere with this serious choice.

§ 259

Considering the minuteness of the doses necessary and proper in homoeopathic treatment, we can easily understand that during the treatment everything must be removed from the diet and regimen which can have any medicinal action, in order that the small dose may not be overwhelmed and extinguished or disturbed by any foreign medicinal irritant.1

1. The softest tones of a distant flute that in the still midnight hours would inspire a tender heart with exalted feelings and dissolve it in religious ecstasy, are inaudible and powerless amid discordant cries and the noise of day.

§ 260 FIFTH EDITION

Hence the careful investigation into such obstacles to cure is so much the more necessary in the case of patients affected by chronic diseases, as their diseases are usually aggravated by such noxious influences and other disease-causing errors in the diet and regimen, which often pass unnoticed.1

1. Coffee; fine Chinese and other herb teas; beer prepared with medicinal vegetable substances unsuitable for the patient's state; so-called fine liquors made with medicinal spices; all kinds of punch; spiced chocolate; odorous waters and perfumes of many kinds; strong-scented flowers in the apartment; tooth powders and essences and perfumed sachets compounded of drugs; highly spiced dishes and sauces; spiced cakes and ices; crude medicinal vegetables for soups; dishes of

herbs, roots and stalks of plants possessing medicinal qualities; old cheese, and meats that are in a state of decomposition, or that passes medicinal properties (as the flesh and fat of pork, ducks and geese, or veal that is too young and sour viands), ought just as certainly to be kept from patients as they should avoid all excesses in food, and in the use of sugar and salt, as also spirituous drinks, heated rooms, woollen clothing next the skin, a sedentary life in close apartments, or the frequent indulgence in mere passive exercise (such as riding, driving or swinging), prolonged suckling, taking a long siesta in a recumbent posture in bed, sitting up long at night, uncleanliness, unnatural debauchery, enervation by reading obscene books, subjects of anger, grief or vexation, a passion for play, over-exertion of the mind or body, especially after meals, dwelling in marshy districts, damp rooms, penurious living, etc. All these things must be as far as possible avoided or removed, in order that the cure may not be obstructed or rendered impossible. Some of my disciples seem needlessly to increase the difficulties of the patient's dietary by forbidding the use of many more, tolerably indifferent things, which is not to be commended.

§ 260 SIXTH EDITION

Hence the careful investigation into such obstacles to cure is so much the more necessary in the case of patients affected by chronic diseases, as their diseases are usually aggravated by such noxious influences and other disease-causing errors in the diet and regimen, which often pass unnoticed.1

1. Coffee; fine Chinese and other herb teas; beer prepared with medicinal vegetable substances unsuitable for the patient's state; so-called fine liquors made with medicinal spices; all kinds of punch; spiced chocolate; odorous waters and perfumes of many kinds; strong-scented flowers in the apartment; tooth powders and essences and perfumed sachets compounded of drugs; highly spiced dishes and sauces; spiced cakes and ices; crude medicinal vegetables for soups; dishes of herbs, roots and stalks of plants possessing medicinal qualities; asparagus with long green tips, hops, and all vegetables possessing medicinal properties, celery, onions; old cheese, and meats that are in a state of decomposition, or that passes medicinal properties (as the flesh and fat of pork, ducks and geese, or veal that is too young and sour viands), ought just as certainly to be kept from patients as they should avoid all excesses in food, and in the use of sugar and salt, as also spirituous drinks, undiluted with water, heated rooms, woollen clothing next the skin, a sedentary life in close apartments, or the frequent indulgence in mere passive exercise (such as riding, driving or swinging), prolonged suckling, taking a long siesta in a recumbent posture in bed, sitting up long at night, uncleanliness, unnatural debauchery, enervation by reading obscene books, reading while lying down, Onanism or imperfect or suppressed intercourse in order to prevent conception, subjects of anger, grief or vexation, a passion for play, over-exertion of the mind or body, especially after meals, dwelling in marshy districts, damp rooms, penurious living, etc. All these things must be as far as possible avoided or removed, in order that the cure may not be obstructed or rendered impossible. Some of my disciples seem needlessly to increase the difficulties of the patient's dietary by forbidding the use of many more, tolerably indifferent things, which is not to be commended.

§ 261

The most appropriate regimen during the employment of medicine in chronic diseases consists in the removal of such obstacles to recovery, and in supplying where necessary the reverse: innocent moral and intellectual recreation, active exercise in the open air in almost all kinds of weather (daily walks, slight manual labor), suitable, nutritious, unmedicinal food and drink, etc.

§ 262

In acute diseases, on the other hand – except in cases of mental alienation – the subtle, unerring internal sense of the awakened life-preserving faculty determines so clearly and precisely, that the physician only requires to counsel the friends and attendants to put no obstacles in the way of this voice of nature by refusing anything the patient urgently desires in the way of food, or by trying to persuade him to partake of anything injurious.

§ 263

The desire of the patient affected by an acute disease with regard to food and drink is certainly chiefly for things that give palliative relief: they are, however, not strictly speaking of a medicinal character, and merely supply a sort of want. The slight hindrances that the gratification of this desire, within moderate bounds, could oppose to the radical removal of the disease1 will be amply counteracted and overcome by the power of the homoeopathically suited medicine and the vital force set free by it, as also by the refreshment that follows from taking what has been so ardently longed for. In like manner, in acute diseases the temperature of the room and the heat or coolness of the bed-coverings must also be arranged entirely in conformity with the patients' wish. He must be kept free from all over-exertion of mind and exciting emotions.

1. This is, however, rare. Thus, for instance, in pure inflammatory diseases, where aconite is so indispensable, whose action would be destroyed by partaking of vegetable acids, the desire of the patient is almost always for pure cold water only.

§ 264

The true physician must be provided with genuine medicines of unimpaired strength, so that he may be able to rely upon their therapeutic powers; he must be able, himself, to judge of their genuineness.

§ 265 FIFTH EDITION

It should be a matter of conscience with him to be thoroughly convinced in every case that the patient always takes the right medicine.

§ 265 SIXTH EDITION

It should be a matter of conscience with him to be thoroughly convinced in every case that the patient always takes the right medicine and therefore he must give the patient the correctly chosen medicine prepared, moreover, by himself.

§ 266

Substances belonging to the animal and vegetable kingdoms possess their medicinal qualities most perfectly in their raw state.1

1. All crude animal and vegetable substances have a greater or less amount of medicinal power, and are capable of altering man's health, each in its own peculiar way. Those plants and animals used by the most enlightened nations as food have this advantage over all others, that they contain a larger amount of nutritious constituents; and they differ from the others in this that their medicinal powers in their raw state are either not very great in themselves, or are diminished by the culinary processes they are subjected to in cooking for domestic use, by the expression of the pernicious juice (like the cassava root of South America), by fermentation (of the rye-flour in the dough for making bread, sour-crout prepared without vinegar and pickled gherkins), by smoking and by the action of heat (in boiling, stewing, toasting, roasting, baking), whereby the medicinal parts of many of these substances are in part destroyed and dissipated. By the addition of salt (pickling) and vinegar (sauces, salads) animal and vegetable substances certainly lose much of their injurious medicinal qualities, but other disadvantages result from these additions.

But even those plants that possess most medicinal power lose that in part or completely by such processes. By perfect desiccation all the roots of the various kinds of iris, of the horseradish, of the different species or arum and the peonies lose almost all their medicinal virtue. The juice of the most virulent plants often becomes inert, pitch-like mass, from the heat employed in preparing the ordinary extracts. By merely standing a long time, the expressed juice of the most deadly plants becomes quite powerless; even at moderate atmospheric temperature it rapidly takes on the vinous fermentation (and thereby loses much of its medicinal power), and immediately thereafter the acetous and putrid fermentation, whereby it is deprived of all peculiar medicinal properties; the fecula that is then deposited, if well washed, is quite innocuous, like ordinary starch. By the transudation that takes place when a number of green plants are laid one above the other, the greatest part of their medicinal properties is lost.

§ 267

We gain possession of the powers of indigenous plants and of such as may be had in a fresh state in the most complete and certain manner by mixing their freshly expressed juice immediately with equal parts of spirits of wine of a strength sufficient to burn in a lamp. After this has stood a day and a night in a close stoppered bottle and deposited the fibrinous and albuminous matters, the clear superincumbent fluid is then to be decanted off for medicinal use.1 All fermentation of the vegetable juice will be at once checked by the spirits of wine mixed with it and rendered impossible for the future, and the entire medicinal power of the vegetable juice is thus retained (perfect and uninjured) for ever by keeping the preparation in well-corked bottles and excluded from the sun's light.2

1. Buchholz (Taschenb. f. Scheidek. u. Apoth. a. d. J., 1815, Weimar, Abth. I, vi) assures his readers (and his reviewer in the Leipziger Literaturzeitung, 1816, No. 82, does not contradict him) that for this excellent mode of operating medicines we have to thank the campaign in Russia, whence it was (in 1812) imported into Germany. According to the noble practice of many Germans to be unjust towards their own countrymen, he conceals the fact that this discovery and those directions, which he quotes in my very words from the first edition of the Organon of Rational Medicine, § 230 and note, proceed from me, and that I first published them to the world two years before the Russian campaign (the Organon appeared in 1810). Some folks would rather assign the origin of a discovery to the deserts of Asia than to a German to whom the honor belongs. O tempora! O mores!
   Alcohol has certainly been sometimes before this used for mixing with vegetable juices, e.g., to preserve them some time before making extracts of them, but never with the view of administering them in this form.
2. Although equal parts of alcohol and freshly expressed juice are usually the most suitable proportion for affecting the deposition of the fibrinous and albuminous matters, yet for plants that contain much thick mucus (e.g. Symphytum officinale, Viola tricolor, etc.), or an excess of albumen (e.g., Aethusa cynapium, Solanum nigrum, etc.), a double proportion of alcohol is generally required for this object. Plants that are very deficient in juice, as Oleander, Buxus, Taxus, Ledum, Sabina, etc., must first be pounded up alone into a moist, fine mass and the stirred up with a double quantity of alcohol, in order that the juice may combine with it, and being thus extracted by the alcohol, may be pressed out; these latter may also when dried be brought with milk-sugar to the millionfold trituration, and then be further diluted and potentized (v. § 271)

§ 268

The other exotic plants, barks, seeds and roots that cannot be obtained in the fresh state the sensible practitioner will never take in the pulverized form on trust, but will first convince himself of their genuineness in their crude, entire state before making any employment of them.1

1. In order to preserve them in the form of powder, a precaution is requisite that has hitherto been usually neglected by druggists, and hence powders, even of well-dried animal and vegetable substances could not be preserved uninjured even in well-corked bottles. The entire crude vegetable substances, though perfectly dry, yet contain, as an indispensable condition of the cohesion of their texture, a certain quantity of moisture, which dose not indeed prevent the unpulverized drug from remaining in as dry a state as is requisite to preserve it from corruption, but which is quite too much for the finely pulverized state. The animal or vegetable substance which in its entire state was perfectly dry, furnishes, therefore, when finely pulverized, a somewhat moist powder, which without rapidly becoming spoilt and mouldy, can yet not be preserved in corked bottles if not previously freed from this superfluous moisture. This is the best effected by spreading out the powder in a flat tin saucer with a raised edge, which floats in a vessel full of boiling water (i.e. a water-bath), and, by means of stirring it about, drying it to such a degree that all the small atoms of it (no longer stick together in lumps, but) like dry, fine sand, are easily separated from each other, and are readily converted into dust. In this dry state the fine powders may be kept forever uninjured in well-corked and sealed bottles, in all their original complete medicinal power, without ever being injured by mites or mould; and they are best preserved when the bottles are kept protected from the daylight (in covered boxes, chests, cases). If not shut up in air-tight vessels, and not preserved from the access of the light of the sun and day, all animal and vegetable substances in time gradually lose their medicinal power more and more, even in the entire state, but still more in the form of powder.

§ 269 FIFTH EDITION

The homoeopathic system of medicine develops for its use, to a hitherto unheard-of degree, the spirit-like medicinal powers of the crude substances by means of a process peculiar to it and which has hitherto never been tried, whereby only they all become penetratingly efficacious1 and remedial, even those that in the crude state give no evidence of the slightest medicinal power on the human body.

§ 269 SIXTH EDITION

The homoeopathic system of medicine develops for its special use, to a hitherto unheard-of degree, the inner medicinal powers of the crude substances by means of a process peculiar to it and which has hitherto never been tried, whereby only they all become immeasurably and penetratingly efficacious1 and remedial, even those that in the crude state give no evidence of the slightest medicinal power on the human body.

This remarkable change in the qualities of natural bodies develops the latent, hitherto unperceived, as if slumbering2 hidden, dynamic (§ 11) powers which influence the life principle, change the well-being of animal life.3 This is effected by mechanical action upon their smallest particles by means of rubbing and shaking and through the addition of an indifferent substance,

dry of fluid, are separated from each other. This process is called dynamizing, potentizing (development of medicinal power) and the products are dynamizations4 or potencies in different degrees.

1. Long before this discovery of mine, experience had taught several changes which could be brought about in different natural substances by means of friction, for instance, warmth, heat, fire, development of odor in odorless bodies, magnetization of steel, and so forth. But all these properties produced by friction were related only to physical and inanimate things, whereas it is a law of nature according to which physiological and pathogenic changes take place in the body's condition by means of forces capable of changing the crude material of drugs, even in such as had never shown any medicinal properties. This is brought about by trituration and succussion, but under the condition of employing an indifferent vehicle in certain proportions. this wonderful physical and especially physiological and pathogenic law of nature had not been discovered before my time. No wonder then, that the present students of nature and physicians (so for unknowing) cannot have faith in the magical curative powers of the minute doses of medicines prepared according to homoeopathic rules (dynamized).

2. The same thing is seen in a bar of iron and steel where a slumbering trace of latent magnetic force cannot but be recognized in their interior. Both, after their completion by means of the forge stand upright, repulse the north pole of a magnetic needle with the lower end and attract the south pole, while the upper end shows itself as the south pole of the magnetic needle. But this is only a latent force; not even the finest iron particles can be drawn magnetically or held on either end of such a bar.
   Only after this bar of steel is dynamized, rubbing it with a dull file in one direction, will it become a true active powerful magnet, one able to attract iron and steel to itself and impart to another bar of steel by mere contact and even some distance away, magnetic power and this in a higher degree the more it has been rubbed. In the same way will triturating a medicinal substance and shaking of its solution (dynamization, potentation) develop the medicinal powers hidden within and manifest them more and more or if one may say so, spiritualizes the material substance itself.

3. On this account it refers to the increase and stronger development of their power to cause changes in the health of animals and men if these natural substances in this improved state, are brought very near to the living sensitive fibre or come in contact with it (by means of intake or olfaction). Just as a magnetic bar especially if its magnetic force is increased (dynamized) can show magnetic power only in a needle of steel whose pole is near or touches it. The steel itself remains unchanged in the remaining chemical and physical properties and can bring about no changes in other metals (for instance, in brass), just as little as dynamized medicines can have any action upon lifeless things.

4. We hear daily how homoeopathic medicinal potencies are called mere dilutions, when they are the very opposite, i.e., a true opening up of the natural substances bringing to light and revealing the hidden specific medicinal powers contained within and brought forth by rubbing and shaking. The aid of a chosen, unmedicinal medium of attenuation is but a secondary condition.
   Simple dilution, for instance, the solution of a grain of salt will become water, the grain of salt will disappear in the dilution with much water and will never develop into medicinal salt which by means of our well prepared dynamization, is raised to most marvellous power.

§ 270 FIFTH EDITION

Thus two drops of the fresh vegetable juice mingled with equal parts of alcohol are diluted with ninety-eight drops of alcohol and potentized by means of two succussions, whereby the first development of power is formed and this process is repeated through twenty-nine more phials, each of which is filled three-quarters full with ninety-nine drops of alcohol, and each succeeding phial is to be provided with one drop from the preceding phial (which has already been shaken twice) and is in its turn twice shaken,1 and in the same manner at last the thirtieth development of power (potentized decillionth dilution X) which is the one most generally used.

1. In order to maintain a fixed and measured standard for developing the power of liquid medicines, multiplied experience and careful observation have led me to adopt two successions for each phial, in preference to the greater number formerly employed (by which the medicines were too highly potentized). There are, however, homoeopathists who carry about with them on their visits to patients homoeopathic medicines in the fluid state, and who yet assert that they do not become more highly potentized in the course of time, but they thereby show their want of ability to observe correctly. I discovered a grain of soda in half an once of water mixed with alcohol in a phial, which was thereby filled two-thirds full, and shook this solution continuously for half an hour, and this fluid was in potency and energy equal to the thirtieth development of power.

§ 270 SIXTH EDITION

In order to best obtain this development of power, a small part of the substance to be dynamized, say one grain, is triturated for three hours with three times one hundred grains sugar of milk according to the method described below1 up to the one-millionth part in powder form. For reasons given below (b) one grain of this powder is dissolved in 500 drops of a mixture of one part of alcohol and four parts of distilled water, of which one drop is put in a vial. To this are added 100 drops of pure alcohol2 and given one hundred strong succussions with the hand against a hard but elastic body.3 This is the medicine in the first degree of dynamization with which small sugar globules4 may then be moistened5 and quickly spread on blotting paper to dry and kept in a well-corked vial with the sign of (I) degree of potency. Only one6 globule of this is taken for further dynamization, put in a second new vial (with a drop a water in order to dissolve it) and then with 100 powerful succussions.

With this alcoholic medicinal fluid globules are again moistened, spread upon blotting paper and dried quickly, put into a well-stoppered vial and protected from heat and sun light and given the sign (II) of the second potency. And in this way the process is continued until the twenty-ninth is reached. Then with 100 drops of alcohol by means of 100 succussions, an alcoholic medicinal fluid is formed with which the thirtieth dynamization degree is given to properly moistened and dried sugar globules.

By means of this manipulation of crude drugs are produced preparations which only in this way reach the full capacity to forcibly influence the suffering parts of the sick organism. In this way, by means of similar artificial morbid affection, the influence of the natural disease on the life principle present within is neutralized. By means of this mechanical procedure, provided it is carried out regularly according to the above teaching, a change is effected in the given drug, which in its crude state shows itself only as material, at times as unmedicinal material but by means of such higher and higher dynamization, it is changed and subtlized at last into spirit-like7 medicinal power, which, indeed, in itself does not fall within our senses but for which the medicinally prepared globule, dry, but more so when dissolved in water, becomes the carrier, and in this condition, manifests the healing power of this invisible force in the sick body.

1. One-third of one hundred grains sugar of milk is put in a glazed porcelain mortar, the bottom dulled previously by rubbing it with fine, moist sand. Upon this powder is put one grain of the powdered drug to be triturated (one drop of quicksilver, petroleum, etc.). The sugar of milk used for dynamization must be of that special pure quality that is crystallized on strings and comes to us in the shape of long bars. For a moment the medicines and powder are mixed with a porcelain spatula and triturated rather strongly, six to seven minutes, with the pestle rubbed dull, then the mass is scraped from the bottom of the mortar and from the pestle for three to four minutes, in order to make it homogeneous. This is followed by triturating it in the same way 6 – 7 minutes without adding anything more and again scraping 3 – 4 minutes from what adhered to the mortar and pestle. The second third of the sugar of milk is now added, mixed with the spatula and again triturated 6 – 7 minutes, followed by the scraping for 3 – 4 minutes and trituration without further addition for 6 – 7 minutes. The last third of sugar of milk is then added, mixed with the spatula and triturated as before 6 -7 minutes with most careful scraping together. The powder thus prepared is put in a vial, well corked, protected from direct sunlight to which the name of the substance and the designation of the first product marked /100 is given. In order to raise this product to /10000, one grain of the powdered /100 is mixed with the third part of 100 grains of powdered sugar of milk and then proceed as before, but every third must be carefully triturated twice thoroughly each time for 6 -7 minutes and scraped together 3 -4 minutes before the second and last third of sugar of milk is added. After each third, the same procedure is taken. When all is finished, the powder is put in a well corked vial and labelled /10000, i.e., (I), each grain containing 1/1,000,000 the original substance. Accordingly, such a trituration of the three degrees requires six times six to seven minutes for triturating and six times 3 -4 minutes for scraping, thus one hour for every degree. After one hour such trituration of the first degree, each grain will contain 1/000; of the second 1/10,000; and in the third 1/1,000,000 of the drug used.*
Mortar and spatula must be cleaned well before they are used for another medicine. Washed first with warm water and dried, both mortar and pestle, as well as spatula are then put in a kettle of boiling water for half an hour. precaution might be used to such an extent as to put these utensils on a coal fire exposed to a glowing heat.
* These are the three degrees of the dry powder trituration, which if carried out correctly, will effect a good beginning for the dynamization of the medicinal substance.
2. The vial used for potentizing is filled two-thirds full.
3. Perhaps on a leather bound book.
4. They are prepared under supervision by the confectioner from starch and sugar and the small globules freed from fine dusty parts by passing them through a sieve. Then they are put through

a strainer that will permit only 100 to pass through weighing one grain, the most serviceable size for the needs of a homoeopathic physician.

5. A small cylindrical vessel shaped like a thimble, made of glass, porcelain or silver, with a small opening at the bottom in which the globules are put to be medicated. They are moistened with some of the dynamized medicinal alcohol, stirred and poured out on blotting paper, in order to dry them quickly.

6. According to first directions, one drop of the liquid of a lower potency was to be taken to 100 drops of alcohol for higher potentiation. This proportion of the medicine of attenuation to the medicine that is to be dynamized (100:1) was found altogether too limited to develop thoroughly and to a high degree the power of the medicine by means of a number of such successions without specially using great force of which wearisome experiments have convinced me.

But if only one such globule be taken, of which 100 weigh one grain, and dynamize it with 100 drops of alcohol, the proportion of 1 to 50,000 and even greater will be had, for 500 such globules can hardly absorb one drop, for their saturation. With this disproportionate higher ratio between medicine and diluting medium many successive strokes of the vial filled two-thirds with alcohol can produce a much greater development of power. But with so small a diluting medium as 100 to 1 of the medicine, if many successions by means of a powerful machine are forced into it, medicines are then developed which, especially in the higher degrees of dynamization, act almost immediately, but with furious, even dangerous violence, especially in weakly patients, without having a lasting, mild reaction of the vital principle. But the method described by me, on the contrary, produces medicines of highest development of power and mildest action, which, however, if well chosen, touches all suffering parts curatively.* In acute fevers, the small doses of the lowest dynamization degrees of these thus perfected medicinal preparations, even of medicines of long continued action (for instance, belladonna) may be repeated in short intervals. In the treatment of chronic diseases, it is best to begin with the lowest degrees of dynamization and when necessary advance to higher, even more powerful but mildly acting degrees.

* In very rare cases, notwithstanding almost full recovery of health and with good vital strength, an old annoying local trouble continuing undisturbed it is wholly permitted and even indispensably necessary, to administer in increasing doses the homoeopathic remedy that has proved itself efficacious but potenized to a very high degree by means of many successions by hand. Such a local disease will often then disappear in a wonderful way.

7. This assertion will not appear improbable, if one considers that by means of this method of dynamization (the preparations thus produced, I have found after many laborious experiments and counter-experiments, to be the most powerful and at the same time mildest in action, i.e., as the most perfected) the material part of the medicine is lessened with each degree of dynamization 50,000 times yet incredibly increased in power, so that the further dynamization of 125 and 18 ciphers reaches only the third degree of dynamization. The thirtieth thus progressively prepared would give a fraction almost impossible to be expressed in numbers. It becomes uncommonly evident that the material part by means of such dynamization (development of its true, inner medicinal essence) will ultimately dissolve into its individual spirit-like, (conceptual) essence. In its crude state therefore, it may be considered to consist really only of this underdeveloped conceptual essence.

§ 271 FIFTH EDITION

All other substances adapted for medicinal use – except sulphur, which has of late years been only employed in the form of a highly diluted (X) tincture – as pure or oxidized and sulphuretted metals and other minerals, petroleum, phosphorus, as also parts and juices of plants that can only be obtained in the dry state, animal substances, neutral salts, etc., all these are first to be potentized by trituration for three hours, up to the millionfold pulverulent attenuation, and of this one grain is to be dissolved, and brought to the thirtieth development of power through twenty-seven attenuating phials, in the same manner as the vegetable juices.1

1. As is still more circumstantially described in the prefaces to Arsenic and Pulsatilla in the Materia Medica Pura.

§ 271 SIXTH EDITION

If the physician prepares his homoeopathic medicines himself, as he should reasonably do in order to save men from sickness,1 he may use the fresh plant itself, as but little of the crude article is required, if he does not need the expressed juice perhaps for purposes of healing. He takes a few grains in a mortar and with 100 grains sugar of milk three distinct times brings them to the one-millionth trituration (§ 270) before further potentizing of a small portion of this by means of shaking is undertaken, a procedure to be observed also with the rest of crude drugs of either dry or oily nature.

1. Until the State, in the future, after having attained insight into the indispensability of perfectly prepared homoeopathic medicines, will have them manufactured by a competent impartial person, in order to give them free of charge to homoeopathic physicians trained in homoeopathic hospitals, who have been examined theoretically and practically, and thus legally qualified. The physician may then become convinced of these divine tools for purposes of healing, but also to give them free of charge to his patients – rich and poor.

§ 272 FIFTH EDITION

In no case is it requisite to administer more than one single, simple medicinal substance at one time.1

1. Some homoeopathists have made the experiment, in cases where they deemed one remedy homoeopathically suitable for one portion of the symptoms of a case of disease, and a second for another portion, of administering both remedies at the same time; but I earnestly deprecate such a hazardous experiment, which can never be necessary, though it may sometimes seem to be of use.

§ 272 SIXTH EDITION

Such a globule,1 placed dry upon the tongue, is one of the smallest doses for a moderate recent case of illness. Here but few nerves are touched by the medicine. A similar globule, crushed with some sugar of milk and dissolved in a good deal of water (§ 247) and stirred well before every administration will produce a far more powerful medicine for the use of several days. Every dose, no matter how minute, touches, on the contrary, many nerves.

1. These globules (§ 270) retain their medicinal virtue for many years, if protected against sunlight and heat.

§ 273 FIFTH EDITION

It is not conceivable how the slightest dubiety could exist as to whether it was more consistent with nature and more rational to prescribe a single well-known medicine at one time in a disease, or a mixture of several differently acting drugs.

§ 273 SIXTH EDITION

In no case under treatment is it necessary and therefore not permissible to administer to a patient more than one single, simple medicinal substance at one time. It is inconceivable how the slightest doubt could exist as to whether it was more consistent with nature and more rational to prescribe a single, simple1 medicine at one time in a disease or a mixture of several differently acting drugs. It is absolutely not allowed in homoeopathy, the one true, simple and natural art of healing, to give the patient at one time two different medicinal substance.

1. Two substances, opposite to each other, united into neutral Natrum and middle salts by chemical affinity in unchangeable proportions, as well as sulphurated metals found in the earth and those produced by technical art in constant combining proportions of sulphur and alkaline salts and earths, for instance (natrum sulph. and calcarea sulph.) as well as those ethers produced by distillation of alcohol and acids may together with phosphorus be considered as simple medicinal substances by the homoeopathic physician and used for patients. On the other hand, those extracts obtained by means of acids of the so-called alkaloids of plants, are exposed to great variety in their preparation (for instance, chinin, strychnine, morphine), and can, therefore, not be accepted by the homoeopathic physician as simple medicines, always the same, especially as he possesses, in the plants themselves, in their natural state (Peruvian bark, nux vomica, opium) every quality necessary for healing. Moreover, the alkaloids are not the only constituents of the plants.

§ 274

As the true physician finds in simple medicines, administered singly and uncombined, all that he can possibly desire (artificial disease-force which are able by homoeopathic power completely to overpower, extinguish, and permanently cure natural diseases), he will, mindful of the wise maxim that "it is wrong to attempt to employ complex means when simple means suffice," never think of giving as a remedy any but a single, simple medicinal substance; for these reasons also, because even though the simple medicines were thoroughly proved with respect to their pure peculiar effects on the unimpaired healthy state of man, it is yet impossible to foresee how two and more medicinal substances might, when compounded, hinder and alter each other's actions on the human body; and because, on the other hand, a simple medicinal substance when used in diseases, the totality of whose symptoms is accurately known, renders efficient aid by itself alone, if it be homoeopathically selected; and supposing the worst case to happen, that it was not chosen in strict conformity to similarity of symptoms, and therefore does no good, it is yet so far useful that it promoted our knowledge of therapeutic agents, because, by the new symptoms excited by it in such a case, those symptoms which this medicinal substance had already shown in experiments on the healthy human body are confirmed, an advantage that is lost by the employment of all compound remedies.[1]

1. When the rational physician has chosen the perfectly homoeopathic medicine for the well-considered case of disease and administered it internally, he will leave to irrational allopathic routine the practice of giving drinks or fomentations of different plants, of injecting medicated glysters and of rubbing in this or the other ointment.

§ 275

The suitableness of a medicine for any given case of disease does not depend on its accurate homoeopathic selection alone, but likewise on the proper size, or rather smallness, of the dose. If we give too strong a dose of a medicine which may have been even quite homoeopathically chosen for the morbid state before us, it must, notwithstanding the inherent beneficial character of its nature, prove injurious by its mere magnitude, and by the unnecessary, too strong impression which, by virtue of its homoeopathic similarity of action, it makes upon the vital force which it attacks and, through the vital force, upon those parts of the organism which are the most sensitive, and are already most affected by the natural disease.

§ 276 FIFTH EDITION

For this reason, a medicine, even though it may be homoeopathically suited to the case of disease, does harm in every dose that is too large, the more harm the larger the dose, and by the magnitude of the dose it does more harm the greater its homoeopathicity and the higher the potency1 selected, and it does much more injury than any equally large dose of a medicine that is unhomoeopathic, and in no respect adapted (allopathic) to the morbid state; for in the former case the so-called homoeopathic aggravation (§§157-160) – that is to say, the very analogous medicinal disease produced by the vital force stirred up by the excessively large dose of medicine, in the parts of the organism that are most suffering and most irritated by the original disease – which medicinal disease, had it been of appropriate intensity, would have gently effected a cure – rises to an injurious height;2 the patient, to be sure, no longer suffers from the original disease, for that has been homoeopathically eradicated, but he suffers all the more from the excessive medicinal disease and from useless exhaustion of his strength.

1. The praise bestowed of late years by some few homoeopathists on the larger doses is owing to this, either that they chose low dynamizations of the medicines to be administered, as I myself used to do twenty years ago, from not knowing any better, or that the medicines selected were not perfectly homoeopathic.
2. See note to §246

§ 276 SIXTH EDITION

For this reason, a medicine, even though it may be homoeopathically suited to the case of disease, does harm in every dose that is too large, the more harm the larger the dose, and by the magnitude of the dose and in strong doses' it does more harm the greater its homoeopathicity and the higher the potency1 selected, and it does much more injury than any equally large dose of a medicine that is unhomoeopathic, and in no respect adapted to the morbid state (allopathic).

Too large doses of an accurately chosen homoeopathic medicine, and especially when frequently repeated, bring about much trouble as a rule. They put the patient not seldom in danger of life or make this disease almost incurable. They do indeed extinguish the natural disease so far as the sensation of the life principle is concerned and the patient no longer suffers from the original disease from the moment the too strong dose of the homoeopathic medicine acted upon him but he is in consequence more ill with the similar but more violent medicinal disease which is most difficult to destroy.2

1. The praise bestowed of late years by some homoeopathists on the larger doses is owing to this, either that they chose low dynamizations of the medicine to be administered (as I myself used to do twenty years ago, from nor knowing any better), or that the medicines selected were not homoeopathic and imperfectly prepared by their manufacturers.
2. Thus, the continuous use of aggressive allopathic large doses of mercurials against syphilis develops almost incurable maladies, when yet one or several doses of a mild but active mercurial preparation would certainly have radically cured in a few days the whole venereal disease, together with the chancre, provided it had not been destroyed by external measures (as is always done by allopathy). In the same way, the allopath gives Peruvian bark and quinine in intermittent fever daily in very large doses, where they are correctly indicated and where one very small dose of a highly potentized China would unfailingly help (in marsh intermittents and even in persons who were not affected by any evident psoric disease). A chronic China malady (coupled at the

same time with the development of psora) is produced, which, if it dose not gradually kill the patient by damaging the internal important vital organs, especially spleen and liver, will put him, nevertheless suffering for years in a sad state of health. A homoeopathic antidote for such a misfortune produced by abuse of large doses of homoeopathic remedies is hardly conceivable.

§ 277

For the same reason, and because a medicine, provided the dose of it was sufficiently small, is all the more salutary and almost marvellously efficacious the more accurately homoeopathic its selection has been, a medicine whose selection has been accurately homoeopathic must be all the more salutary the more its dose is reduced to the degree of minuteness appropriate for a gentle remedial effect.

§ 278 FIFTH EDITION

Here the question arises, what is this most suitable degree of minuteness for sure and gentle remedial effect; how small, in other words, must be the dose of each individual medicine, homoeopathically selected for a case of disease, to effect the best cure? To solve this problem, and to determine for every particular medicine, what dose of it will suffice for homoeopathic therapeutic purposes and yet be so minute that the gentlest and most rapid cure may be thereby obtained – to solve this problem is, as may easily be conceived, not the work off theoretical speculation; not by fine-spun reasoning, not by specious sophistry can we expect to obtain the solution of this problem. Pure experiment, careful observation, and accurate experience can alone determine this; and it were absurd to adduce the large doses of unsuitable (allopathic) medicines of the old system, which do not touch the diseased side of the organism homoeopathically, but only attack the parts unaffected by the disease, in opposition to what pure experience pronounces respecting the smallness of the doses required for homoeopathic cures.

§ 278 SIXTH EDITION

Here the question arises, what is this most suitable degree of minuteness for sure and gentle remedial effect; how small, in other words, must be the dose of each individual medicine, homoeopathically selected for a case of disease, to effect the best cure? To solve this problem, and to determine for every particular medicine, what dose of it will suffice for homoeopathic therapeutic purposes and yet be so minute that the gentlest and most rapid cure may be thereby obtained – to solve this problem is, as may easily be conceived, not the work off theoretical speculation; not by fine-spun reasoning, not by specious sophistry can we expect to obtain the solution of this problem. It is just as impossible as to tabulate in advance all imaginable cases. Pure experiment, careful observation of the sensitiveness of each patient, and accurate experience can alone determine this; and it were absurd to adduce the large doses of unsuitable (allopathic) medicines of the old system, which do not touch the diseased side of the organism homoeopathically, but only attack the parts unaffected by the disease, in opposition to what pure experience pronounces respecting the smallness of the doses required for homoeopathic cures.

§ 279 FIFTH EDITION

This pure experience shows UNIVERSALLY, that if the disease do not manifestly depend on a considerable deterioration of an important viscus (even though it belong to the chronic and complicated diseases), and if during the treatment all other alien medicinal influences are kept away from the patients, the dose of the homoeopathically selected remedy can never be prepared so small that it shall not be stronger than the natural disease, and shall not be able to overpower, extinguish and cure it, at least in part as long as it is capable of causing some, though but a slight preponderance of its own symptoms over those of the disease resembling it (slight homoeopathic aggravation, (§§ 157-160) immediately after its ingestion.

§ 279 SIXTH EDITION

This pure experience shows UNIVERSALLY, that if the disease do not manifestly depend on a considerable deterioration of an important viscus (even though it belong to the chronic and complicated diseases), and if during the treatment all other alien medicinal influences are kept away from the patients, the dose of the homoeopathically selected and highly potentized remedy for the beginning of treatment of an important, especially chronic disease can never be prepared so small that it shall not be stronger than the natural disease and shall not be able to overpower it, at least in part and extinguish it from the sensation of the principle of life and thus make a beginning of a cure.

§ 280 FIFTH EDITION

This incontrovertible axiom of experience is the standard of measurement by which the doses of all homoeopathic medicines, without exception, are to be reduced to such an extent that after their ingestion, they shall excite a scarcely observable homoeopathic aggravation, let the diminution of the dose go ever so far, and appear ever so incredible to the materialistic ideas of ordinary physicians;1 their idle declamations must before the verdict of unerring experience.

1. Let them learn from the mathematicians how true it is that a substance divided into ever so many parts must still contain in its smallest conceivable parts always some of this substance, and that the smallest conceivable part does not cease to be some of this substance and cannot possibly become nothing; – let them, if they are capable of being taught, hear from natural philosophers that there are enormously, powerful things (forces) which are perfectly destitute of weight, as,

for example, caloric, light, etc., consequently infinitely lighter than the medicine contained in the smallest doses used in homoeopathy; – let them, if they can, weigh the irritating words that bring on a bilious fever, or the mournful intelligence respecting her only son that kills the mother; let them touch, for a quarter of an hour, a magnet capable of lifting a hundred pounds weight, and learn from the pain it excites that even imponderable agencies can produce the most violent medicinal effects upon man; – and let the weak ones among them allow the pit of the stomach to be slightly touched by the thumb's point of a strong-willed mesmeriser for a few minutes, and the disagreeable sensations they then suffer will make them repent of attempting to set limits to the boundless activity of nature; the weak-minded creatures!

If the allopathist who is trying the homoeopathic system imagine he cannot bring himself to give such small and profoundly attenuated doses, let him only ask himself what risk he runs by so doing? If the scepticism which holds what is ponderable only to be real, and all that is imponderable to be nothing, be right, nothing worse could result from a dose that appears to him to be nothing, than that no effect would ensue – and consequently this would be always much more innocuous than what must result from his too large doses of allopathic medicine. Why will he consider his inexperience, coupled with prejudice, more reliable than an experience of many years corroboration by facts? And, moreover, the homoeopathic medicine becomes potentized at every division and diminution by trituration or succussion! – a development of the inherent powers of medicinal substances which was never dreamed of before my time, and which is of so powerful a character that of late I have been compelled by convincing experience to reduce the ten succussions formerly directed to be given after each attenuation, to two.

§ 280 SIXTH EDITION

The dose of the medicine that continues serviceable without producing new troublesome symptoms is to be continued while gradually ascending, so long as the patient with general improvement, begins to feel in a mild degree the return of one or several old original complaints. This indicates an approaching cure through a gradual ascending of the moderate doses modified each time by succussion (§ 247). It indicates that the vital principal no longer needs to be affected by the similar medicinal disease in order to lose the sensation of the natural disease (§ 148). It indicates that the life principle now free from the natural disease begins to suffer only something of the medicinal disease hitherto known as homoeopathic aggravation.

§ 281 FIFTH EDITION

Every patient is, especially in his diseased point, capable of being influenced in an incredible degree by medicinal agents corresponding by similarity of action; and there is no person, be he ever so robust, and even though he be affected only with a chronic or so-called local disease, who will not soon experience the desired change in the affected part, if he take the salutary, homoeopathically suited medicine in the smallest conceivable dose, who, in a word, will not

thereby be much more altered in his health than a healthy infant of but a day old would be. How insignificant and ridiculous is mere theoretical scepticism in opposition to this unerring, infallible experimental proof!

§ 281 SIXTH EDITION

In order to be convinced of this, the patient is left without any medicine for eight, ten of fifteen days, meanwhile giving him only some powders of sugar of milk. If the few last complaints are due to the medicine simulating the former original disease symptoms, then these complaints will disappear in a few days or hours. If during these days without medicine, while continuing good hygienic regulations nothing more of the original disease is seen, he is probably cured. But if in the later days traces of the former morbid symptoms should show themselves, they are remnants of the original disease not wholly extinguished, which must be treated with renewed higher potencies of the remedy as directed before. If a cure is to follow, the first small doses must likewise be again gradually raised higher, but less and more slowly in patients where considerable irritability is evident than in those of less susceptibility, where the advance to higher dosage may be more rapid. There are patients whose impressionability compared to that of the insusceptible ones is like the ratio as 1000 to 1.

§ 282 FIFTH EDITION

The smallest possible dose of homoeopathic medicine capable of producing only the very slightest homoeopathic aggravation, will, because it has the power of exciting symptoms bearing the greatest possible resemblance to the original disease (but yet stronger even in the minute dose), attack principally and almost solely the parts in the organism that are already affected, highly irritated, and rendered excessively susceptible to such a similar stimulus, and will alter the vital force that rules in them to a state of very similar artificial disease, somewhat greater in degree than the natural one was; this artificial disease will substitute itself for the natural (the original) disease, so that the living organism now suffers from the artificial medicinal disease alone, which, from its nature and owing to the minuteness of the dose, will soon be extinguished by the vital force that is striving to return to the normal state, and (if the disease were only an acute one) the body is left perfectly free from disease – that is to say, quite well.

§ 282 SIXTH EDITION

It would be a certain sign that the doses were altogether too large, if during treatment, especially in chronic disease, the first dose should bring forth a so-called homoeopathic aggravation, that is, a marked increase of the original morbid symptoms first discovered and in the same way every

repeated dose (§ 247) however modified somewhat by shaking before its administration (i.e., more highly dynamized).1

1, The rule to commence the homoeopathic treatment if chronic diseases with the smallest possible doses and only gradually to augment them is subject to a notable exception in the treatment of the three great miasms while they still effloresce on the skin, i.e., recently erupted itch, the untouched chancre (on the sexual organs, labia, mouth or lips, and so forth), and the figwarts. These not only tolerate, but indeed require, from the very beginning large doses of their specific remedies of ever higher and higher degrees of dynamization daily (possibly also several times daily). If this course be pursued, there is no danger to be feared as is the case in the treatment of diseases hidden within, that the excessive dose while it extinguishes the disease, initiates and by continued usage possible produces a chronic medicinal disease. During external manifestations of these three miasms this is not the case; for from the daily progress of their treatment it can be observed and judged to what degree the large dose withdraws the sensation of the disease from the vital principle day by day; for none of these three can be cured without giving the physician the conviction through their disappearance that there is no longer any further need of these medicines.

Since diseases in general are but dynamic attacks upon the life principle and nothing material – no materia peccans – as their basis (as the old school in its delusion has fabulated for a thousand years and treated the sick accordingly to their ruin) there is also in these cases nothing material to take away, nothing to smear away, to burn or tie or cut away, without making the patient endlessly sicker and more incurable (Chron. Dis. Part 1), than he was before local treatment of these three miasms was instituted. The dynamic, inimical principle exerting its influence upon the vital energy is the essence of these external signs of the inner malignant miasms that can be extinguished solely by the action of a homoeopathic medicine upon the vital principle which affects it in a similar but stronger manner and thus extracts the sensation of internal and external spirit-like (conceptual) disease enemy in such a way that it no longer exists for the life principle (for the organism) and thus releases the patient of his illness and he is cured.

Experience, however, teaches that the itch, plus its external manifestations, as well as the chancre, together with the inner venereal miasm, can and must be cured only by means of specific medicines taken internally. But the figwarts, if they have existed for some time without treatment, have need for their perfect cure, the external application of their specific medicines as well as their internal use at the same time.

§ 283 FIFTH EDITION

Now, in order to act really in conformity with nature, the true physician will prescribe his well-selected homoeopathic medicine only in exactly as small a dose as will just suffice to over power and annihilate the disease before him – in a dose of such minuteness, that if human fallibility should betray him into administering an inappropriate medicine, the injury, accruing from its nature being unsuited to the disease will be diminished to a mere trifle; moreover the harm done

by the smallest possible dose is so slight, that it may be immediately extinguished and repaired by the natural vital powers, and by the speedy administration of a remedy more suitable selected according to similarity of action, and given also in the smallest dose.

§ 283 SIXTH EDITION

In order to work wholly according to nature, the true healing artist will prescribe the accurately chosen homoeopathic medicine most suitable in all respects in so small a dose on account of this alone. For should he be misled by human weakness to employ an unsuitable medicine, the disadvantage of its wrong relation to the disease would be so small that the patient could through his own vital powers and by means of early opposition (§ 249) of the correctly chosen remedy according to symptom similarly (and this also in the smallest dose) rapidly extinguish and repair it.

§ 284 FIFTH EDITION

The action of a dose, moreover, dose not diminish in the direct ratio of the quantity of material medicine contained in the dilutions used in homoeopathic practice. Eight drops of the tincture of a medicine to the dose do not produce four times as much effect on the human body as two drops, but only about twice the effect that is produced by two drops to the dose. In like manner, one drop of a mixture of a drop of the tincture with ten drops of some unmedicinal fluid, when taken, will not produce ten times more effect than one drop of mixture ten times more attenuated, but only about (scarcely) twice as strong an effect, and so on, in the same ratio – so that a drop of the lowest dilution must, and really does, display still a very considerable action.1

1. Supposing one drop of a mixture that contains 1/10 of a grain of medicine produces an effect = a; one drop of a more diluted mixture containing 1/100th of a grain of the medicine will only produce an effect = a/2; if it contain 1/10000th of a grain of medicine, about = a/4; if it contain 1/100000000th of a grain of medicine it will produce and effect = a/8; and thus it goes on, the volume of the doses being equal, with every (perhaps more than) quadratic diminution of the quantity of medicine, the action on the human body will be diminished each time to only about one-half. I have very often seen a drop of the decillion-fold dilution of tincture of nux vomica produce pretty nearly just half as much effect as a drop of the quintillion-fold dilution, under the same circumstances and in the same individual.

§ 284 SIXTH EDITION

Besides the tongue, mouth and stomach, which are most commonly affected by the administration of medicine, the nose and respiratory organs are receptive of the action of medicines in fluid form by means of olfaction and inhalation through the mouth. But the whole remaining skin of the body clothed with epidermis, is adapted to the action of medicinal solutions, especially if the inunction is connected with simultaneous internal administration.1

1. The power of medicines acting upon the infant through the milk of the mother or wet nurse is wonderfully helpful. Every disease in a child yields to the rightly chosen homoeopathic medicines given in moderate doses to the nursing mother and so administered, is more easily and certainly utilized by these new world-citizens than is possible in later years. Since most infants usually have imparted to them psora through the milk of the nurse, if they do not already possess it through heredity from the mother, they may be at the same time protected antipsorically by means of the milk of the nurse rendered medicinally in this manner. But the case of mothers in their (first) pregnancy by means of a mild antipsoric treatment, especially with sulphur dynamizations prepared according to the directions in this edition (§ 270), is indispensable in order to destroy the psora – that producer of most chronic diseases – which is given them hereditarily; destroy it both within themselves and in the foetus, thereby protecting posterity in advance. This is true of pregnant women thus treated; they have given birth to children usually more healthy and stronger, to the astonishment of everybody. A new confirmation of the great truth of the psora theory discovered by me.

§ 285 FIFTH EDITION

The diminution of the dose essential for homoeopathic use, will also be promoted by diminishing its volume, so that, if, instead of a drop of a medicinal dilution, we take but quite a small part1 of such a drop for a dose, the object of diminishing the effect still further will be very effectually attained; and that this will be the case may be readily conceived for this reason, because with the smaller volume of the dose but few nerves of the living organism can be touched, whereby the power of the medicine is certainly also communicated to the whole organism, but it is a weaker power.

1. For this purpose it is most convenient to employ fine sugar globules of the size of poppy seeds, one of which imbibed with the medicine and put into the dispensing vehicle constitutes a medicinal dose, which contains about the three hundredth part of a drop, for three hundred such small globules will be adequately moistened by one drop of alcohol. The dose is vastly diminished by laying one such globule alone upon the tongue and giving nothing to drink. If it be necessary, in the case of a very sensitive patient, to employ the smallest possible dose and to bring about the most rapid result, one single olfaction merely will suffice (see note to §288).

§ 285 SIXTH EDITION

In this way, the cure of very old disease may be furthered by the physician applying externally, rubbing it in the back, arms, extremities, the same medicine he gives internally and which showed itself curatively. In doing so, he must avoid parts subject to pain or spasm or skin eruption.1

1. From this fact may be explained those marvellous cures, however infrequent, where chronic deformed patients, whose skin nevertheless was sound and clean, were cured quickly and permanently after a few baths whose medicinal constituents (by, chance) were homoeopathically related. On the other hand, the mineral baths very often brought on increased injury with patients, whose eruptions on the skin were suppressed. After a brief period of well-being, the life principle allowed the inner, uncured malady to appear elsewhere, more important for life and health.

At times, instead, the ocular nerve would become paralyzed and produce amaurosis, sometimes the crystalline lens would become clouded, hearing lost, mania or suffocating asthma would follow or an apoplexy would end the sufferings of the deluded patient.

A fundamental principle of the homoeopathic physician (which distinguishes him from every physician of all older schools) is this, that he never employs for any patient a medicine, whose effects on the healthy human has not previously been carefully proven and thus made known to him (§§ 20,21). To prescribe for the sick on mere conjecture of some possible usefulness for some similar disease or from hearsay "that a remedy has helped in such and such a disease" – such conscienceless venture the philanthropic homoeopathist will leave to the allopath. A genuine physician and practitioner or our art will therefore never send the sick to any of the numerous mineral baths, because almost all are unknown so far as their accurate, positive effects on the healthy human organism is concerned, and when misused, must be counted among the most violent and dangerous drugs. In this way, out of a thousand sent to the most celebrated of these baths by ignorant physicians allopathically uncured and blindly sent there perhaps one or two are cured by chance more often return only apparently cured and the miracle is proclaimed aloud. Hundreds, meanwhile sneak quietly away, more or less worse and the rest remain to prepare themselves for their eternal resting place, a fact that is verified by the presence of numerous well-filled graveyards surrounding the most celebrated of these spas.*

* A true homoeopathic physician, one who never acts without correct fundamental principles, never gambles with the life of the sick entrusted to him as in a lottery where the winner is in the ratio of 1 to 500 or 1000 (blanks here consisting of aggravation or death), will never expose any one of his patients to such danger and send him for good luck to a mineral bath, as is done so frequently by allopaths in order to get rid of the sick in an acceptable manner spoiled by him or others.

§ 286 FIFTH EDITION

For the same reason the effect of a homoeopathic dose of medicine increases, the greater the quantity of fluid in which it is dissolved when administered to the patient, although the actual amount of medicine it contains remains the same. For in this case, when the medicine is taken, it comes in contact with a much larger surface of sensitive nerves responsive to the medicinal action. Although theorists may imagine there should be a weakening of the action of dose of medicine by its dilution with a large quantity of liquid, experience asserts exactly the opposite, at all events when the medicines are employed homoeopathically.1

1. It is only the most simple of stimulants, wine and alcohol, that have their heating and intoxicating action diminished by dilution with much water.

§ 286 SIXTH EDITION

The dynamic force of minerals magnets, electricity and galvanism act no less powerfully upon our life principle and they are not less homoeopathic than the properly so-called medicines which neutralize disease by taking them through the mouth, or by rubbing them on the skin or by olfaction. There may be diseases, especially diseases of sensibility and irritability, abnormal sensations, and involuntary muscular movements which may be cured by those means. But the more certain way of applying the last two as well as that of the so-called electromagnetic lies still very much in the dark to make homoeopathic use of them. So far both electricity and Galvanism have been used only for palliation to the great damage of the sick. The positive, pure action of both upon the healthy human body have until the present time been but little tested.

§ 287 FIFTH EDITION

But in this increase of action by the mixture of the dose of medicine with a larger quantity of liquid (before its ingestion), the result is vastly different whether the mixture of the dose of medicine with a certain quantity of liquid is performed merely superficially and imperfectly, or so uniformly and intimately1 that the smallest portion of the diluting fluid received the same quantity of medicine in proportion as all the rest; for the latter becomes much more medicinally powerful by the diluting mixture than the former. From this every one will be able to judge for himself how to proceed with the regulation of the homoeopathic medicinal doses when he desires to diminish their medicinal action as much as possible, in order to make them suitable for the most sensitive patients.2

1. By the word intimately I mean this: that when, for instance, the drop of a medicinal fluid has been shaken up once with one hundred drops of spirits of wine; that is to say, the phial containing both, held in the hand, has been rapidly moved from above downwards with a single smart jerk of the arm, there certainly ensues a thorough mixture of the whole, but with two, three, ten and more such strokes, this mixture becomes much more intimate; that is to say, the medicinal power becomes much more potentized, and the spirit of this medicine, so to speak, becomes much more unfolded, developed and rendered much more penetrating in its action on the nerves. If, then, the required object we wish to attain with the low dilutions be the diminution of the doses for the purpose of moderating their powers upon the organism, we would do well to give no more than two such succussion-jerks to each of the twenty, thirty, etc., dilution phials, and thus to develop the medicinal power only moderately. It is also advisable, in attenuating the medicine in the state of dry powder by trituration in a porcelain mortar, to keep within certain limits, and, for example, to triturate strongly, for one hour only, one grain of the crude entire medical substance, mixed with the first hundred grains of milk-sugar (to the 1/10000th attenuation) likewise only for one hour, and to make the third attenuation (to 1/1000000) also by one hour of strong trituration of one grain of the previous mixture with one hundred grains of milk-sugar, in order to bring the medicine to such an attenuation that its development of power shall remain moderate.

A more exact description of this process will be found in the prefaces to Arsenic and Pulsatilla in the Materia Medica Pura.

2. The higher we carry the attenuation accompanied by dynamization (by two succession strokes), with so much the more rapid and penetrating action does the preparation seem to affect the vital force and to alter the health, with but slight diminution of strength even when this operation is carried very far, – in place, as is usual (and generally sufficient) to X when it is carried up to XX, L, C, and higher; only that then the action always appears to last a shorter time.

§ 287 SIXTH EDITION

The powers of the magnet for healing purposes can be employed with more certainty according to the positive effects detailed in the Materia Medica Pura under north and south pole of a powerful magnetic bar. Though both poles are alike powerful, they nevertheless oppose each other in the manner of their respective action. The doses may be modified by the length of time of contact with one or the other pole, according as the symptoms of either north or south pole are indicated. As antidote to a too violent action the application of a plate of polished zinc will suffice.

§ 288 FIFTH EDITION

The action of medicines in the liquid from1 upon the living human body takes place in such a penetrating manner, spreads out from the point of the sensitive fibers provided with nerves whereto the medicine is first applied with such inconceivable rapidity and so universally through all parts of the living body, that this action of the medicine must be denominated a spirit-like (a dynamic, virtual) action.

1. It is especially in the form of vapour, by olfaction and inhalation of the medicinal aura that is always emanating from a globule impregnated with a medicinal fluid in a high development of power, and placed, dry, in a small phial, that the homoeopathic remedies act most surely and most powerfully. The homoeopathic physician allows the patient to hold the open mouth of the phial first in one nostril, and in the act of inspiration draw the air out of it into himself and then if he wished to give a stronger dose, smell in the same manner with the other nostril, more or less strongly, according to the strength it is intended the dose should be, he then corks up the phial and replaces it in his pocket case to prevent any misuse of it, and unless he wishes it he has no occasion for an apothecary's assistance in his practice. A globule of which ten, twenty or one hundred weigh one grain, impregnated with the thirtieth potentized dilution, and then dried, retains for this purpose all its power undiminished for at least eighteen or twenty years (my experience extends this length of time), even though the phial be opened a thousand times during that period, if it be but protected from heat and the sun's light. Should both nostrils be stopped up by coryza or polypus, the patient should inhale by the mouth, holding the orifice of the phial betwixt his lips. In little children it may be applied close to their nostrils whilst they are asleep

with the certainty of producing an effect. The medicinal aura thus inhaled comes in contact with the nerves in the walls of the spacious cavities it traverses without obstruction, and thus produces a salutary influence on the vital force, in the mildest yet most powerful manner, and this is much preferable to every other mode of administering the medicament in substance by the mouth. All that homoeopathy is capable of curing (and what can it not cure beyond the domain of mere manual surgery affections?) among the most severe chronic diseases that have not been quite ruined by allopathy, as also among acute disease, will be most safely and certainly cured by this olfaction. I can scarcely name one in a hundred out of the many patients that have sought the advice of myself and my assistant during the past year, whose chronic or acute disease we have not treated with the most happy results, solely by means of this olfaction; during the latter half of this year, moreover, I have become convinced (of what I never could previously have believed) that by this olfaction the power of the medicines is exercised upon the patient in, at least, the same degree of strength, and that more quietly and yet just as long as when the dose of medicine is taken by the mouth, and that, consequently, the intervals at which the olfaction should be repeated should not be shorter than in the ingestion of the material dose by the mouth.

§ 288 SIXTH EDITION

I find it yet necessary to allude here to animal magnetism, as it is termed, or rather Mesmerism (as it should be called in deference to Mesmer, its first founder) which differs so much in its nature from all other therapeutic agents. This curative force, often so stupidly denied and disdained for a century, acts in different ways. It is a marvellous, priceless gift of God to mankind by means of which the strong will of a well intentioned person upon a sick one by contact and even without this and even at some distance, can bring the vital energy of the healthy mesmerizer endowed with this power into another person dynamically (just as one of the poles of a powerful magnetic rod upon a bar of steel).

It acts in part by replacing in the sick whose vital force within the organism is deficient here and there, in part also in other parts where the vital force has accumulated too much and keeps up irritating nervous disorders it turns it aside, diminishes and distributes it equally and in general extinguishes the morbid condition of the life principle of the patient and substitutes in its place the normal of the mesmerist acting powerfully upon him, for instance, old ulcers, amaurosis, paralysis of single organs and so forth. Many rapid apparent cures performed in all ages, by mesmerizers endowed with great natural power, belong to this class. The effect of communicated human power upon the whole human organism was most brilliantly shown, in the resuscitation of persons who had lain some time apparently dead, by the most powerful sympathetic will of a man in full vigor of vital energy,1 and of this kind of resurrection history records many undeniable examples.

If the mesmerizing person of either sex capable at the same time of a good-natured enthusiasm (even its degeneration into bigotry, fanaticism, mysticism or philanthropic dreaming) will be empowered all the more with this philanthropic self-sacrificing performance to direct exclusively the power of his commanding good will to the recipient requiring his help and at the same time to concentrate these, he may at times perform apparent miracles.

1. Especially of one of such persons, of whom there are not many, who, along with great kindness of disposition and perfect bodily powers, possesses but a very moderate desire for sexual intercourse, which it would give him very little trouble wholly to suppress, in whom, consequently, all the fine vital spirits that would otherwise be employed in the production of the semen, are ready to be communicated to others, by touching them and powerfully exerting the will. Some powerful mesmerisers, with whom I have become aquatinted, had all this peculiar character.

§ 289 FIFTH EDITION

Every part of our body that possesses the sense of touch is also capable of receiving the influences, and of propagating their power to all other parts.1

1. A patient even destitute of the sense of smell may expect an equally perfect action and cure from the medicine by olfaction.

§ 289 SIXTH EDITION

All the above-mentioned methods of practicing mesmerism depend upon influx of more or less vital force into the patient, and hence are termed positive mesmerism.1 An opposite mode of employing mesmerism, however, as it produces just the contrary effect, deserves to be termed negative mesmerism. To this belong the passes which are used to rouse from the somnambulic sleep, as also all the manual processes known by the names of soothing and ventilating. This discharge by means of negative mesmerism of the vital force accumulated to excess in individual parts of the system of undebilitated persons is most surely and simply performed by making a very rapid motion or the flat extended hand, held parallel to, and about an inch distant from the body, from the top of the head to the tips of the toes.2 The more rapidly this pass is made, so much the more effectually will the discharge be effected. Thus, for instance, in the case where a previously healthy woman,3 from the sudden suppression of her catamenia by a violent mental shock, lies to all appearance dead, the vital force which is probably accumulated in the precordial region, will, by such a rapid negative pass, be discharged and its equilibrium throughout the whole organism restored. So that the resuscitation generally follows, immediately.4 In like manner, a gentle, less rapid, negative pass diminishes the excessive restlessness and sleeplessness accompanied with anxiety sometimes produced in very irritable persons by a too powerful positive pass, etc.

1. When I here speak of the decided and certain curative power of positive mesmerism, I most assuredly do not mean that abuse of it, where, by repeated passes of this kind, continued for half an hour or a whole hour at a time, and, even day after day, performed on weak, nervous patients, that monstrous revolution of the whole human system is effected which is termed somnambulism, wherein the human being is ravished from the world of sense and seems to belong more to the world of spirits – a highly unnatural and dangerous state, by means of which it has not infrequently been attempted to cure chronic diseases.

2. It is a well known rule that a person who is either to be positively or negatively mesmerised, should not wear silk on any part of the body.
3. Hence a negative pass, especially if it be very rapid, is extremely injurious to a delicate person affected with a chronic ailment and deficient in vital force.
4. A strong country lad, ten years of age, received in the morning, on account of slight indisposition, from a professed female mesmeriser, several very powerful passes with the points of both thumbs, from the pit of the stomach along the lower edge of the ribs, and he instantly grew deathly pale, and fell into such a state of unconsciousness and immobility that no effort could arouse him, and he was almost given up for dead. I made his eldest brother give him a very rapid negative pass from the crown of the head over the body to the feet, and in one instance he recovered his consciousness and became lively and well.

§ 290 FIFTH EDITION*

Besides the stomach, the tongue and the mouth are the parts most susceptible to the medicinal influences; but the interior of the nose is more especially so, and the rectum, the genitals, as also all particularly sensitive parts of our body are almost equally capable of receiving the medicinal action; hence also, parts that are destitute of skin, wounded or ulcerated spots permit the powers of medicines to exercise almost as penetrating an action upon the organism as if the medicine had been taken by the mouth or still better by olfaction and inhalation.

* § 290 corresponds to some extent to § 284 of the Sixth Edition.

§ 290 SIXTH EDITION

Here belongs also the so-called massage of vigorous good-natured person given to a chronic invalid, who, though cured, still suffers from loss of flesh, weakness of digestion and lack of sleep due to slow convalescence. The muscles of the limbs, breast and back, separately grasped and moderately pressed and kneaded arouse the life principle to reach and restore the tone of the muscles and blood and lymph vessels. The mesmeric influences of this procedure is the chief feature and it must not be used to excess in patients still hypersensitive.

§ 291 FIFTH EDITION

Even those organs which have lost their peculiar sense, e.g., a tongue and palate that have lost the faculty of tasting, or a nose that has lost the faculty of smelling, communicate the power of the medicine that acts first on them alone not less perfectly to all the other organs of the body.

§ 291 SIXTH EDITION

Baths of pure water prove themselves partly palliative, partly as homoeopathic serviceable aids in restoring health in acute diseases as well as in convalescence of cured chronic patients with proper consideration of the conditions of the convalescent and the temperature of the bath, its duration and repetition. But even if well applied, they may bring only physically beneficial changes in the sick body, in themselves they are no true medicine. The lukewarm baths at 25 to 27? serve to arouse the slumbering sensibility of fibre in the apparent dead (frozen, drowned, suffocated) which benumbed the sensation of the nerves. Though only palliative, still they often prove themselves sufficiently active, especially when given in conjunction with coffee and rubbing with the hands. They may give homoeopathic aid in cases where the irritability is very unevenly distributed and accumulated too unevenly in some organs as is the case in certain hysteric spasms and infantile convulsions. In the same way, cold baths 10 to 6? in persons cured medically of chronic diseases and with deficiency of vital heat, act as an homoeopathic aid. By instantaneous and later with repeated immersions they act as a palliative restorative of the tone of the exhausted fibre. For this purpose, such baths are to be used for more than momentary duration, rather for minutes and of gradually lowered temperature, they are a palliative, which, since it acts only physically has no connection with the disadvantage of a reverse action to be feared afterwards, as takes place with dynamic medicinal palliatives.

§ 292 FIFTH EDITION

Even the external surface of the body, covered as it is with skin and epidermis, is not insusceptible of the powers of medicines, especially those in a liquid form, but the most sensitive parts are also the most susceptible.1

1. Rubbing-in appears to favour the action of the medicines only in this way, that the friction makes the skin more sensitive, and the living fibres thereby more capable of feeling, as it were, the medicinal power and of communicating to the whole organism this health-affecting sensation. The previous employment of friction to the inside of the thigh makes the mere laying on the mercurial ointment afterwards quite as powerfully medicinal as if the ointment itself had been rubbed upon that part, a process which is termed rubbing-in, but it is very doubtful whether the mental itself can penetrate in substance into the interior of the body, or be taken up by the absorbent vessels by means of this so-called rubbing-in. Homoeopathy, however, hardly ever requires for its cures the rubbing-in of any medication, nor does it need any mercurial ointment.

§ 293 FIFTH EDITION

I find it necessary to allude here to animal magnetism, as it is termed, or rather mesmerism (as it should be called, out of gratitude to Mesmer, its first founder), which differs so much in its nature from all other therapeutic agents. This curative power, often so stupidly denied, which streams upon a patient by the contact of a well-intentioned person powerfully exerting his will, either acts homoeopathically, by the production of symptoms similar to those of the diseased state to be cured; and for this purpose a single pass made, without much exertion of the will, with the palms of the hands not too slowly from the top of the head downwards over the body to the tips of the toes,1 is serviceable in, for instance, uterine haemorrhages, even in the last stage when death seems approaching; or it is useful by distributing the vital force uniformly throughout the organism, when it is in abnormal excess in one part and deficient in other parts, for example, in rush of blood to the head and sleepless, anxious restlessness of weakly persons, etc., by means of a similar, single, but somewhat stronger pass; or for the immediate communication and restoration of the vital force to some one weakened part or to the whole organism, – an object that cannot be attained so certainly and with so little interference with the other medicinal treatment by any other agent besides mesmerism. If it is wished to supply a particular part with the vital force, this is effected by concentrating a very powerful and well-intentioned will for the purpose, and placing the hands or tips of the fingers on the chronically weakened parts, whither an internal chronic dyscrasia has transferred its important local symptom, as, for example, in the case of old ulcers, amaurosis, paralysis of certain limbs, etc.2 Many rapid apparent cures performed in all ages, by mesmerizers endowed with great natural power, belong to this class. The effect of communicated human power upon the whole human organism was most brilliantly shown, in the resuscitation of persons who had lain some time apparently dead, by the most powerful sympathetic will of a man in full vigor of vital force,3 and of this kind of resurrection history records many undeniable examples.

1. The smallest homoeopathic dose, which however, often effects wonders when used on proper occasions. Imperfect homoeopathists, who think themselves monstrously clever, not infrequently deluge their patients in difficult diseases with doses of different medicines, given rapidly one after the other, which, although they may have been homoeopathically selected and given in highly potentized attenuation, bring the patients into such an over-excited state that life and death are struggling for the mastery, and the least additional quantity of medicine would infallibly kill them. In such cases a mere gentle mesmeric pass and the frequent application, for a short time of the hand of a well-intentioned person to the part that is particularly affected, produce the harmonious uniform distribution of the vital force throughout the organism, and therewith rest, sleep and recovery.
2. Although by this restoration of the vital force, which ought to be repeated from time to time, no permanent cure can be effected in cases where, as has been taught above, a general internal dyscrasia lies at the root of the old local affection, as it always does, yet this positive strengthening and immediate saturation with the vital force (which no more belongs to the category of palliatives than does eating and drinking when hunger and thirst are present) is no mean auxiliary to the actual treatment of the whole disease by homoeopathic medicines.
3. Especially of one of those persons, of whom there are not many who, along with great kindness of disposition and perfect bodily powers, possesses but a very moderate desire for sexual intercourse, which it would give him very little trouble to suppress, in whom, consequently, all the fine vital spirits that would otherwise be employed in the preparation of the semen, are ready to be

communicated to others, by touching them and powerfully exerting the will. Some powerful mesmerisers, with whom I have become acquainted, has all this peculiar character.

§ 294 FIFTH EDITION*

All the above-mentioned methods of practicing mesmerism depend upon an influx of more or less vital force into the patient, and hence are termed positive mesmerism.1 An opposite mode of employing mesmerism, however, as it produces just the contrary effect, deserves to be termed negative mesmerism. To this belong the passes which are used to rouse from the somnambulic sleep, as also all the manual processes known by the names of soothing and ventilating. This discharge by means of negative mesmerism of the vital force accumulated to excess in individual parts of the system of undebiliated persons is most surely and simply performed by making a very rapid motion of the flat extended hand, held parallel to, and about an inch distant from the body, from the top of the head to the tips of the toes.2 The more rapidly this pass is made, so much the more effectually will the discharge be effected. Thus, for instance, in the case where a previously healthy woman,3 from the sudden suppression of her catamenia by a violent mental shock, lies to all appearance dead, the vital force which is probably accumulated in the precordial region, will by such a rapid negative pass, be discharged and its equilibrium throughout the whole organism restored, so that the resuscitation generally follows immediately.4 In like manner, a gentle, less rapid, negative pass diminishes the excessive restlessness and sleeplessness accompanied with anxiety sometimes produced in very irritable persons by a too powerful positive pass, etc.

* This Section corresponds to § 289 of the Sixth Edition.

1. When I here speak of the decided and certain curative power of positive mesmerism, I most assuredly do not mean the abuse of it, where, by repeated passes of this kind, continued for half an hour or a whole hour at a time, and, even day after day, performed on weak, nervous patients, that monstrous revolution of the whole human system is effected which is termed somnambulism, wherein the human being is ravished from the world of sense and seems to belong more to the world of spirits – a highly unnatural and dangerous state, by means of which it has not infrequently been attempted to cure chronic diseases.
2. It is a well known rule that a person who is either to be positively or negatively mesmerised, should not wear silk on any part of the body.
3. Hence a negative pass, especially if it be very rapid, is extremely injurious to a delicate person affected with a chronic ailment and deficient in vital force.
4. A strong country lad, ten years of age, received in the morning, on account of slight indisposition, from a professed female mesmeriser, several very powerful passes with the points of both thumbs, from the pit of the stomach along the lower edge of the ribs, and he instantly grew pale, and fell into such a state of unconsciousness and immobility that no effort could arouse him, and he was almost given up for dead. I made his eldest brother give him a very rapid negative pass from the crown of the head over the body to the feet, and in one instant he recovered his consciousness and became lively and well.

§ 1

MISSION OF PHYSICIAN

The physician's high and only mission is to restore the sick to health, to cure, as it is termed(1).

German – {" Die höchste und einzige Mission des Arztes ist es, die Gesundheit der Kranken wiederherzustellen und sie zu heilen, wie es als " bezeichnet wird.}

[Footnote – His mission is not, however, to construct so-called systems, by interweaving empty speculations and hypotheses concerning the internal essential nature of the vital processes and the mode in which diseases originate in the interior of the organism, (whereon so many physicians have hitherto ambitiously wasted their talents and their time); nor is it to attempt to give countless explanations regarding the phenomena in diseases and their proximate cause (which must ever remain concealed), wrapped in unintelligible words and an inflated abstract mode of expression, which should sound very learned in order to astonish the ignorant – whilst sick humanity sighs in vain for aid. Of such learned reveries (to which the name of theoretic medicine is given, and for which special professorships are instituted) we have had quite enough, and it is now high time that all who call themselves physicians should at length cease to deceive suffering mankind with mere talk, and begin now, instead, for once to act, that is, really to help and to cure.]

EXPLANATION

- *THE* — Used to indicate that someone or something is the best known or most important of that name or type.

(origin):	**German**	**Latin**	**English**
	Das/ Die/Der	QUOD	THE

- *PHYSICIAN'S* — A person who cures moral or spiritual ills; a healer.

(origin):	**Old French**	**Latin**	**English**
	Fisicien	Physica	Physician

- *HIGH* — A state of high spirits
- *ONLY* — And no one or nothing more besides; solely.
- *MISSION* — A strongly felt aim, ambition.
- *RESTORE* — Repair or renovate, so as to return it to its original condition.

(origin):	**Latin**	**Old French**	**English**
	Restaurare	Restorer	Restore

- **SICK** — Affected by physical or mental illness

(origin):	**Dutch**	**German**	**English**
	Ziek	Siech	Sick

- **HEALTH** — The state of being free from illness or injury.
- **TO CURE** — Relieve of the symptoms of a disease or condition.
- **TERMED** — Give a descriptive name to; call by a specified term.

(origin):	**Latin**	**Old French**	**English(Modern)**
	Terminus	Terme	Termed

Hahnemann says that the "The physician's high and only mission is to restore the sick to health &, cure the patient

Footnote:-

1. Hahnemann says that his Mission is not to construct any systems. The system which is made by empty Speculations & Hypothesis about the internal essential nature of vital processes in the body & mode in which diseases originate. This is waste of talent & time.
2. He also say that his mission is not to give countless explanations regarding the disease processes & their causes, This is explained by unintelligible words which sounds very learned to surprise the ignorant-but in reality the sick humanity (Human-Beings) while what they actually need is aid.
3. Till now many such theories to which the name theoretic medicine are given & for which special professorships are instituted. Now what is needed is that physician should stop mere talks & begin to act, really to help & to Cure the sick mankind.

§ 2

HIGHEST IDEAL OF CURE

The highest ideal of cure is rapid, gentle and permanent restoration of the health, or removal and annihilation of the disease in its whole extent, in the shortest, most reliable, and most harmless way, on easily comprehensible principles.

German – (Das höchste Ideal der Heilung ist die schnelle, sanfte und dauerhafte Wiederherstellung der Gesundheit, oder Beseitigung und Vernichtung der Krankheit in ihrem gesamten Ausmaß auf kürzeste, zuverlässigste und harmloseste Weise nach leicht verständlichen Grundsätzen")

EXPLANATION

- **THE** — Used to indicate that someone or something is the best known or most important of that name or type.
- **Highest** — Great, or greater than normal, in quality or intensity.

  (origin): | **Dutch** | **German** | **English** |
  |---|---|---|
  | Hoog | Hoch | Highest |

- **Ideal** — A standard or principle to be aimed at.

  (origin): | **Late** | **Latin German = English** |
  |---|---|
  | Idealis | Ideal = Idea |

- **Cure** — Relieve of the symptoms of a disease or condition.
- **Rapid** — Happening in a short time or at a great rate.

  (origin): | **Latin** | **German** | **English** |
  |---|---|---|
  | Rapere | Rapide | Rapid |

- **Gentle** — Having or showing a mild or gradual.

  (origin): | **Latin** | **German** | **Old English** | **English** |
  |---|---|---|---|
  | Gentilis | SANFT | Gentile | Gentle |

- **Permanent** — Remaining to the end.

  (origin): **Latin** Permanere = per + manere = **Permanent**
  (through) (remain) (Remaining to the end)

- **Restoration** — Denoting the action of restoring to a former state

  (origin): **late 15th century (denoting the action of restoring to a former state) partly from Old French, partly an alteration of obsolete restauration from late Latin restauratio, suggested by restore.**

- **Health** -- The state of being free from illness or injury.
- **Removal** — The action of taking away or abolishing something unwanted.
- **Anihilation** — Complete destruction or obliteration.

  (origin): **Latin** = Annihilare
  German = Vernichtung
  English = Anihilation

- **Disease** — A disorder of structure or function, especially one that produces specific.
- **Symptoms** — A physical or mental feature which is regarded as indicating a condition of d/s, particularly such a feature that is apparent to the patient.

  (origin): **Old French** = des + aise = desaise
  (Lack of ease) (expressing reversal) (ease).

- **Whole extent** — All of; entire area is covered by something.
- **Whole** — All of; Entire.
- **Extent** — The area covered by something

(origin):	**Latin**	**French**	**English Middle**	**English**
	Extendere	Extente	Extend	Extent

- **Shortest** — Small amount of time.
- **Most Reliable** — Consistently good in quality or performance.
- **Most Harmless** — Not able or likely to cause harm.
- **Way-** A method, style, or manner of doing something; an optional or alternative form of action.

    (origin): {Germanic origin; related to Dutch -weg and German-Weg, from a base meaning= 'move, carry'}.

- **Easily-** Without difficulty or effort
- **Comprehensible-** Able to be understood; intelligible.
- **Principles-** A fundamental truth or proposition that serves as the foundation for a system of belief or behaviour or for a chain of reasoning.

(origin):	**Latin**	**German**	**French**	**English**
	Principium	Prinzipien	Des Principles	Principles
	(source)	(First, chief)	(Foundation)	(the basic principles of justice)

According to Dr. Hahnemann, the best perfect treatment is when it is less time consuming, painless, irreversible change so that his signs and symptoms will never reappear in future. Internally dynamic vital force is in harmonious flow without any deviation. Not only external visible signs & symptoms are gone but internally body is in state of perfect harmony. No discomfort either external or internal.

Both internal & external that is whole body, fully has recovered with No side effects. By giving remedy which is proven based on universal principles without any pain and without any side effects. Homoeopathy do not suppress the symptoms and give temporary relief but it completely treats the patient, without any side effects in a painless way through medicines which are based on universal laws of nature, in minimum time as possible.

§ 3

KNOWLEDGE OF PHYSICIAN

If the physician clearly perceives what is to be cured in diseases, that is to say, in every individual case of disease (knowledge of disease, indication), if he clearly perceives what is curative in medicines, that is to say, in each individual medicine (knowledge of medical powers), and if he

knows how to adapt, according to clearly defined principles, what is curative in medicines to what he has discovered to be undoubtedly morbid in the patient, so that the recovery must ensue – to adapt it, as well in respect to the suitability of the medicine most appropriate according to its mode of action to the case before him (choice of the remedy, the medicine indicated), as also in respect to the exact mode of preparation and quantity of it required (proper dose), and the proper period for repeating the dose; – if, finally, he knows the obstacles to recovery in each case and is aware how to remove them, so that the restoration may be permanent, then he understands how to treat judiciously and rationally, and he is a true practitioner of the healing art.

EXPALANATION

If the physician knows what is to be cured in every individual case of disease I.e.

Knowledge of disease, indication

- If he has knowledge of medicinal powers
- If he knows how to act according to the defined principles, so that recovery must ensue
- If he knows most appropriate mode of medicine in every individual case I.e choice of remedy indicated in the case
- If he knows the exact mode of preparation & quantity of remedy required i.e proper dose.
- If he knows when to repeat the dose.
- If he knows, what can be obstacles to recovery in each case & how to remove them So that restoration is permanent.

Then he understand how to treat patient judiciously & rationally And He is the true practitioner of the healing art.

Dr. Hahnemann explains what knowledge is required to be a true practitioner of healing art, so that he can achieve his mission of ideal cure.

Second way to understand:

TRUE PRACTITIONER OF HEALING ART

1] KNOWLEDGE OF DISEASE:
- Physician should understand meaning of disease.
- Physician should clearly perceive,, what is to be cured in diseases, that is to say, in every individual case of disease.
- it is internal deviation of normal harmonious vital force.
- Physician should understand concept of dynamic vital force.
- Physician should have knowledge of basic science like
  - ✦ Anatomy, physiology, pathology, etc & uncommon symptoms.

2] KNOWLEDGE OF MEDICINAL POWERS:

- Physician should understand the dynamic power of medicines that it is not the quantity of drug which will bring cure but its potential dynamic powers.

3] KNOWLEDGE OF MEDICINE:

- Physician should know similia similibus curantur.
- Physician should know laws on basis of which medicines are prescribed.
- Physician should be able to match the totality of symptoms in each individual case with that of the medicine
- Physician should have good knowledge of materia medica so that he can select exact similimum.

4] KNOWLEDGE OF PROPER DOSE:

- Physician should understand how much dose is required to just arouse the vitality and cure the patient.
- Exact mode of preparation and quantity of it required.
- Knowledge of Homoeopathy pharmacy & posology is required'
- How to choose potency
- More potency means more dynamic
- Less potency means less dynamic
- Physician should have knowledge when to prescribe for more dynamic and when for the less dynamic dose.

5] KNOWLEDGE OF REPETITION OF DOSE:

- Physician should not repeat the medicine unnecessary in order to avoid aggravation.
- He should know the correct time to repeat the remedy
- Physician should observe that same medicine required repetition or a different one and the same potency or different.

6] KNOWLEDGE OF OBSTACLES TO RECOVERY:

- Knowledge of miasms
- He should know the obstacles to recovery in each case & how to remove them, so that the restoration may be permanent.

7] KNOWLEDGE OF CAUSE OF DISEASE:

- Causative factors like internal & external.

8] KNOWLEDGE OF LAWS OF HOMOEOPATHY:

- similia similibus curantur.

§ 4

PRESERVER OF HEALTH

He is likewise a preserver of health if he knows the things that derange health and cause disease, and how to remove them from persons in health.

German:- Er ist auch ein Bewahrer der Gesundheit, wenn er die Dinge, die derange Gesundheit und Ursache Vonse krank, und wie man sie von Menschen in der Gesundheit zu entfernen.

EXPLANATION

- **Likewise** { In like wise} -- In a similar way.
- **Preserver** -- Maintain in its original or existing state

  (Origin): **Late latin**

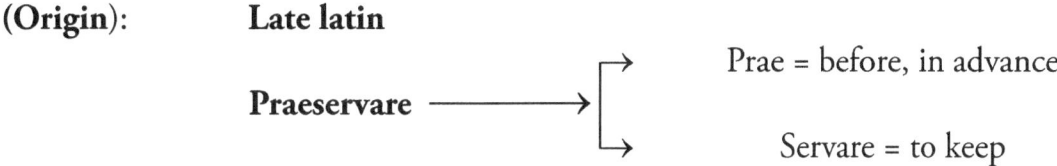

- **Health** - The state of being free from illness or injury
- **Things-** Factors
- **Derange-** Disturb

  (Origin):

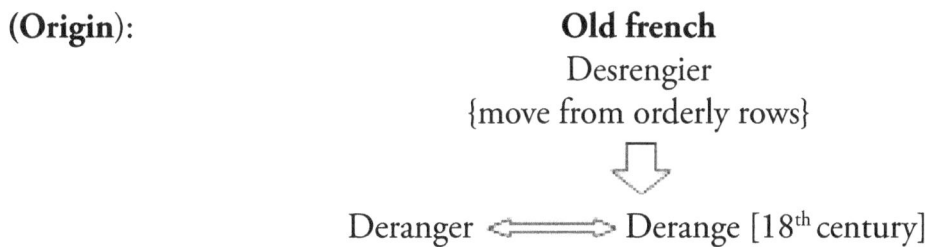

- **Cause-** Reason
- **Disease-** A disorder of structure or function, especially one that produces specific.
- **Remove-** Away

  (Origin):   **Latin - Removere**

   RE + MOVERE = REMOVE
   [BACK] + [TO MOVE]

If the physician has the knowledge of the things which derange health & cause disease.
  If he knows how to remove them from persons who are in health.

HE IS A PRESERVER OF HEALTH

182 | SOUL OF THE ORGANON – II

Dr. Hahnemann instructs us that being a doctor does not means only to treat diseased individuals but physician is also a preserver of health.

It is the responsibility of the physician to help society in preservation of health. Physician should have knowledge of preventive & social medicine & also knowledge of exciting and maintaining causes.

He should aware those who are in the state of health, about things which can bring deviation from the state of health. E.g.-Diet, hygiene, exercise, miasms etc.

§ 5

EXCITING & FUNDAMENTAL CAUSE

Useful to the physician in assisting him to cure are the particulars of the most probable exciting cause of the acute disease, as also the most significant points in the whole history of the chronic disease, to enable him to discover its fundamental cause, which is generally due to a chronic miasm. In these investigations, the ascertainable physical constitution of the patient (especially when the disease is chronic), his moral and intellectual character, his occupation, mode of living and habits, his social and domestic relations, his age, sexual function, etc., are to be taken into consideration.

EXPLANATION

- **Useful** — In several ways
- **Physician** — A person who cures moral or spiritual ills; a healer.

  (origin): | **Old French** | **Latin** | **English** |
  |---|---|---|
  | Fisicien | Physica | Physician |

- **Assisting** — Be present as a helper

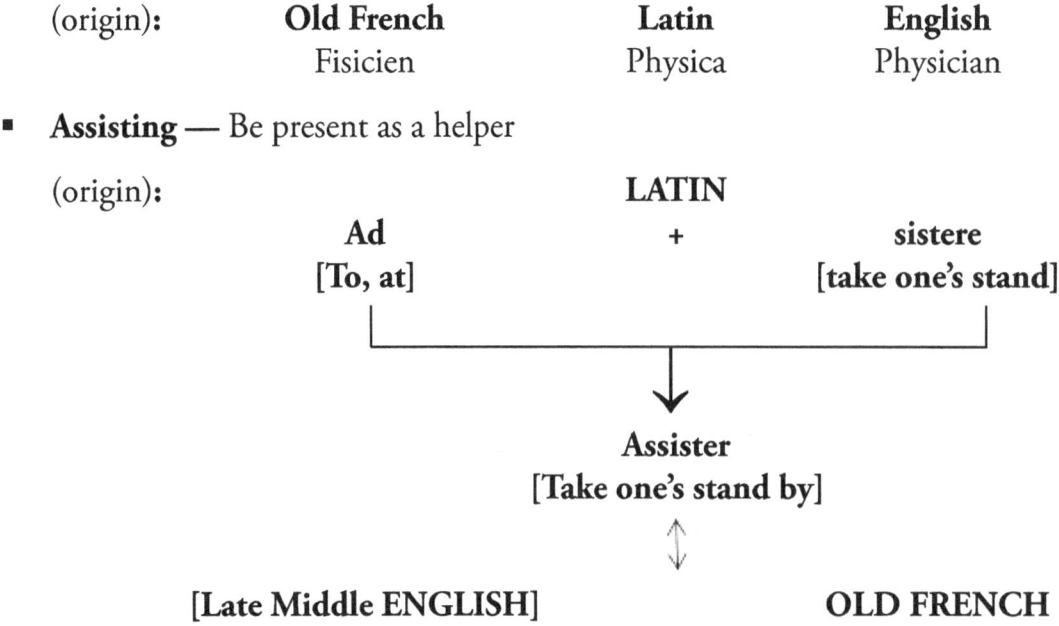

- **Particulars** — A detail
- **Probable** — Likely to happen or be in the case

  (origin):   **LATIN:**   Probare {to test, demonstrate}
                OLD FRENCH: Probable {worthy of belief}

- **Significant** — Indicative of something.
- **Ascertainable** — Capable of being determined or limited or fixed.
- **Constitution** — A person's physical state as regards vitality health & strength.

For Acute diseases the most probable exciting cause and
- In Chronic diseases -the most important points in the whole history, the fundamental cause(which is mainly due to a chronic miasm) are useful in assisting the physician to cure.

In these in investigations-
- Physical constitution of the patient
- Moral & Intellectual character
- His occupation
- His mode of living & habits
- His social & domestic relations

→ All are to be considered

Dr. Hahnemann teaches us about case taking, according to him there are 2 types of cases:-

1. ACUTE CASES - Exciting cause is important and prescribe on the basis of that to cure the patient.
2. CHRONIC CASES - Fundamental cause is important I.e. Miasmatic cause along with his physical constitution, moral and intellectual character, occupation, mode of living and habits, social and domestic relation, sexual function, age, etc

§ 6

FOR THE PHYSICIAN THE DISEASE CONSISTS OF THE TOTALITY OF SYMPTOMS

The unprejudiced observer – well aware of the futility of transcendental speculations which can receive no confirmation from experience – be his powers of penetration ever so great, takes note of nothing in every individual disease, except the changes in the health of the body and of the mind (morbid phenomena, accidents, symptoms) which can be perceived externally by means of the senses; that is to say, he notices only the deviations from the former healthy state of the now diseased individual, which are felt by the patient himself, remarked by those around him and observed by the physician. All these perceptible signs represent the disease in its whole extent, that is, together they form the true and only conceivable portrait of the disease.2

In Organon 6th Edition, Aphrosims 6 is same but the footnote is different from 5th Edition.

Disease 1*-

In 5th Edition footnote	In 6th Edition footnote
1. I know not, therefore, how it was possible for physicians at the sick-bed to allow themselves to suppose that, without most carefully attending to the symptoms and being guided by them in the treatment, they ought to seek and could discover, only in the hidden and unknown interior, what there was to be cured in the disease, arrogantly and ludicrously pretending that they could, without paying much attention to the symptoms, discover the alteration that had occurred in the invisible interior, and set it to rights with (unknown!) medicines, and that such a procedure as this could alone be called radical and rational treatment. Is not, then, that which is cognizable by the senses in diseases through the phenomena it displays, the disease itself in the eyes of the physician, since he never can see the spiritual being that produces the disease, the vital force? nor is it necessary that he should see it, but only that he should ascertain its morbid actions, in order that he may thereby be enabled to cure the disease. What else will the old school search for in the hidden interior of the organism, as a prima causa morbi, whilst they reject as an object of cure and contemptuously despise the sensible and manifest representation of the disease, the symptoms, that so plainly address themselves to us? What else do they wish to cure in disease but these?* * The physician whose researches are directed towards the hidden relations in the interior of the organism, may daily err; but the homoeopathist who grasps with requisite carefulness the whole group of symptoms, possesses a sure guide; and if he succeed in removing the whole group of symptoms he has likewise most assuredly destroyed the internal, hidden cause of the disease.	1. I know not, therefore, how it was possible for physicians at the sick-bed to allow themselves to suppose that, without most carefully attending to the symptoms and being guided by them in the treatment, they ought to seek and could discover, only in the hidden and unknown interior, what there was to be cured in the disease, arrogantly and ludicrously pretending that they could, without paying much attention to the symptoms, discover the alteration that had occurred in the invisible interior, and set it to rights with (unknown!) medicines, and that such a procedure as this could alone be called radical and rational treatment. Is not, then, that which is cognizable by the senses in diseases through the phenomena it displays, the disease itself in the eyes of the physician, since he never can see the spiritual being that produces the disease, the vital force? nor is it necessary that he should see it, but only that he should ascertain its morbid actions, in order that he may thereby be enabled to cure the disease. What else will the old school search for in the hidden interior of the organism, as a prima causa morbi, whilst they reject as an object of cure and contemptuously despise the sensible and manifest representation of the disease, the symptoms, that so plainly address themselves to us? What else do they wish to cure in disease but these?

EXPLANATION

* 'THE UNPREJUDICED OBSERVER "- Dr. Hahnemann describes another quality of Homoeopathic physician -Physician should be unprejudiced observer.

- ✦ Physician should carefully with his keen observation and perception notice and prescribe on the basis of the totality of symptoms.
- ✦ Physician should individualize each case.
- ✦ Physician should not jump to conclusions on the basic of his past experience.
- ✦ Physician should know the real cause of the symptoms.
- ✦ Physician should understand that the exterior visible and perceptible signs & symptoms are reflection of internally deranged vital force.

- Always learn this that Each case is different
- We should not be prejudiced I.e. biased in our option while prescribing the medicine.

Footnote 1:

Hahnemann says that he does not know how the physicians without carefully attending to the symptoms and observing can guide the treatment.

Their focus is to find and discover what is there inside the body interior which has to be cured and without paying much attention to the symptoms, discover only the alterations that has occurred in the invisible interior and try to set it right with unknown medicines and such a procedure was called radical and rational treatment.

Since these physicians can never observe the spiritual being that produces the disease i.e. the vital force.

If they cannot see the spiritual being what else do they wish to cure in diseases?

What else the old school will search for in the hidden interior of the organism, as a prima causa morbi when they reject the main object of cure, the deranged vital force.

§ 7

TOTALITY OF SYMPTOMS

Now, as in a disease, from which no manifest exciting or maintaining cause (causa occasionalis) has to be removed1, we can perceive nothing but the morbid symptoms, it must (regard being had to the possibility of a miasm, and attention paid to the accessory circumstances, § 5) be the symptoms alone by which the disease demands and points to the remedy suited to relieve it – and, moreover, the totality of these its symptoms, of this outwardly reflected picture of the internal essence of the disease, that is, of the affection of the vital force, must be the principal, or the sole means, whereby the disease can make known what remedy it requires – the only thing that can determine the choice of the most appropriate remedy – and thus, in a word, the totality2 of the symptoms must be the principal, indeed the only thing the physician has to take note of in every case of disease and to remove by means of his art, in order that it shall be cured and transformed into health.

[**Footnote-1** It is not necessary to say that every intelligent physician would first remove this where it exists; the indisposition thereupon generally ceases spontaneously. He will remove from the room strong-smelling flowers, which have a tendency to cause syncope and hysterical sufferings; extract from the cornea the foreign body that excites inflammation of the eye; loosen the over-tight bandage on a wounded limb that threatens to cause mortification, and apply a more suitable one; lay bare and put ligature on the wounded artery that produces fainting; endeavour to promote the expulsion by vomiting of belladonna berries etc., that may have been swallowed; extract foreign substances that may have got into the orifices of the body (the nose, gullet, ears, urethra, rectum, vagina); crush the vesical calculus; open the imperforate anus of the newborn infant, etc.

2 In all times, the old school physicians, not knowing how else to give relief, have sought to combat and if possible to suppress by medicines, here and there, a single symptom from among a number in diseases – a one-sided procedure, which, under the name of symptomatic treatment, has justly excited universal contempt, because by it, not only was nothing gained, but much harm was inflicted. A single one of the symptoms present is no more the disease itself than a foot is the man himself. This procedure was so much the more reprehensible, that such a single symptom was only treated by an antagonistic remedy (therefore only in an enantiopathic and palliative manner), whereby, after a slight alleviation, it was subsequently only rendered all the worse.]

EXPLANATION

In this Aphrosim, Hahnemann begins to outline the importance of symptoms themselves in the understanding of disease & for identifying a therapeutic medicine.

His preposition is that the totality of the symptoms of the patient are the outwardly reflected picture of the internal essence of the disease, that is, of the affection of the vital force.

In case where any exciting or maintaining cause is not to be removed.

The symptoms alone I.e the totality of symptoms, is the principal & only thing physician should take note in every case of disease & to remove it in order that the disease shall be cured & transformed into health

Because the symptoms are the only outwardly reflected picture of internal diseases, of affection of the vital force.

Hahnemann Mentions 4 Qualifications For Understanding -

1. Any exciting 0r Maintaining cause have been removed,& the symptoms experienced are not attributable to these aggravators.
2. Accessory circumstances are understood, such as those due to the patient lifestyle
3. Some or more of the symptoms may be attributable to a miasm -the deeper roots which predispose us to disease, such as genetics.
4. Totality of symptoms:- Hahnemann states that this is the principal, whereby the disease can make us known what remedy it requires'., so symptoms are information rich and meaningful for the Homoeopathic physician.

Hahnemann opposes the study of medicine where only a single symptom is treated, as he considers this antagonistic to the goal of the complete symptom picture. Hahnemann states that; **A SINGLE ONE OF THE SYMPTOMS PRESENT IS NO MORE THE DISEASE ITSELF THAN A SINGLE FOOT IS THE MAN HIMSELF'**.

Footnote 1:
In a disease, from which manifest exciting or Maintaining cause{Causa Occasionalis} has to be removed, after removal of this where it exists, the indisposition thereupon generally ceases spontaneously.

Like:
[a] Remove strong -smelling flowers from the room which can cause syncope & hysterical sufferings
[b] Remove foreign body from cornea that causes inflammation of the eye.
[c] Loose the bandage on wounded limb, if it is over-tight — it can cause necrosis.
[d] Promote expulsion of belladonna berries etc which may have been swallowed, by vomiting.
[e] Remove foreign substances that may have got into vagina, nose, gullet, ears, urethra, rectum etc
[f] Open imperforate anus of new-born infant etc.

Footnote 2:
The old school physicians do not know how else to give relief to the patient, they suppress a single symptom from among a number of symptoms by medicines and follow a one-sided procedure called symptomatic treatment. By it nothing was gained but much harm was inflicted.

Hahnemann opposes the study of medicine where only a single symptom is treated, as he considers this antagonistic to the goal of the complete symptom picture. Here after a slight alleviation, it was subsequently only rendered all the worse.

Hahnemann states that; **A SINGLE ONE OF THE SYMPTOMS PRESENT IS NO MORE THE DISEASE ITSELF THAN A SINGLE FOOT IS THE MAN HIMSELF'**.

§ 8

ONCE SYMPTOMS ARE ERADICATED DISEASE IS CURED

It is not conceivable, not can it be proved by any experience in the world, that, after removal of all the symptoms of the disease and of the entire collection of the perceptible phenomena, there should or could remain anything else besides health, or that the morbid alteration in the interior could remain uneradicated.1

[FOOTNOTE-1 When a patient has been cured of his disease by a true physician, in such a manner that no trace of the disease, no morbid symptom, remains, and all the signs of health have permanently returned, how can anyone, without offering an insult to common sense, affirm in such an individual the whole bodily disease still remains interior? And yet the chief of the old school, Hufeland, asserts this in the following words: "Homoeopathy can remove symptoms, but the disease remains." (Vide Homoopathie, p.27, 1, 19.) This he maintains partly from mortification at the progress made by homoeopathy to the benefits of mankind, partly because he still holds thoroughly material notions respecting disease, which he is still unable to regard as a state of being of the organism wherein it is dynamically altered by the morbidly deranged vital force, as an altered state of health, but he views the disease as a something material, which after the cure is completed, may still remain lurking in some corner in the interior of the body, in order, some day during the most vigorous health, to burst forth at its pleasure with its material presence! So dreadful is still the blindness of the old pathology!

No wonder that it could only produce a system of therapeutics which is solely occupied with scouring out the poor patient.]

EXPLANATION

In the previous aphrosim, Hahnemann describes the significance of the totality of symptoms, that of being the outward reflection of the inner essence of disease; the affection of the vital force.

In this aphorism, Hahnemann proposition is that the removal of these symptoms means the disease has been eradicated.

It is not imaginable, nor it can be proved, that after removal of all the symptoms of the disease & noticeable phenomena, there should remain anything else besides health (means health is attained as all the symptoms have been removed) or that the morbid alteration in the interior could remain uneradicated(otherwise the morbid changes would still be present).

Footnote:
When a patient is cured of his disease by a true physician in such a manner that No morbid symptom remains and All the signs of health have returned permanently.

How can anyone say that the whole bodily disease still remains in the interior?

*[The chief of the old school, Hufeland says,"Homoeopathy can remove the symptoms, but the disease remains."Because according to him the disease is something material, which after, the cure is completed, May remain in some corner in the body & appear with its material presence some day. They are still unable to regard dynamically deranged vital force, as an altered state of health.

This above system of therapeutics is only scouring out the poor patient.

§ 9

VITAL FORCE

In the healthy condition of man, the spiritual vital force (autocracy), the dynamis that animates the material body (organism), rules with unbounded sway, and retains all the parts of the organism in admirable, harmonious, vital operation, as regards both sensations and functions, so that our indwelling, reason-gifted mind can freely employ this living, healthy instrument for the higher purpose of our existence.

EXPLANATIONS

In the healthy condition of man ————-

The spiritual Vital force (Autocracy), the dynamis that animates the organism, rules the body unrestrained. Vital force has unrestrained influence over the material organism & keeps all the parts of the organism in harmony to each other. So that our mind can freely, employ this living, healthy body for the higher purpose of our existence.

Hahnemann believed that the purpose of the regulatory systems of our organism is to maintain harmonious, vital operation of the senses and functions of the body -or create a state of health & that with our health, we are able to focus on the higher purpose of our existence.

However, it does highlight how important health is, as well as the journey to health and that when we are feeling vital & well, we have the energy to apply ourselves to this higher purpose, whatever it maybe.

§ 10

WITHOUT VITAL FORCE ORGANISM IS DEAD

The material organism, without the vital force, is capable of no sensation, no function, no self-preservation1, it derives all sensation and performs all the functions of life solely by means of the immaterial being (the vital principle) which animates the material organism in health and in disease.

[FOOTNOTE:- 1 It is dead, and only subject to the power of the external physical world; it decays, and is again resolved into its chemical constituents.]

EXPLANATION

In this Aphorism Hahnemann says that without the vital force our body cannot have any sensation, function or self preservation. Our body is governed by vital force in both health & in disease.

All sensations & All functions of life are governed by this vital principle.

1. Let us take an example: you have a toy, this toy is useless without a battery. As soon as you insert battery the toy comes to life, it moves, produces sound etc.
2. In our body this vital force is just like a battery without this battery the body is lifeless & useless.
3. This vital force carries out all the sensations, functions & working of the body.
4. When vital force is healthy the body is healthy

When vital force is disturbed, it produces some unpleasent sensations in body as symptoms & signs and **Disease occurs.**

Footnote 1:
Without vital force, the physical body is dead, its organs & tissue start to die & decay. Without vital force the body cannot be preserved, it decays into its chemical constituents.

§ 11

ILLNESS MEANS THE VITAL FORCE IS DISTURBED/DERANGED

When a person falls ill, it is only this spiritual, self acting (automatic) vital force, everywhere present in his organism, that is primarily deranged by the dynamic1 influence upon it of a morbific agent inimical to life; it is only the vital force, deranged to such an abnormal state, that can furnish the organism with its disagreeable sensations, and incline it to the irregular processes which we call disease; for, as a power invisible in itself, and only cognizable by its effects on the organism, its morbid derangement only makes itself known by the manifestation of disease in the sensations and functions of those parts of the organism exposed to the senses of the observer and physician, that is, by morbid symptoms, and in no other way can it make itself known.2

[FOOTNOTE:-1 Materia peccans!

2 What is dynamic influence, – dynamic power? Our earth, by virtue of a hidden invisible energy, carries the moon around her in twenty-eight days and several hours, and the moon alternately, in definite fixed hours (deducting certain differences which occur with the full and new moon) raises our northern seas to flood tide and again correspondingly lowers them to ebb. Apparently this takes place not through material agencies, not through mechanical contrivances, as are used for products of human labor; and so we see numerous other events about us as results of the action of one substance on another substance without being able to recognize a sensible connection between cause and effect. Only the cultured, practised in comparison and deduction, can form for himself a kind of supra-sensual idea sufficient to keep all that is material or mechanical in his thoughts from such concepts. He calls such effects dynamic, virtual, that is, such as result from absolute, specific, pure energy and action of he one substance upon the other substance.

For instance, the dynamic effect of the sick-making influences upon healthy man, as well as the dynamic energy of the medicines upon the principle of life in the restoration of health is nothing else than infection and so not in any way material, not in any way mechanical. Just as the energy of a magnet attracting a piece of iron or steel is not material, not mechanical. One sees that the piece of iron is attracted by one pole of the magnet, but how it is done is not seen. This invisible energy of the magnet does not require mechanical (material) auxiliary means, hook or lever, to attract the iron. The magnet draws to itself and this acts upon the piece of iron or upon a steel needle by means of a purely immaterial invisible, conceptual, inherent energy, that is, dynamically, and communicates to the steel needle the magnetic energy equally invisibly (dynamically). The steel needle becomes itself magnetic, even at a distance when the magnet does not touch it, and magnetises other steel needles with the same magnetic property (dynamically) with which it had been endowed previously by the magnetic rod, just as a child with small-pox or measles communicates to a near, untouched healthy child in an invisible manner (dynamically) the small-pox or measles, that is, infects it at a distance without anything material from the infective child going or capable of going to the one to be infected.

A purely specific conceptual influence communicated to the near child small-pox or measles in the same way as the magnet communicated to the near needle the magnetic property.

In a similar way, the effect of medicines upon living man is to be judged. Substances, which are used as medicines, are medicines only in so far as they possess each its own specific energy to alter the well-being of man through dynamic, conceptual influence, by means of the living sensory fibre, upon the conceptual controlling principle of life. The medicinal property of those material substances which we call medicines proper, relates only to their energy to call out alterations in the well-being of animal life. Only upon this conceptual principle of life, depends their medicinal health-altering, conceptual (dynamic) influence. Just as the nearness of a magnetic pole can communicate only magnetic energy to the steel (namely, by a kind of infection) but cannot communicate other properties (for instance, more hardness or ductility, etc.). And thus every special medicinal substance alters through a kind of infection, that well-being of man in a peculiar manner exclusively its own and not in a manner peculiar to another medicine, as certainly as the nearness of the child ill with small-pox will communicate to a healthy child only small-pox and not measles. These medicines act upon our well-being wholly without communication of material parts of the medicinal substances, thus dynamically, as if through infection. Far more healing energy is expressed in a case in point by the smallest dose of the best dynamized medicines, in which there can be, according to calculation, only so little of material substance that its minuteness cannot be thought and conceived by the best arithmetical mind, than by large doses of the same medicine in substance. That smallest dose can therefore contain almost entirely only the pure, freely-developed, conceptual medicinal energy, and bring about only dynamically such great effects as can never be reached by the crude medicinal substances itself taken in large doses.

It is not in the corporal atoms of these highly dynamized medicines, nor their physical or mathematical surfaces (with which the higher energies of the dynamized medicines are being interpreted but vainly as still sufficiently material) that the medicinal energy is found. More likely, there lies invisible in the moistened globule or in its solution, an unveiled, liberated, specific, medicinal force contained in the medicinal substance which acts dynamically by contact with the living animal fibre upon the whole organism (without communicating to it anything material however highly attenuated) and acts more strongly the more free and more immaterial the energy has become through the dynamization.

Is it then so utterly impossible for our age celebrated for its wealth in clear thinkers to think of dynamic energy as something non-corporeal, since we see daily phenomena which cannot be explained in any other manner? If one looks upon something nauseous and becomes inclined to vomit, did a material emetic come into his stomach which compels him to this anti-peristaltic movement? Was it not solely the dynamic effect of the nauseating aspect upon his imagination? And if one raises his arm, does it occur through a material visible instrument? a lever? Is it not solely the conceptual dynamic energy of his will which raises it?]

EXPLANATION

1. In a healthy person the vital force like power is invisible & is present everywhere.
2. It carries out all the sensations &functions of organism in order.
3. When any harmful agent acts on this vital principle

This self-acting vital force is disturbed or deranged

This produces disagreeable sensations & irregular processes in the body.

The disturbed vital force makes itself visible only by its effects on organisms I.e.by producing morbid symptoms.

Otherwise in a healthy person it can not make itself known & is invisible.

Example - 1] A patient comes to you & tells his symptoms,

Now as a physician you should know that his vital force has been disturbed.

Now based on his totality of symptoms [Explained Later]you give the remedy & bring this vital force to normal state **And hence the patient is cured**.

Footnote 1:
What is dynamic influence-dynamic power?

A Magnet attracts the piece of iron but how it is done, cannot be seen, this invisible energy of the magnet do not require hook or lever to attract the iron. It means it do not require any mechanical means, it attracts iron by a purely immaterial, invisible, conceptual energy I.e.dynamically

In similar way a child suffering from measles infects other child at a distance without anything going from the infective child to the other one.

In the similar way, the medicines have their effect upon living man, dynamically, by contact with the living animal fibre upon the whole organism without communicating to it anything material however highly attenuated medicinal forces.. These medicines act upon our well-being wholly without communication of material parts of the medicinal substance, dynamically.

§ 12

DISEASE MEANS VITAL FORCE IS DERANGED BY A MORBIFIC AGENT

It is the morbidly affected vital energy alone that produces disease1, so that the morbid phenomena perceptible to our senses express at the same time all the internal change, that is to say, the whole morbid derangement of the internal dynamis; in a word, they reveal the whole disease; consequently, also, the disappearance under treatment of all the morbid phenomena and of all the morbid alterations that differ from the healthy vital operations, certainly affects and necessarily implies the restoration of the integrity of the vital force and, therefore, the recovered health of the whole organism.

1 How the vital force causes the organism to display morbid phenomena, that is, how it produces disease, it would be of no practical utility to the physician to know, and will forever remain concealed from him; only what it is necessary for him to know of the disease and what is fully sufficient for enabling him to cure it, has the Lord of life revealed to his senses

EXPLANATION

In the healthy state of an organism all the sensations & functions are under control of a healthy vital force.

When this vital force is deranged (disturbed) by any harmful agent, Internal changes or derangement of internal dynamics occurs.

It Appears as signs & symptoms

* Now when a proper homoeopathic remedy is given and is followed by the Disappearance of all morbid phenomena & alternations it means that the healthy vital operations are restored. This means restoration of the vital force has occured & therefore, the recovery of health of the whole organism.

Footnote 1:

Hahnemann says that, how the vital force causes the organism to display morbid phenomenon i.e., how it produces disease, is of no practical use to the physician. It is not necessary to know it.

Only the thing that is necessary for him to know about the disease is what is sufficient to enable him to cure it, not how a disease is caused..

§ 13

MATERIAL THINGS/SPIRITUAL THINGS

Therefore disease (that does not come within the province of manual surgery) considered, as it is by the allopathists, as a thing separate from the living whole, from the organism and its animating vital force, and hidden in the interior, be it ever so subtle a character, is an absurdity, that could only be imagined by minds of a materialistic stamp, and has for thousands of years given to the prevailing system of medicine all those pernicious impulses that have made it a truly mischievous (non-healing) art.

EXPLANATION

Therefore disease[that do not come under manual surgery] as allopathists, describe as a thing that is separate from the living organism and it's animating vital force.

- ✦ They only believe in material things & not on spiritual things.
- ✦ They believe that no vital force exists in the body.
- ✦ This belief of allopathic minds is ridiculous as stated by this aphorism.
- ✦ This has lead to a non-healing & harmful art of system of medicine for thousands of years.

Example-

Let us take an example of a stone, one person sees it as a material thing which is visible to eye & can be felt by touch.

Other person goes at spiritual level not material things and believes in the vital force that is not visible to our senses, this person has seen the effect of vital force & seen the patient being cured on this basis.

§ 14

VITAL FORCE EXPRESS ITSELF ONLY BY SIGN& SYMPTOMS

There is, in the interior of man, nothing morbid that is curable and no invisible morbid alteration that is curable which does not make itself known to the accurately observing physicians by means of morbid signs and symptoms – an arrangement in perfect conformity with the infinite goodness of the all-wise Preserver of human life.

EXPLANATION

The Morbid alteration which occur in the vital force ………

1. When the vital force is disturbed by any harmful agent, it expresses itself to the observing physician.
2. It expresses itself by means of morbid signs & symptoms.
3. These morbid signs & symptoms are the only expression of the diseased/disturbed vital force.
4. The vital force can express itself only by these signs & symptoms.
5. Therefore when proper Homeopathic medicine is given, these signs & symptoms disappear.
6. This removal of signs & symptoms from organism means that the vital force has been restored or is back to normal healthy state, without any sufferings.

§15

DYNAMIC PLANE/MATERIAL PLANE OF VITAL FORCE

The affection of the morbidly deranged, spirit-like dynamis (vital force) that animates our body in the invisible interior, and the totality of the outwardly cognizable symptoms produced by it in the organism and representing the existing malady, constitute a whole; they are one and the same. The organism is indeed the material instrument of the life, but it is not conceivable without the animation imparted to it by the instinctively perceiving and regulating dynamis, just as the vital force is not conceivable without the organism, consequently the two together constitute a unity,

although in thought our mind separates this unity into two distinct conceptions for the sake of easy comprehension.

EXPLANATION

1. In the 15th aphorism he says that the deranged vital force & the signs & symptoms which appear are not separate from each other.
2. The outwardly signs &symptoms are the reflection of deranged vital force.
3. The vital force which is deranged internally & the signs & symptoms which are present externally are the same.
4. They are one & the same -
   + One is on the dynamic plane [deranged vital force]
   + Other on the material plane [signs & symptoms]
5. Material body & vital force are not separate from each other.
6. We cannot imagine the material body without the life force I.e.vital force similarly the vital force has no existence without the material body.
7. The material body & the vital force from a unity.
8. If you restore any one, the other is restored too.
9. Just for easy understanding we study them separately.
10. Never study what words are in aphorisms, study true way what it means in life, in person.

§ 16

VITAL FORCE IS DYNAMIC IN NATURE

Our vital force, as a spirit-like dynamis, cannot be attacked and affected by injurious influences on the healthy organism caused by the external inimical forces that disturb the harmonious play of life, otherwise than in a spirit-like (dynamic) way, and in like manner, all such morbid derangements (diseases) cannot be removed from it by the physician in any other way than by the spirit-like (dynamic1, virtual) alterative powers of the serviceable medicines acting upon our spirit-like vital force, which perceives them through the medium of the sentient faculty of the nerves everywhere present in the organism, so that it is only by their dynamic action on the vital force that remedies are able to re-establish and do actually re-establish health and vital harmony, after the changes in the health of the patient cognizable by our senses (the totality of the symptoms) have revealed the disease to the carefully observing and investigating physician as fully as was requisite in order to enable him to cure it.

[**FOOTNOTE**-1 Most severe disease may be produced by sufficient disturbance of the vital force through the imagination and also cured by the same means.]

EXPLANATION

i. In this aphorism, Hahnemann says that our vital force is dynamic in nature.
ii. Therefore it can only be affected by the dynamic influence of external inimical forces to cause disease
iii. Similarly the dynamic power, the energy in our remedies can correct this dynamic disturbance at the dynamic level of energy only.
iv. Let us see how these remedies affect the vital force.
v. Hahnemann says that the energy in our remedies is taken up by the nerves which are present everywhere in our body.
vi. Thus our remedies act as signals
vii. The remedies provide some information to the body to correct the disturbance & restoration work is done by the body itself.
viii. Hahnemann says that even serious diseases with advanced pathologies can be caused by non-material I.e.dynamic causes

E.g. Asthma, Hypertension that are caused or affected by mental, emotional & environment factors.

§ 17

WHAT HAPPEN TO THE V.F &D/S PROCESS AFTER REMEDY INTAKE

Now, as in the cure effected by the removal of the whole of the perceptible signs and symptoms of the disease the internal alteration of the vital principle to which the disease is due – consequently the whole of the disease – is at the same time removed,1 it follows that the physician has only to remove the whole of the symptoms in order, at the same time, to abrogate and annihilate the internal change, that is to say, the morbid derangement of the vital force – consequently the totality of the disease, the disease itself.2 But when the disease is annihilated the health is restored, and this is the highest, the sole aim of the physician who knows the true object of his mission, which consists not in learned – sounding prating, but in giving aid to the sick.

1 A warning dream, a superstitious fancy, or a solemn prediction that death would occur at a certain day or at a certain hour, has not unfrequently produced all the signs of commencing and increasing disease, of approaching death and death itself at the hour announced, which could not happen without the simultaneous production of the inward change (corresponding to the state observed internally); and hence in such cases all the morbid signs indicative of approaching death have frequently been dissipated by an identical cause, by some cunning deception or persuasion to a belief in the contrary, and health suddenly restored, which could not have happened without the removal, by means of this mortal remedy, of the internal and external morbid change that threatened death.

2 It is only thus that God the preserver of mankind, could reveal His wisdom and goodness in reference to the cure of the disease to which man is liable here below, by showing to the physician what he had to remove in disease in order to annihilate them and thus re-establish health. But what would we think of His wisdom and goodness if He has shrouded in mysterious obscurity that which was to be cured in diseases (as is asserted by the dominant school of medicine, which affects to possess a supernatural insight into the nature of things), and shut it up in the hidden interior, and thus rendered it impossible for man to know the malady accurately, consequently impossible for him to cure it?

EXPLANATION

I. In aphroism 17, he explains that when the correct remedy is given what happens to the vital force & the disease process
II. We know that disturbance of vital force by harmful agents causes disease.
III. This disturbance of vital force manifests itself in the form of signs & symptoms that can be perceived by our senses.
IV. Under the action of a suitable homoeopathic remedy, the signs &symptoms are removed.
V. Some of the opponents of Hahnemann used to say that under the action of a homoeopathic remedy, the symptoms may disappear but the disease remains.
VI. To which the answer is, the disease manifests in the form of abnormal sign & symptoms,
VII. The physician has to remove the totality of the sign &symptoms to remove the disease.
VIII. If these sign & symptoms are removed means the deranged vital force & the health are restored, otherwise the symptoms would not go.
IX. To such people he says that the sole aim, of the physician is to restore the sick to health.
X. He is not supposed to make comments on hidden dynamics of disease because he cannot see the internal dynamics of the disease process.
XI. In the footnote he says that the physician should not make predictions about the nature of disease or the time of death, because we cannot predict such things
XII. The main aim of physician should be to focus on the sign & symptoms & understand the sick body & use these gifts to help the sick.

Footnote 1:
A warning prediction that death would occur at a certain day or at a certain hour has produced all the signs of commencing and increasing disease and of approaching death and death itself. This would not happen without the simultaneous production of the inward change and in such cases all the morbid signs indicative of approaching death have frequently been dissipated by an identical cause and health is suddenly restored, by means of this moral remedy, by means of removal of the internal and external morbid change that threatened death.

Footnote 2:
God, the preserver of mankind can reveal his wisdom and goodness for the cure of the diseases by showing to the physician what he has to remove in diseases in order to annihilate and thus re-establish health. But what would we think of his wisdom and goodness if the physician (of the dominant school of medicine) was uncertain what is to be cured in diseases and thus render it impossible for man to know the malady accurately, consequently impossible for him to cure it.

§ 18

TOTALITY IS THE SOLE GUIDE TO THE CHOICE OF RIGHT REMEDY

From this indubitable truth, that besides the totality of the symptoms with consideration of the accompanying modalities (§ 5) nothing can by any means be discovered in disease wherewith they could express their need of aid, it follows undeniably that the sum of all the symptoms and conditions in each individual case of disease must be the sole indication, the sole guide to direct us in the choice of a remedy.

EXPLANATION

- In this aphorism he says that the totality of the symptoms is the only way by means of which body signals the need of aid.
- The signs & symptoms are usually the first reason for contacting a physician
- The diagnostic tools can discover & only enhances our understanding of the disease process. They cannot reduce the importance of the sign & symptoms.
- The totality of symptoms [I.e.the sum total of all the alteration from health]is the sole guide for selecting a remedy.

§ 19

MEDICINAL POWER TO ALTER OUR HEALTH

Now, as diseases are nothing more than alterations in the state of health of the healthy individual which express themselves by morbid signs, and the cure is also only possible by a change to the healthy condition of the state of health of the diseased individual, it is very evident that medicines could never cure disease if they did not possess the power of altering man's state of health which depends on sensations and functions; indeed, that their curative power must be owing solely to this power they possess of altering man's state of health.

EXPLANATION

- In aphorism 19, Hahnemann says that medicines have power of altering man's state of health, they are not inert.

- The sources of these medicines could be inert but the potentized form has curative power.
- Thus medicines have power of altering man's state from diseased to healthy state, which depends on sensations & functions.
- Disease is just alterations in the state of health of healthy individual which expresses itself by morbid signs & symptoms.
- Cure means change of health of the diseased individual to healthy condition. It means total removal off signs & symptoms of disease by proper remedy.
- Thus medicines help in alternations of diseased state to healthy states, thus bringing cure.

§20

MEDICINAL POWERS OF A SUBSTANCES

This spirit-like power to alter man's state of health (and hence to cure diseases) which lies hidden in the inner nature of medicines can in itself never be discovered by us by a mere effort of reason; it is only by experience of the phenomena it displays when acting on the state of health of man that we can become clearly cognizant of it.

EXPLANATION

- Now as in aphorism 19 we read that a medicine should have the power to alter our health.
- In this aphorism 20, Hahnemann tells us how to discover the medicinal powers of a substance.
- We can only find out the medicine's effectiveness by understanding its effect on human body.
- The power of medicines to alter man's state of health is "Spirit-like" as it is invisible.
- Hahnemann says that the medicinal properties of a substance are hidden in its interior.
- They cannot be seen by just seeing the substance or by making theoretical assumptions.
- The only way to find the curative powers of a substance is to find out its effect on healthy human being.

§ 21

MEDICINES PRODUCE SYMPTOMS IN HEALTHY INDIVIDUAL

Now, as it is undeniable that the curative principle in medicines is not in itself perceptible, and as in pure experiments with medicines conducted by the most accurate observers, nothing can be observed that can constitute them medicines or remedies except that power of causing distinct alterations in the state of health of the human body, and particularly in that of the healthy individual, and of exciting in him various definite morbid symptoms; so it follows that when medicines act as remedies, they can only bring their curative property into play by means of this their power of altering man's state of health by the production of peculiar symptoms; and that, therefore, we have only to rely on the morbid phenomena which the medicines produce in the healthy body as the sole possible revelation of their in-dwelling curative power, in order to learn what disease-producing power, and at the same time what disease-curing power, each individual medicine possesses.

EXPLANATION

- In aphorism 20 we read that, the medicinal power of a substance is its power to alter the state of health
- This study of alterations which are produced on a healthy body are the most useful in finding out the therapeutic sphere of a medicine.
- As we know sick body is already working in a compromised state, so in them the test medicines often do not reveal their full effect on human body.
- The medicines are able to cure symptoms because of their ability to produce similar symptoms.
- 5]He had tested the medicines with known therapeutic action & had observed that medicines often produce symptoms in healthy individuals, which they are known to cure in sick.

E.g. **A= medicine**
      B = disease
      C =symptoms,

[A] medicine cures [B] disease, [B] disease produces [C] symptoms.
[A] also produces, [C] symptoms.
This means [A] medicine ability to produce [C] symptoms must be the property which helps it to cure the disease [B]..

§ 22

METHODS OF TREATMENT

But as nothing is to be observed in diseases that must be removed in order to change them into health besides the totality of their signs and symptoms, and likewise medicines can show nothing curative besides their tendency to produce morbid symptoms in healthy persons and to remove them in diseased persons; it follows, on the one hand, that medicines only become remedies and capable of annihilating disease, because the medicinal substance, by exciting certain effects and symptoms, that is to say, by producing a certain artificial morbid state, removes and abrogates the symptoms already present, to wit, the natural morbid state we wish to cure. On the other

hand, it follows that, for the totality of the symptoms of the disease to be cured, a medicine must be sought which (according as experience shall prove whether the morbid symptoms are most readily, certainly, and permanently removed and changed into health by similar or opposite medicinal symptoms1) have the greatest tendency to produce similar or opposite symptoms.

[FOOTNOTE:-1 The other possible mode of employing medicines for diseases besides these two is the allopathic method, in which medicines are given, whose symptoms have no direct pathological relation to the morbid state, neither similar nor opposite, but quite heterogeneous to the symptoms of the disease. This procedure plays, as I have shown elsewhere, an irresponsible murderous game with the life of the patient by means of dangerous, violent medicines, whose action is unknown and which are chosen on mere conjectures and given in large and frequent doses. Again, by means of painful operations, intended to lead the disease to other regions and taking the strength and vital juices of the patient, through evacuations above and below, sweat or salivation, but especially through squandering the irreplaceable blood, as is done by the reigning routine practice, used blindly and relentlessly, usually with the pretext that the physician should imitate and further the sick nature in its efforts to help itself, without considering how irrational it is, to imitate and further these very imperfect, mostly inappropriate efforts of the instinctive unintelligent vital energy which is implanted in our organism, so long as it is healthy to carry on life in harmonious development, but not to heal itself in disease. For, were it possessed of such a model ability, it would never have allowed the organism to get sick. When made ill by noxious agents, our life principle cannot do anything else than express its depression caused by disturbance of the regularity of its life, by symptoms, by means of which the intelligent physician is ask for aid. If this is not given, it strives to save by increasing the ailment, especially through violent evacuations, no matter what this entails, often with the largest sacrifices or destruction of life itself.

For the purpose of cure, the morbidly depressed vital energy possesses so little ability worthy of imitation since all changes and symptoms produced by it in the organism are the disease itself. What intelligent physician would want to imitate it with the intention to heal if he did not thereby sacrifice his patient?]

EXPLANATION

- The aphorism 22 states two basic things
- First, if a disease becomes shown through signs & symptoms &the only action of medicines on human being is their ability to produce symptoms.
- This means the ability of a medicines to produce symptoms is the power which cures the sick.
- Now the symptoms that a medicine can produce could be similar or opposite to the symptoms of disease.
- Secondly, Hahnemann says that a remedy must be chosen which has the greatest tendency to produce similar or opposite symptoms.
- Conventional medicine is not able to cure the disease, the anitpathic mode only suppress or palliate symptoms: e.g. the antibiotics, anti-hypertension etc.
- In a long foot -note to aphorism 22, Hahnemann tells us about a third mode of treatment, which he called Allopathic.
- Use of medicine that have similar effect was called Homoeopathy.

- Use of medicines that have opposite action was called Antipathy.
- The use of medicines or treatment that have no similar or opposite action was called Allopathy. Today the conventional medicine is known as Allopathy but today's conventional medicine is primarily antipathic.
- Antipathy & Allopathy have merged to form a conventional medicine or allopathy system.
- When we are sick, our vital force is depressed, when we use allopathic medicines they further decrease the vitality.
  eg- After intake of antibiotics for any acute illness we feel low energy, bad taste & indigestion. The infection goes away but body does not feel fit.
- Body requires many days or weeks to recover its lost vitality.
  This procedure ia ab irresponsible murderous game with the life of the patient by means of dangerous, violent medicines, whose action is unknown and which are chosen on mere opinion based on incomplete information and given in large and frequent doses. They also follow painful operations and lead the disease to other regions more vital and take all the strength and vital juices of the patient.
- Homeopathy medicine bring a change in vitality as the first sign of cure.

§ 23

ANTIPATHIC MEDICINE

All pure experience, however, and all accurate research convince us that persistent symptoms of disease are far from being removed and annihilated by opposite symptoms of medicines (as in the antipathic, enantiopathic or palliative method), that, on the contrary, after transient, apparent alleviation, they break forth again, only with increased intensity, and become manifestly aggravated (see § 58 – 62 and 69).

EXPLANATION

- In aphorism 23, Hahnemann states that the antipathic method always fails in curing the persistent symptoms, that is, the chronic diseases.
- In chronic disease, the symptoms often persists or rebound after an initial amelioration when allopathic medicines are used.
- In acute diseases, the cause of the symptoms [which is usually infection], is often removed by antipathic measures. They usually do not relapse unless patient has low vitality or the case is actually acute exacerbation of underlying chronic complaint.
- Therefore we often do not see a rebound of fever or diarrhoea after a course of antibiotics.
- This does not mean that antipathic mode is good for treating acute conditions.
- In acute diseases we see lowered vitality & increased susceptibility & more suppressions & increased tendency for chronic disease.

- So the antipathic mode maybe useful sometimes but it should not be the preferred first line of treatment in most conditions

§ 24

MERITS OF HOMOEOPATHY

There remains, therefore, no other mode of employing medicines in diseases that promises to be of service besides the homoeopathic, by means of which we seek, for the totality of the symptoms of the case of disease, a medicine which among all medicines (whose pathogenetic effects are known from having been tested in healthy individuals) has the power and the tendency to produce an artificial morbid state most similar to that of the case of disease in question.

EXPLANANTION

- In this aphorism he finally says that on the basis of aphorism 22 & 23, the only acceptable mode of employing medicines on sick is the homoeopathic method.
- Only those medicines should be applied whose action has been proved by testing on healthy individuals.
- Physician should have knowledge of disease also, along with note of mental, emotional & PQRS symptoms of each individual case.
- People often think that thinking about the 'disease' in classical homoeopathy is a crime, but Hahnemann has no where said so.
- Hahnemann never said not to use the information & knowledge about the disease, in curing the patient.
- So the physician should use the knowledge of Disease & take note of mental, emotional & PQRS symptoms of each individual case, then based on totality of symptoms, proper Homoeopathic remedy is given to cure the sick.

§ 25

SIMILAR REMEDY

Now, however, in all careful trials, pure experience,1 the sole and infallible oracle of the healing art, teaches us that actually that medicine which, in its action on the healthy human body, has demonstrated its power of producing the greatest number of symptoms similar to those observable in the case of disease under treatment, does also, in doses of suitable potency and attenuation, rapidly, radically and permanently remove the totality of the symptoms of this morbid state, that is to say (§ 6 – 16), **the whole disease present, and change it into health; and that all medicines cure, without exception, those diseases whose symptoms most nearly resemble their own, and leave none of them uncured.**

1 I do not mean that sort of experience of which the ordinary practitioners of the old school boast, after they have for years worked away with a lot of complex prescriptions on a number of diseases which they never carefully investigate, but which, faithful to their school, they consider as already described in works of systematic pathology, and dreamed that they could detect in them some imaginary morbific matter, or ascribe to them some other hypothetical internal abnormality. They always saw something in them, but knew not what it was they saw, and they got results, from the complex forces acting on an unknown object, that no human being but only a God could have unravelled – results from which nothing can be learned, no experience gained. Fifty years' experience of this sort is like fifty years of looking into a kaleidoscope filled with unknown colored objects, and perpetually turning round; thousands of ever changing figures and no accounting for them!

EXPLANATION

Hahnemann says -
- Pure experience using proved medicines is the only source of knowledge for the healing art.
- A medicine that produced the maximum number of similar symptoms during a drug proving [on a healthy human being], it removes the totality of symptoms of a diseased state.
- After the correct remedy based on totality of symptoms has been found next important step is to give suitable potency & dilution for rapid & total cure which is premanent.
- Proper organon should be studied to decide the potency of remedy.
- The more the similar the medicine, the more rapid the cure.
- If the remedy is 'the simillium', we will see radical & rapid cure.
- If it is a very close simillium the cure will not be as rapid as is the ideal one.
- If it is still less similar, it will only be able to palliate or remove partial set of symptoms.
- When the symptoms are removed in totality, no part of disease remains & the health is restored.
- Symptoms are indicators of the disharmony in the body, they are the language of disease.
- This means if there are no symptoms the disease has been cured totally & health has been restored.

Footnote 1:
Hahnemann says that he does not mean with experience of the ordinary practitioner of the old school, who have worked for years with a lot of complex prescriptions on a number of diseases which they never investigated carefully. They work only on systematic pathology and dream that they can detect some imaginary morbific matter or some other hypothetical internal abnormality. They got results from which nothing can be learned, no experience gained. Fifty years experience of this sort is like looking into a kaleidoscope filled with unknown coloured objects for 50 years., Getting nothing.

§ 26

NATURE'S LAW OF CURE

This depends on the following homoeopathic law of nature which was sometimes, indeed, vaguely surmised but not hitherto fully recognized, and to which is due every real cure that has ever taken place:

A weaker dynamic affection is permanently extinguished in the living organism by a stronger one, if the latter (whilst differing in kind) is very similar to the former in its manifestations.1

1 Thus are cured both physical affections and moral maladies. How is it that in the early dawn the brilliant Jupiter vanishes from the gaze of the beholder? By a stronger very similar power acting on his optic nerve, the brightness of approaching day! – In situations replete with foetid odors, wherewith is it usual to soothe effectually the offended olfactory nerves? With snuff, that affects the sense of smell in a similar but stronger manner! No music, no sugared cake, which act on the nerves of other senses, can cure this olfactory disgust. How does the soldier cunningly stifle the piteous cries of him who runs the gauntlet from the ears of the compassionate bystanders? By the shrill notes of the fife commingled with the roll of the noisy drum! And the distant roar of the enemy's cannon that inspires his army with fear? By the loud boom of the big drum! For neither the one nor the other would the distribution of a brilliant piece of uniform nor a reprimand to the regiment suffice. In like manner, mourning and sorrow will be effaced from the mind by the account of another and still greater cause for sorrow happening to another, even though it be a mere fiction. The injurious consequences of too great joy will be removed by drinking coffee, which produces an excessive joyous state of mind. Nations like the Germans, who have for centuries been gradually sinking deeper and deeper in soulless apathy and degrading serfdom, must first be trodden still deeper in the dust by the Western Conqueror, until their situation became intolerable; their mean opinion of themselves was thereby over-strained and removed; they again became alive to their dignity as men, and then, for the first time, they raised their heads as Germans.

EXPLANATION

A] In this aphorism he says how the similar remedy is able to cure the patient.
B] In nature also it has been observed that a weaker disease is removed automatically if patient has a similar but stronger disease.
C] This phenomenon is called-- " The Homoeopathic law of nature" or "The nature's law of cure.
D] The conditions for this law to become applicable are:-

1. Both the affections should be dynamic in nature.
2. They both should be similar in their manifestations.
3. But they should differ in kind
4. The later {second disease}should be stronger than the former one.

E] "Dynamic in nature" -

1. Means affection which primarily starts as derangement of the vital force.
2. Sickness that arises from injury or accident may need allopathic or antipathic intervention.
3. It does not mean that Homoeopathic remedies will not work in sickness arising from injuries
4. They will often do but in many cases non-homoeopathic primary intervention may be required.
5. Hahnemann has clearly written in the organon that sometimes surgery & antipathic measures are required to save the life of a person.

F] Differing in kind--Means

1. Use of 'similar' influence not 'same'

E.g.- A hard substances hits the forehead.
We press the spot for a period with thumb strongly at first & then gradually less forcibly, Homoeopathically, it will soon diminish the pain & swelling

- Here we have not used equally hard blow with an equally hard body, this will increase the evil isopathically {isopathy means same}
- This Homoeopathically means "similar' not same"
- In his footnote Hahnemann has explained how a strong similar affection overshadows or annihilates a weaker similar affection

e.g-
A] The jupiter is bright appears at night but when sun shines the Jupiter disappears in sun's brightness [sun brightness is stronger than jupiter]
B] A patient had following symptoms since last six years
- burning miliary rash on face, neck & arms.

It was aggravated by change of weather, when the patient had another disease measles.
This rash was cured & did not return.
- while nature has shown the way but it has its limitation too.

1. Occurance of natural similar cures is very rare.
2. The later disease might remove the first disease but the later one can be more dangerous than former.
3. The body cannot regulate the later disease & it takes its own time to go.

It is where the Homoepathic medicines are needed, they produce similar condition and is in our hand.

So, the second dynamic disease[by Homoepathic medicine]also passes away more swiftly, without causing any harm.

This law of nature was known to many people before Hahnemann but could not be put into practice.

Footnote 1:
Thus both physical affections and moral maladies are cured by this nature's law of cure. To understand this various examples are there.

The jupiter is bright and appears at night but when the sun shines the Jupiter disappears in sun's brightness [sun brightness is stronger than jupiter]

B] A patient had following symptoms since last six years
  + burning miliary rash on face, neck & arms.

It was aggravated by change of weather, when the patient had another very similar but differing in kind disease, i.e., measles.
This rash was cured & did not return.
In the same manner, mourning and sorrow will be effaced from the mind if another and still greater sorrow happens.
The injurious consequences of too great joy will be removed by drinking coffee, which produces excessively joyous state of mind.

§ 27

CURATIVE POWER OF DRUG

The curative power of medicines, therefore, depends on their symptoms, similar to the disease but superior to it in strength (§ 12 – 26), so that each individual case of disease is most surely, radically, rapidly and permanently annihilated and removed only by a medicine capable of producing (in the human system) in the most similar and complete manner the totality of its symptoms, which at the same time are stronger than the disease.

EXPLANATION

In this aphorism Hahnemann again stresses on "Individualization" of the case.
This means taking note of common symptoms of a nosological d/s entity will not be sufficient to decide the remedy for a case.

+ The individualizing characteristic symptoms of the case must be noted & then based on totality of symptoms, remedy should be given. This way each individual case of disease is most surely, rapidly, radically and permanently annihilated and removed by a medicine capable of producing in the most similar & complete manner the totality of its symptoms, which are stronger than the disease.

- The Homoepathic therapeutics books should be used as filter simillimum & not as a definite guide for remedy selection.
- The remedy might not even be listed among the therapeutics of the disease that the patient is suffering from.

e.g – For every injury don't prescribe Arnica all time
 – For every muscle ache don't prescribe Rhus-tox

We have already read in aphorism 26 about Nature's law of cure & how it relates to Homoepathic principle of 'Simila Similbus Curantur'.

§ 28

MODUS OPERANDI OF CURE

As this natural law of cure manifests itself in every pure experiment and every true observation in the world, the fact is consequently established; it matters little what may be scientific explanation of how it takes place; and I do not attach much importance to the attempts made to explain it. But the following view seems to commend itself as the most probable one, as it is founded on premises derived from experience.

EXPLANATION

In this aphorism Hahnemann says that when the truth is clearly visible, he does not give much importance to how internal dynamics of the body & the remedy are working & interacting with each other.

- He wanted that everyone should focus on the clinical application of the remedies.
- Hahnemann wrote these lines 200 years back & today Homeopathy has a wide & growing user base & its clinical efficacy is also fairly well documented.

Now two fundamental questions arise:-

1. How is information stored & transmitted in Homoepathic remedies?
2. How do the remedies interact with biological systems?

After saying this he also gives an explanation to answer the people, who always wanted to know how Homeopathic remedies worked. let us read aphorism 29 & find out what Hahnemann said.

§ 29

HOW HOMEOPATHIC REMEDIES CURE D/S?

As every disease (not entirely surgical) consists only in a special, morbid, dynamic alteration of our vital energy (of the principle of life) manifested in sensation and motion, so in every homoeopathic cure this principle of life dynamically altered by natural disease is seized through the administration of medicinal potency selected exactly according to symptom-similarity by a somewhat stronger, similar artificial disease-manifestation. By this the feeling of the natural (weaker) dynamic disease-manifestation ceases and disappears. This disease-manifestation no longer exists for the principle of life which is now occupied and governed merely by the stronger, artificial disease-manifestation. This artificial disease-manifestation has soon spent its force and leaves the patient free from disease, cured. The dynamis, thus freed, can now continue to carry life on in health. This most highly probable process rests upon the following propositions.

EXPLANATION

Hahnemann says that diseases are mainly of 2 types:-

1. Surgical
2. Dynamic

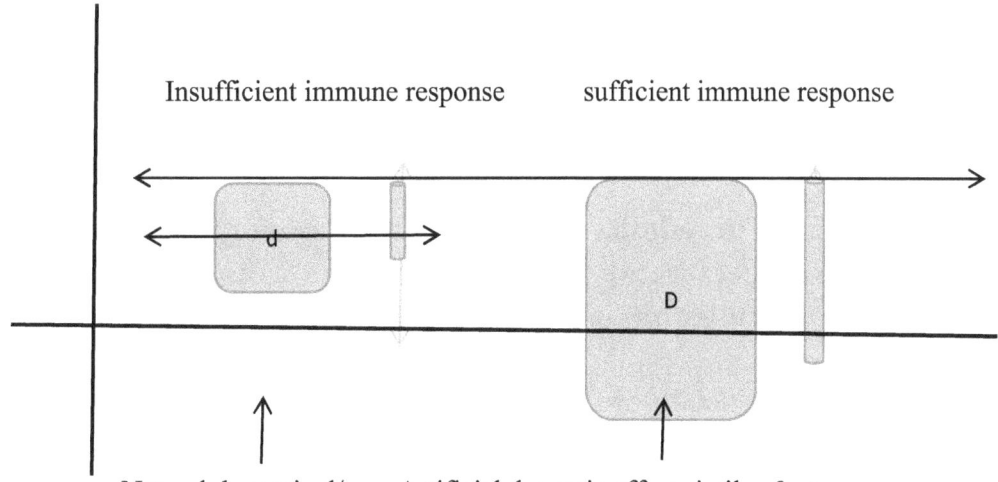

Dynamic diseases are those that start with the derangement of the vital force or disturbance in the biological thermodynamic equilibrium.

✦ We know that the curative power of Homoeopathic medicines lies in their ability to produce similar symptoms.

- So it means when a Homoepathic remedy is given to a patient, it produces symptoms similar to the existing disease condition.
- Hahnemann says that when the body is affected by a similar but stronger dynamic disturbance, the weaker dynamic disturbance stops to have an effect on the body & disappears.

HOW DOES THIS HAPPEN?

1. Suppose a dynamic disturbance is affecting a body to a level 'd'
   The body is putting in 'v' resources to get the equilibrium back, now this 'v' resources are insufficient because the vital force is deranged & it needs more effort to get rid of the disturbance 'd', hence the disease state is still present.
2. Now when we give a Homeopathic remedy that produces a similar but stronger state 'D' in the body.
   The body perceives it as a greater threat & mounts greater defense using its reserves.

   - The new defense 'V' is stronger than the previous one.
   - The disease 'd' will now cease to exist if the new defense is sufficient to get rid of the disturbance 'D'
   - Now the artificial disturbance "D" produced by medicine is in control of physician & is short lived & disappears on its own & the body is now healthy once again.

§ 30

THREE STATEMENTS

The human body appears to admit of being much more powerfully affected in its health by medicines (partly because we have the regulation of the dose in our own power) than by natural morbid stimuli – for natural diseases are cured and overcome by suitable medicines.1

1 The short duration of the action of the artificial morbific forces, which we term medicines, makes it possible that, although they are stronger than the natural diseases, they can yet be much more easily overcome by the vital force than can the weaker natural diseases, which solely in consequence of the longer, generally lifelong, duration of their action (psora, syphilis, sycosis), can never be vanquished and extinguished by it alone, until the physician affects the vital force in a stronger manner by an agent that produces a disease very similar, but stronger to wit a homoeopathic medicine. The cures of diseases of many years' duration (§ 46), by the occurrence of smallpox and measles (both of which run a course of only a few weeks), are processes of a similar character.

EXPLANATION

Here Hahnemann makes three statements:-

1. Human body is more powerfully affected by medicines than disease causing stimuli.
2. When suitable remedies are given, they are able to remove the diseased state
3. The ability of physician to control power /dose of the medicines is one of the reasons for this greater effect.

{The first point comes from our observation that in nature every d/s is unable to affect every person, also even during drug provings, every person is not able to produce symptoms in high attenuations.

But when we prove a remedy in low attenuations or give a remedy to a sick person, the possibility of getting an effect is much higher.

There are 2 reasons for this:-

1. Every disease causing stimuli does not affect the people in health hence disease usually does not affect us unconditionally.
2. The doses of medicine can be regulated so that body produce an effect in response to the stimulus. This second point is explained in the footnote to aphorism 30.

* *Hahnemann in his footnote says:--*

1. The natural disease state is created by either -psora, syphilis or sycosis miasms, these states are usually life-long
2. As we know in diseased state the vital force is debilitated [its strength is reduced], so these natural disease state cannot be overcome by vital force itself.
3. Here body needs aid of Homeopathic remedies.
4. The medicines creates an artificial state which is short-lived.
5. The artificial disease state, which is stronger than the natural disease are overcome by the vital force because of their short duration.
6. When a physician excites the vital force with a similar artificial disease state. The natural disease state is removed.
7. The similarity is essential.

§ 31

D3 [DISEASE, DYNAMIC, DERANGEMENT]

The inimical forces, partly psychical, partly physical, to which our terrestrial existence is exposed, which are termed morbific noxious agents, do not possess the power of morbidly deranging the health of man unconditionally1; but we are made ill by them only when our organism is

sufficiently disposed and susceptible to attack of the morbific cause that may be present, and to be altered in its health, deranged and made to undergo abnormal sensations and functions – hence they do not produce disease in every one nor at all times.

1 When I call a disease a derangement of man's state of health, I am far from wishing thereby to give a hyperphysical explanation of the internal nature of disease generally, or of any case of disease in particular. It is only intended by this expression to intimate, what it can be proved diseases are not and cannot be, that they are not mechanical or chemical alterations of material substance of the body, and not dependant on a material morbific substance, but that they are merely spirit-like (conceptual) dynamic derangements of the life.

EXPLANATION

- Dr. Hahnemann says that diseases are not mere pathological changes in our body.
- Diseases are 'dynamic' derangement of our vital force.

For the disease to affect or manifest in an organism the organism must be predisposed to & must be in a susceptible state for the disease to affect it.

- Disposed means having an inclination towards something.
- Susceptible means 'easily influenced or affected"
- Most of the chronic d/s are somewhere governed by our genetics.
- The d/s tendency that we are genetically born with is what the word 'disposition' refers to

Whereas susceptibility refers to a prone to acquire a d/s

e.g- suppose 5 people in a, family get wet by rain.one of them develops fever another develops running nose another develops headache, another develops joint pain & the fifth one remains unaffected all 5 people are exposed to the same meteoric influence.

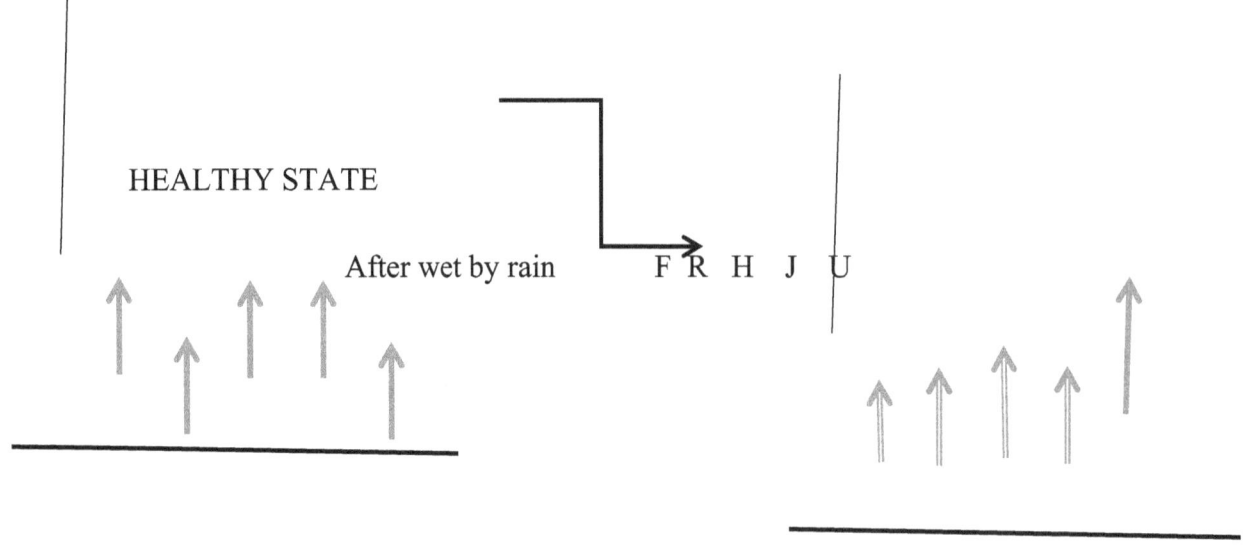

Family Memeber   *Family Memeber*

F = fever
R = Running nose
H = Headache
J = Joint pain
U = Unaffected

The first & second people are relatively healthy, they are not 'disposed' to chronic d/s or that tendency is not active yet.

The third & fourth person have a disposition that affects joints & muscles.

The fifth person is either very healthy or has a disposition to deep seated mental /neurological / hormonal pathologies & thus does not produce an acute d/s easily.

So, one is born with 'disposition' & the disposition manifests when we are in a susceptible state.

E.g- Let us take another example:-

Diseases like diabetes, hypertension, depression & cancer etc run in the families. people are born with those genes. but these genes or at a young age, something has to work as a trigger to switch on those genes. trigger can be anything like wrong life-style or excessive physical, mental or emotional stress. these triggers switch on those genes.

A father with a hypertension gene might develop hypertension at age of 50 yrs while his son with same gene develops it at 40years

* Now lets come to susceptibility being susceptible means that you are in a state where you can easily be affected by an external stimulus.

In above example 'the rain' was that stimulus. This stimulus decreased the vitality of these men & allowed their disposition or secondary causes of d/s [bacteria /viruses] to affect the body. In life, any mental, emotional or physical stress can decrease the vitality & make person susceptible.

If you are born with a healthy disposition You will resist chronic d/s for long. here even under stress, the body is likely to produce acute ailments that can be easily overcome. But if the d/s disposition is strong even minor stress can start the chronic d/s process & it never stops on its own, the chronic d/s dispositions will only start manifesting if there is a susceptible state & then only we suffer from acute conditions.

Disposition + Susceptibility = Chronic d/s

Disposition + Susceptibility + Infectious agents = Acute d/s

Footnote 1:
When he calls disease a Derangement of man's State of health, he means diseases are not mechanical or chemical alterations of the material substance of the body and are not dependent on a material morbific substance, but they are spirit-like dynamic Derangements of the life.

§ 32

REAL MEDICINE

But it is quite otherwise with the artificial morbific agents which we term medicines. Every real medicine, namely, acts at all times, under all circumstances, on every living human being, and produces in him its peculiar symptoms (distinctly perceptible, if the dose be large enough), so that evidently every living human organism is liable to be affected, and, as it were, inoculated with the medicinal disease at all times, and absolutely (unconditionally), which, as before said, is by no means the case with the natural diseases.

EXPLANATION

In this aphorism Hahnemann says:-

1. Any medicine can affect any person at any time.
2. When a remedy is given to a person, it produces in him its peculiar symptoms
3. But these symptoms or artificial morbific d/s is perceptible only if the dose be large enough.

So, every medicine:-

- Acts at all times
- Under all circumstances
- On every living human being & produces peculiar symptoms

So medicine affects every living human organism but natural diseases do not effect every living human organism at all times.

§ 33

MEDICINAL AGENTS HAVE UNCONDITIONAL POWER

In accordance with this fact, it is undeniably shown by all experience1 that the living organism is much more disposed and has a greater liability to be acted on, and to have its health deranged by medicinal powers, than by morbific noxious agents and infectious miasms, or, in order words, that the morbific noxious agents possess a power of morbidly deranging man's health that is subordinate and conditional, often very conditional; whilst medicinal agents have an absolute unconditional power, greatly superior to the former.

1 A striking fact in corroboration of this is, that whilst previously to the year 1801, when the smooth scarlatina of Sydenham still occasionally prevailed epidemically among children, it attacked without exception all children who had escaped it in a former epidemic; in a similar epidemic which I witnessed in Konigslutter, on the contrary, all the children who took in time a very small dose of belladonna remained unaffected by this highly infectious infantile disease. If medicines can protect from a disease that is raging around, they must possess a vastly superior power of affecting our vital force.

EXPLANATION

* In aphorism 33 Hahnemann explains with example in his footnote that medicinal agents have unconditional power, superior to the morbific noxious agents & infectious miasms which are inferior in power & are conditional.

The morbific noxious agents posses a power of morbidly deranging health of man and is inferior and conditional, while the medicinal agents have an unconditional power, which is greatly superior to the morbific noxious agents.

In his footnote he shares his experience:-
In sydenham the smooth scarlatina prevailed epidemically among children, it attacked without exception all the children.

In konigslutter, all the children who took in time a very small dose of belladonna were unaffected by this highly infectious infantile d/s, it means if medicines can protect from a d/s it posses a vastly superior power than d/s & has more power of affecting our vital force.

§ 34

SIMILARITY

The greater strength of the artificial diseases producible by medicines is, however, not the sole cause of their power to cure natural disease. In order that they may effect a cure, it is before all things requisite that they should be capable of producing in the human body an artificial disease as similar as possible to the disease to be cured, which, with somewhat increased power, transforms to a very similar morbid state the instinctive life principle, which in itself is incapable of any reflection or act of memory. It not only obscures, but extinguishes and thereby annihilates the derangement caused by the natural disease. This is so true, that no previously existing disease can be cured, even by Nature herself, by the accession of a new dissimilar disease, be it ever so strong, and just as little can it be cured by medical treatment with drugs which are incapable of producing a similar morbid condition in the healthy body.

EXPLANATION

Hahnemann here says that the more symptoms & the underlying susceptibility covered by the remedy the better is the chance for cure. The lesser the similarity is the lesser the chance of cure. So it means 'similarity' is the first pre-requisite for a cure to take place.

Now what should be the strength of the dose? He says" 'with some what increased power'

That means the remedy should be able to produce a slightly stronger & similar artificial d/s.

In india there is a common myth that disease first increase under homoeopathic treatment.

If the patient aggravates seriously than the prescription is not homoeopathic either in remedy or in dose.

An aggravation is Homoeopathic, only if it is mild, very slight.

If the d/s aggravates so much that the patient is troubled by it, then how can this cure be gentle? Hahnemann in his aphorism says that cure should be gentle.

Similar dose in our body produces a similar morbid state. Dissimilar morbific state, however strong it may be, which is produced either by nature or through allopathic drugs, can never result in a cure.

§ 35

3 STAGES OF DISEASE

In order to illustrate this, we shall consider in three different cases, as well what happens in nature when two dissimilar natural diseases meet to in one person, as also the result of the ordinary medical treatment of diseases with unsuitable allopathic drugs, which are incapable of producing an artificial morbid condition similar to the disease to be cured, whereby it will appear that even Nature herself is unable to remove a dissimilar disease already present by one that is unhomoeopathic, even though it be stronger, and just as little is the unhomoeopathic employment of even the strongest medicines ever capable of curing any disease whatsoever.

EXPLANATION

To illustrate what is said in aphorism 34 we will consider 3 different cases:-

1. When the second dissimilar d/s is weaker or of same strength, it is repelled.
2. When the second dissimilar d/s is stronger, it suspends the earlier one temporarily & completes its course & then the former comes back again.
3. When the second dissimilar d/s is of similar strength, chronic in nature & with different organ affinity, they may joint to form a complex d/s

    (i) First d/s + second dissimilar d/s [weaker or same strength]
    Second d/s is repelled & not allowed

(ii) First d/s + second dissimilar d/s
Second one suspends the first, completes its duration & then first appears back
(iii) First d/s + second dissimilar d/s [same & chronic in nature + different organ affinity]— Complex d/s

- We will also consider what happens in nature when two dissimilar natural diseases meet together in one person.
- We will also see result of ordinary medical treatment of d/s with unsuitable allopathic drugs. * These are not able to produce an artificial morbid condition similar to the d/s to be cured.
- Even nature herself is not able to remove a dissimilar disease by one that is unhomoeopathic.
- If the d/s is dissimilar than even if it is stronger it is not able to remove the d/s already present, similar is the case with unhomoeopathic use of even the strongest medicine which are not able of curing any d/s

§ 36

EXISTING STRONGER REPELS THE WEAKER

I. If the two dissimilar diseases meeting together in the human being be of equal strength, or still more if the older one be the stronger, the new disease will be repelled by the old one from the body and not allowed to affect it. A patient suffering from a severe chronic disease will not be infected by a moderate autumnal dysentery or other epidemic disease. The plague of the Levant, according to Larry,1 does not break out where scurvy is prevalent, and persons suffering from eczema are not infected by it. Rachitis, Jenner alleges, prevents vaccination from taking effect. Those suffering from pulmonary consumption are not liable to be attacked by epidemic fevers of a not very violent character, according to Von Hildenbrand.

1 "Memoires et Observations," in the Description de l' Egpte, tom. i.

EXPLANATION

If the two dissimilar d/s meet in the human body & they are of equal strength or if the older one is stronger then the new d/s will be repelled by the old one from the body & the new d/s will not affect it.

E.g- A patient who is already suffering from a severe chronic d/s will not be infected by a moderate dysentery

E.g - In places where scurvy is already prevalent, plaque does not break out

First d/s +second d/s dissimilar &equal or weaker — The new d/s will not affect the body

Von hildenbrand said --
Those person suffering from pulmonary consumption are not attacked by epidemic fever of moderate character.

§ 37

ALLOPATHY CHRONIC D/S

So, also under ordinary medical treatment, an old chronic disease remains uncured and unaltered if it is treated according to the common allopathic method, that is to say, with medicines that are incapable of producing in healthy individuals a state of health similar to the disease, even though the treatment should last for years and is not of too violent character.1 This is daily witnessed in practice, it is therefore unnecessary to give any illustrative examples.

1 But if treated with violent allopathic remedies, other diseases will be formed in its place which are more difficult and dangerous to life.

EXPLANATION

In aphorism 37, He says that if a person is suffering from an old chronic d/s & is treated according to the common allopathic method with medicines that are incapable of producing a state of health similar to the d/s, the d/s remains uncured & unaltered.

This allopathic treatment usually would last for years & is not of too violent character.

Footnote 1:
But if the patient is treated with violent allopathic remedies, other d/s will be formed in its place. these new d/s are more difficult & dangerous to life

Thus common allopathic method according to Hahenemann fails to cure the patient.

§ 38

NEW STRONGER SUSPENDS

II. Or the new dissimilar disease is the stronger. In this case the disease under which the patient originally labored, being the weaker, will be kept back and suspended by the accession of the stronger one, until the latter shall have run its course or been cured, and then the old one reappears uncured. Two children affected with a kind of epilepsy remained free from epileptic attacks after infection with ringworm (tinea) but as soon as the eruption on the head was gone the epilepsy returned just as before, as Tulpius1 observed. The itch, as Schopf2 saw, disappeared on the occurrence of the scurvy, but after the cure of the latter it again broke out. So, also the pulmonary phthisis remained stationary when the patient was attacked by a violent typhus, but went on again after the latter had run its course.3 If mania occur in a consumptive patient, the phthisis with all its symptoms is removed by the former; but if that go off, the phthisis returns immediately and proves fatal.4 When measles and smallpox are prevalent at the same time, and both attack the same child, the measles that had already broken out is generally checked by the smallpox that came somewhat later; nor does the measles resume its course until after the cure of the smallpox; but it not infrequently happens that the inoculated smallpox is suspended for four days by the supervention of the measles, as observed by Manget,5 after the desquamation of which the smallpox completes its course. Even when the inoculation of the smallpox had taken effect for six days, and the measles then broke out, the inflammation of the inoculation remained stationary and the smallpox did not ensue until the measles had completed its regular course of seven days.6 In an epidemic of measles, that disease attacked many individuals on the fourth or fifth day after the inoculation of smallpox and prevented the development of the smallpox until it had completed its own course, whereupon the smallpox appeared and proceeded regularly to its termination.7 The true, smooth, erysipelatous-looking scarlatina of Sydenham, with sore throat, was checked on the fourth day by the eruption of cow-pox, which ran its regular course, and not till it was ended did the scarlatina again establish itself; but on another occasion, as both diseases seem to be of equal strength, the cow-pox was suspended on the eighth day by the supervention of the true, smooth scarlatina of Sydenham,8 and the red areola of the former disappeared until the scarlatina was gone, wherein the cow-pox immediately resumed its course, and went on its regular termination.9 The measles suspended the cow-pox; on the eighth day, when the cow-pox had nearly attained its climax, the measles broke out; the cow-pox now remained stationary, and did not resume and complete its course until the desquamation of the measles, had taken place, so that on the sixteenth day it presented the appearance it otherwise would have shown on the tenth day, as Kortum10 observed. Even after the measles had broken out the cow-pox inoculation took effect, but did not run its course until these measles had disappeared, as Kortum likewise witnessed.11I myself saw the mumps (angina parotidea) immediately disappear when the cow-pox inoculation had taken effect and had nearly attained its height; it was not until the complete termination of the cow-pox and the disappearance of its red areola that this febrile tumefaction of the parotid and submaxillary glands, that is caused by a peculiar miasm, reappeared and ran its regular course of seven days.

And thus it is with all dissimilar disease; the stronger suspends the weaker (when they do not complicate one another, which is seldom the case with acute disease), but they never cure one another.

1 Obs., lib. I, obs. 8.
2 In Hufeland's Journal, xv, 2.
3 Chevalier, in Hufeland's Neuesten Annalen der franzosichen Heikunde, ii, p.192.
4 Mania phthisi superveniens eam cum omnibus suis phaenomenis auffert, verum mox redit phthisis et occidit, abeunte mania. Reil Memorab., fasc. iii, v, p.171.
5 In the Edinb. Med. Comment., pt. i, 1.
6 John Hunter, On the veneral Disease, p.5.
7 Rainey, in the Edinb. Med. Comment., iii, p.480.

8 Very accurately described by Withering and Plenciz, but differing greatly from the purpura (or Roodvonk), which is often erroneously denominated scarlet fever. It is only of late year that the two, which were originally very different diseases, have come to resemble each other in their symptoms.

9 Jenner, in Medicinische Annalen, August, 1800, p.747.

10 In Hufeland's Journal der praktischen Arzneikunde, xx, 3, p.50.

11 Loc. cit.

EXPLANATION

II-Now if the new dissimilar d/s is stronger. In this case the former d/s which is weaker is suspended by the stronger one.

The new d/s runs its course or is been cured & then the old one reappear uncured.

E.g - As Tulpius observed, when two children were affected with epilepsy, when they were infected with ringworm [a stronger d/s], they remained free from epilepsy during the infection with ringworm.

But as soon as the eruption of ringworm on head was gone the epilepsy returned as it was in the starting.

This means the new stronger dissimilar d/s runed its full course & when it was gone the earlier weaker d/s appeared again.

Schopf saw that the itch disappeared on the occurence of the scurvy but after the cure of scurvy the itch again broke out.

Pulmonary phthisis remained stationary when the patient was attacked by a violent typhus, but went on again after the typhus had run its course.

E.g- In a patient with phthisis if mania occurs, the pthisis with all its symptoms is removed but when mania goes off, the phthisis returns immediately & proves fatal.

When measles and smallpox are prevalent at the same time, and both attack the same child. The measles that had already broken out is generally checked by the smallpox that came later; the smallpox come again later after measles subside, but it not infrequently happens that the inoculated smallpox is suspended for four days by the supervention of the measles, as observed by Manget, after the desquamation of which the smallpox completes its course. Even when the inoculation of the smallpox had taken effect for six days, and the measles then broke out, the inflammation of the inoculation remained stationary and the smallpox did not ensue until the measles had completed its regular course of seven days.

In an epidemic of measles, that disease attacked many individuals on the fourth or fifth day after the inoculation of smallpox and prevented the development of the smallpox until it had completed its own course, whereupon the smallpox appeared and proceeded regularly to its termination.

The true, smooth, erysipelatous-looking scarlatina of Sydenham, with sore throat, was checked on the fourth day by the eruption of cow-pox, which ran its regular course, and when cow-pox ended, the scarlatina again established itself; but on another occasion, as both diseases seem to be of equal strength, the cow-pox was suspended on the eighth day by the supervention of the true, smooth scarlatina of Sydenham, and the red areola of the former disappeared until the scarlatina was gone, wherein the cow-pox immediately resumed its course, and went on its regular termination.

Kortum observed that the measles suspended the cow-pox; on the eighth day, when the cow-pox had nearly attained its climax, the measles broke out; the cow-pox now remained stationary, and did not resume and complete its course until the desquamation of the measles, had taken place, so that on the sixteenth day it presented the appearance it otherwise would have shown on the tenth day.

Even after the measles had broken out the cow-pox inoculation took effect, but did not run its course until these measles had disappeared, as Kortum likewise witnessed.

* Lets take another example - Hahnemann says that a patient with mumps when cow-pox inoculation had taken effect, the mumps disappeared. On complete termination of cow-pox & disappearance of its red area mumps appeared again with febrile swelling of parotid & submaxillary glands & it ran its regular course of seven days.

Thus in all above examples we can see that with all dissimilar d/s, the stronger suspends the weaker when they do not complicate one another [seldom the case with acute d/s] but they never cure one another.

§ 39

ROUTINE EXAMPLES

Now the adherents of the ordinary school of medicine saw all this for so many centuries; they saw that Nature herself cannot cure any disease by the accession of another, be it ever so strong, if the new disease be dissimilar to that already present in the body. What shall we think of them, that they nevertheless went on treating chronic disease with allopathic remedies, namely, with medicines and prescriptions capable of producing God knows what morbid state – almost invariably, however, one dissimilar to the disease to be cured? And even though physicians did not hitherto observe nature attentively, the miserable results of their treatment should have taught them that they were pursuing an inappropriate, a false path. Did they not perceive when they employed, as was their custom, and aggressive allopathic treatment in a chronic disease, that thereby they only created an artificial disease dissimilar to the original one, which, as long as it was kept up, merely held in abeyance, merely suppressed, merely suspended the original disease, which latter, however, always returned, and must return, as soon as the diminished strength of the patient no longer admitted of a continuance of the allopathic attacks on the life? Thus the itch exanthema certainly disappears very soon from the skin under the employment of violent purgatives, frequently repeated; but when the patient can no longer stand the factitious (dissimilar) disease of the bowels, and can take no more purgatives, then either the cutaneous eruption breaks out as before, or the internal psora displays itself in some bad symptom, and the patient, in addition to his undiminished original disease, has to endure the misery of a painful ruined digestion and impaired strength to boot. So, also, when the ordinary physicians keep up artificial ulcerations of the skin and issues on the exterior of the body, with the view of thereby eradicating a chronic disease, they can NEVER cure them by that means, as such

artificial cutaneous ulcers are quite alien and allopathic to the internal affection; but inasmuch as the irritation produced by several tissues is at least sometimes a stronger (dissimilar) disease than the indwelling malady, the latter is thereby sometimes silenced and suspended for a week or two. But it is only suspended, and that for a very short time, while the patient's powers are gradually worn out. Epilepsy, suppressed for many years by means of issues, invariably recurred, and in an aggravated form, when they were allowed to heal up, as Pechlin[1] and others testify. But purgatives for itch, and issues for epilepsy, cannot be more heterogeneous, more dissimilar deranging agents – cannot be more allopathic, more exhausting modes of treatment – than are the customary prescriptions, composed of unknown ingredients, used in ordinary practice for the other nameless, innumerable forms of disease. These likewise do nothing but debilitate, and only suppress or suspend the malady for a short time without being able to cure it, and when used for a long time always add a new morbid state to the old disease.

1 Obs. phys. med., lib. ii, obs, 30.

EXPLANATION

- The physician of the ordinary school of medicine saw all above incidences for many centuries.
- They saw that nature on its own cannot cure any d/s even if it is very strong, if the new d/s is dissimilar to the d/s already present in the body.
- The physicians of the ordinary school keep on doing the same above thing.
- They keep on treating chronic d/s with allopathic remedies, which produce a morbid state, one dissimilar to the d/s to be cured.
- Hahnemann says that till now the physicians did not observe nature carefully, the results of their treatment should have taught them that they were following an inappropriate & a false path.
- Hahnemann here asks questions to allopathic believers that

A] Don't they feel that when they give an aggressive allopathic treatment in a chronic d/s they create an artificial d/s which is dissimilar to the original one. This artificial d/s created by their medicines only suspend the original d/s which returns as soon as the strength of the patient does not allow continuance of the allopathic attacks on their life.

E.g- if the patient having itch is given allopathic treatment by violent purgatives repeated at short interval, the itch disappear but when the patient can no longer stand the false dissimilar d/s of the bowels & now can not take more purgatives then either eruption come out as they were before or internal psora shows bad symptoms.

So, we see the patient who already had a original d/s now also has a painful impaired digestion.

When the ordinary physician keep up artificial ulcerations of the skin and issues on the exterior of the body, with the view of removing a chronic disease, they can NEVER cure them by that means because such artificial cutaneous ulcers are quite alien and allopathic to the internal affection; but as the irritation produced by several tissues is at least sometimes a stronger (dissimilar) disease than the indwelling malady, the old disease is thereby sometimes silenced and suspended for a week or two.

But it is only suspended, and that also for a very short time, while the patient's powers are gradually worn out.

Epilepsy was suppressed for many years by means of issues but it recurred in an aggravated form, when the issues were allowed to heal up, as Pechlin and others testify

But purgatives for itch, and issues for epilepsy, cannot be more dissimilar deranging agents – cannot be more allopathic, more exhausting modes of treatment than the customary prescriptions used in ordinary practice.

- Allopathic treat is not able to attain their object of eradicating a chronic d/s
- when the patient's power are gradually destroyed the original d/s reappears.
- when these medicine are used for a long time they always add a new morbid state to the old disease.

§ 40

COMPLEX DISEASES

III. Or the new disease, after having long acted on the organism, at length joins the old one that is dissimilar to it, and forms with it a complex disease, so that each of them occupies a particular locality in the organism, namely, the organs peculiarly adapted for it, and, as it were, only the place specially belonging to it, while it leaves the rest to the other disease that is dissimilar to it. Thus a syphilitic patient may become psoric, and vice versa. As two disease dissimilar to each other, they cannot remove, cannot cure one another. At first the venereal symptoms are kept in abeyance and suspended when the psoric eruption begins to appear; in course of time, however (as the syphilis is at least as strong as the psora), the two join together,1 that is, each involves those parts of the organism only which are most adapted for it, and the patient is thereby rendered more diseased and more difficult to cure.

When two dissimilar acute infectious diseases meet, as, for example, smallpox and measles, the one usually suspends the other, as has been before observed; yet there have also been severe epidemics of this kind, where, in rare cases, two dissimilar acute diseases occurred simultaneously in one and the same body, and for a short time combined, as it were, with each other. During an epidemic, in which smallpox and measles were prevalent at the same time, among three hundred cases (in which these diseases avoided or suspended one another, and measles attacked patients twenty days after the smallpox broke out, the smallpox, however, from seventeen to eighteen days after the appearance of the measles, so that the first disease had previously completed its regular course) there was yet one single case in which P. Russell2 met with both these dissimilar diseases in one person at the same time. Rainey3 witnessed the simultaneous occurrence of smallpox and measles in two girls. J. Maurice4, in his whole practice, only observed two such cases. Similar cases are to be found in Ettmuller's5 works, and in the writings of a few others.

Zencker6 saw cow-pox run its regular course along with measles and along with purpura.

The cow-pox went on its course undisturbed during a mercurial treatment for syphilis, as Jenner saw.

1 From careful experiments and cures of complex diseases of this kind, I am now firmly convinced that no real amalgamation of the two takes place, but that in such cases the one exists in the organism besides the other only, each in pairs that are adapted for it, and their cure will be completely effected by a judicious alternation of the best mercurial preparation, with the remedies specific for the psora, each given in the most suitable dose and form

EXPLANATION

III The other condition can be that the new d/s acts for a long time on organism & joins the old dissimilar d/s & forms a complex d/s.

Now both of the d/s occupy a particular organ and leave rest to the other d/s that is dissimilar to it.

- As the two d/s are dissimilar to each other, they cannot remove, cannot cure one another & the patient is rendered more diseased & more difficult to cure.
- One d/s exists in the organism besides the other only, each in the part that is adapted for it. Their cure will be completely effected by a alteration of the best mercurial preparation with the remedies specific for the psora each of which is given in the most suitable dose & form.

E.g. when two dissimilar acute infectious diseases meet, e.g- smallpox & measles. One d/s usually suspends the other but there have also been cases of severe epidemic, in rare cases, where the two dissimilar acute d/s occurred at the same time simultaneously in one and the same body for a short time combined.

During an epidemic, where smallpox & measles were prevalent at the same time.among 300 cases there was one single case in which P. Russell found both smallpox & measles in one person at the same time.

- Rainey says that two cases of girl with both d/s in one person at the same time were found.
- Few others like etimuller etc, have found such cases of complex d/s
- Zencker saw that cow-pox runs its regular course along with measles & along with purpura.

Foot note 1:
From careful experiments and cures of complex diseases of this kind, Hahnemann says that no real amalgamation of the two diseases occurs in the body But in such cases the one exists in the organism besides the other only, each in the part of body adapted for it. Their cure will be effected by a judicious alteration of the best mercurial preparation, with remedies specific for the psora, each of them given in the most suitable dose and form.

§ 41

ALLOPATHIC METHOD

Much more frequent than the natural diseases associating with and complicating one another in the same body are the morbid complication resulting from the art of the ordinary practitioner, which the inappropriate medical treatment (the allopathic method) is apt to produce by the long-continued employment of unsuitable drugs. To the natural disease, which it is proposed to cure, there are then added, by the constant repetition of the unsuitable medical agent, the new, often very tedious, morbid conditions corresponding to the nature of this agent; these gradually coalesce with and complicate the chronic malady which is dissimilar to them (which they were unable to cure by similarity of action, that is, homoeopathically), adding to the old disease a new, dissimilar, artificial malady of a chronic nature, and thus give the patient a double in place of a single disease, that is to say, render him much worse and more difficult to cure, often quite incurable. Many of the cases for which advice is asked in medical journals, as also the records of other cases in medical writings, attest the truth of this. Of a similar character are the frequent cases in which the venereal chancrous disease, complicated especially with psora or with the venereal chancrous disease, complicated especially with psora or with dyscrasia of condylomatous gonorrhoea, is not cured by long-continued or frequently repeated treatment with large doses of unsuitable mercurial preparations, but assumes its place in the organism beside the chronic mercurial affection1 that has been in the meantime gradually developed, and thus along with it often forms a hideous monster of complicated disease (under the general name of masked venereal disease), which then, when not quite incurable, can only be transformed into health with the greatest difficulty.

1 For mercury, besides the morbid symptoms which by virtue of similarity can cure the venereal disease homoeopathically, has among its effects many others unlike those of syphilis, for instance, swelling and ulceration of bones, which, if it be employed in large doses, causes new maladies and commit great ravages in the body, especially when complicated with psora, as is so frequently the case.

EXPLANATION

Hahnemann says that natural d/s forming complex d/s in the human body are rare.
- ✦ But morbid complications due to use of inappropriate medical treatment I.e- the allopathic method is more frequent & leads to complicating the case.
- ✦ This is due to long -continued employment of unsuitable drugs.
- ✦ A case with natural d/s when given this allopathic treatment by constant repetition of the unsuitable medicinal agent, a new: dissimilar artificial malady of a chronic nature is added & it gives the patient a double d/s in place of treating a single d/s.
- ✦ This makes the patient much worse & more difficult to cure & it often make the case incurable.

- When a case is treated by allopathic method, in our body new morbid conditions develops depending on the nature of the agent.
- These gradually combine & complicate the chronic malady which is dissimilar to them & are unable to cure the sick by similarity of action I.e- Homoeopathically.

e.g. A case of veneral chancrous d/s, complicated gonorrhoea when given a long-continued or frequently repeated treatment with large doses of unsuitable mercurial preparations is not cured by it.

- but the d/s be assumes a place in the organism beside the chronic mercurial affection that has developed due to the treatment, it along with the mercurial affection often forms a hideous monster of complicated d/s.
- thus the case becomes quite incurable or is more difficult to cure and can only ne transformed into health with the greatest difficulty.

Footnote 1:
Mercury can cure the venereal disease homoeopathically by virtue of similarity. If it is employed in large doses, it causes new maladies and cause great damage in the body especially when it is complicated with psora, as is so frequently the case.

§ 42

DIS-SIMILAR DISEASES COMPLICATES

Nature herself permits, as has been stated, in some cases, the simultaneous occurrence of two (indeed, of three) natural disease in one and the same body. This complication, however, it must be remarked, happens only in the case of two dissimilar disease, which according to the eternal laws of nature do not remove, do not annihilate and cannot cure one another, but, as it seems, both (or all three) remain, as it were, separate in the organism, and each takes possession of the parts and systems peculiarly appropriate to it, which, on account of the want of resemblance of these maladies to each other, can very well happen without disparagement to the unity of life.

EXPLANATION

In aphorism 42, he says that in some cases nature herself allows the occurrence of two [indeed of three], natural d/s at the same time & in the same body.

- This occurs only in the case of two dissimilar d/s, which according to the eternal laws of nature don't remove, don't annihilate don't cure one another.
- both [or all three] remain separate in the organism by taking possession of the parts & systems appropriate to each.
- thus they dwell in different organs of the human body together at the same time.

§ 43

TO SIMILAR DISEASES CURE

Totally different, however, is the result when two similar disease meet together in the organism, that is to say, when to the disease already present a stronger similar one is added. In such cases we see how a cure can be effected by the operations of nature, and we get a lesson as to how man ought to cure.

EXPLANATION

He says that the result is totally different when two similar d/s meet in the organism.

- ✦ keep in mind now we are talking about similar diseases..

It means a d/s is already present & a new stronger similar one is added to it. In such cases we see that nature cures the earlier or the older d/s already present.

Thus hahnemann tries to say here that a keen observer of nature will know this truth that if similar d/s interact one being stronger than other, the cure occurs.

Thus we should get a lesson how man needs to be cured.

§ 44

THEY NEITHER-REPEL, SUSPEND, COMPLEX

Similar diseases can neither (as is asserted of dissimilar disease in I) repel one another, nor (as has been shown of dissimilar disease in II) suspend on another, so that the old one shall return after the new one has run its course; and just as little can two similar disease (as has been demonstrated in III respecting dissimilar affections) exist beside each other in the same organism, or together form a double complex disease.

EXPLANATION

In this aphorism he says that two similar diseases can neither repel one another nor suspend one another, means they do not suppress or repel each other.

- ✦ Here the old one does not return back after the new one has run its course.
- ✦ Two similar d/s don't exist beside each other in the same organism & at the same time nor they form a double complex d/s.
- ✦ It means that two similar diseases cannot remain in the same body & at the same time.
- ✦ They don't form a double complex d/s

§ 45

HOW 2 D/S WORK?

No! Two diseases, differing, it is true, in kind1 but very similar in their phenomena and effects and in the sufferings and symptoms they severally produce, invariably annihilate one another whenever they meet together in the organism; the stronger disease namely, annihilates the weaker, and that for this simple reason, because the stronger morbific power when it invades the system, by reason of its similarity of action involves precisely the same part of the organism that were previously affected by the weaker morbid irritation, which, consequently, can no longer act on these parts, but is extinguished2, or (in other words), the new similar but stronger morbific potency controls the feelings of the patient and hence the life principle on account of its peculiarity, can no longer feel the weaker similar which becomes extinguished – exists no longer – for it was never anything material, but a dynamic – spirit-like – (conceptual) affection. The life principle henceforth is affected only and this but temporarily by the new, similar but stronger morbific potency.

1 Vide, supra, § 26, note.

2 Just as the image of a lamp's flame is rapidly overpowered and effaced from our retina by the stronger sunbeam impinging on the eye.

EXPLANATION

- ✦ In the aphorism he explains how a new similar d/s cures an existing d/s in the body.
- ✦ When the two similar d/s which differ in kind but are very similar in their phenomena, effects and sufferings & symptoms meet in the body, the stronger d/s completely cures the weaker one.
- ✦ This is because when the stronger morbific power invades the system, [and for the reason that it is similar in action]it involves that same parts of the organism that were affected by the weaker morbid irritation [The d/s person is already suffering]
- ✦ The weaker morbid irritation now cannot act on these parts & is removed.
- ✦ We can also say that the new similar but stronger morbific potency now controls the feelings of the patient.

- The life principle now cannot feel the weaker similar which does not exists now as it was a dynamic spirit-like affection. In other words we can say that now the life principle is affected by the new, similar but stronger d/s.

The stronger, similar d/s completely cures the older d/s & now the person has the new d/s in the body. The older one is cured.

Footnote:
It is just like the image of a lamp flame is overpowered rapidly and fades from our retina by the stronger Sunbeam impinging on the eye.

§ 46

EXAMPLE

Many examples might be adduced of disease which, in the course of nature, have been homoeopathically cured by other diseases presenting similar symptoms, were it not necessary, as our object is to speak about something determinate and indubitable, to confine our attention solely to those (few) disease which are invariably the same, arise from a fixed miasm, and hence merit a distinct name.

Among these the smallpox, so dreaded on account of the great number of its serious symptoms, occupies a prominent position, and it has removed and cured a number of maladies with similar symptoms.

How frequently does smallpox produce violent ophthalmia, sometimes even causing blindness! And see! By its inoculation Dezoteux[1] cured a chronic ophthalmia permanently, and Leroy[2] another.

An amaurosis of two years' duration, consequent on suppressed scald head, was perfectly cured by it, according to Klein.[3]

How often does smallpox cause deafness and dyspnoea! And both these chronic diseases it removed on reaching its acme, as J. Fr. Closs[4] observed.

Swelling of the testicle, even of a very severe character, is a frequent symptom of small-pox, and on this account it was enabled, as Klein[5] observed, to cure, by virtue of similarity, a large hard swelling of the left testicle, consequently on a bruise. And another observer[6] saw a similar swelling of the testicle cured by it.

Among the troublesome symptoms of small-pox is a dysenteric state of the bowels; and it subdued, as Fr. Wendt[7] observed, a case of dysentery, as a similar morbific agent.

Smallpox coming on after vaccination, as well on account of its greater strength as its great similarity, at once removes entirely the cow-pox homoeopathically, and does not permit it to come to maturity; but, on the other hand, the cow-pox when near maturity does, on account of its great similarity, homoeopathically diminish very much the supervening smallpox and make it much milder[8], as Muhry[9] and many others testify.

The inoculated cow-pox, whose lymph, besides the protective matter, contains the contagion of a general cutaneous eruption of another nature, consisting of usually small, dry (rarely large, pustular) pimples, resting on a small red areola, frequently conjoined with round red cutaneous spots and often accompanied by the most violent itching, which rash appears in not a few children several days before, more frequently, however, after the red areola of the cow-pock, and goes off in a few days, leaving behind small, red, hard spots on the skin; – the inoculated cow-pox, I say, after it has taken, cures perfectly and permanently, in a homoeopathic manner, by the similarity of this accessory miasm, analogous cutaneous eruptions of children, often of very long standing and of a very troublesome character, as a number of observers assert.[10]

The cow-pox, a peculiar symptom of which is to cause tumefaction of the arm[11], cured, after it broke out, a swollen half-paralyzed arm.[12]

The fever accompanying cow-pox, which occurs at the time of the production of the red areola, cured homoeopathically intermittent fever in two individuals, as the younger Hardege[13] reports, confirming what J. Hunter[14] had already observed, that two fevers (similar diseases) cannot co-exist in the same body.

The measles bear a strong resemblance in the character of its fever and cough to the whooping-cough, and hence it was that Bosquillon[15] noticed, in an epidemic where both these affections prevailed, that many children who then took measles remained free from whooping-cough during that epidemic. They would all have been protected from, and rendered incapable of being infected by, the whooping-cough in that and all subsequent epidemics, by the measles, if the whooping-cough were not a disease that has only a partial similarity to the measles, that is to say, if it had also a cutaneous eruption similar to what the latter possesses. As it is, however, the measles can but preserve a large number from whooping-cough homoeopathically, and that only in the epidemic prevailing at the time.

If, however, the measles come in contact with a disease resembling it in its chief symptom, the eruption, it can indisputably remove, and effect a homoeopathic cure of the latter. Thus a chronic herpetic eruption was entirely and permanently (homoeopathically) cured[16] by the breaking out of the measles, as Kortum[17] observed. An excessively burning miliary rash on the face, neck, and arms, that had lasted six years, and was aggravated by every change of weather, on the invasion of measles assumed the form of a swelling of the surface of the skin; after the measles had run its course the exanthema was cured, and returned no more.[18]

1 Traite de l'inoculation, p.189.
2 Heilkunde fur Mutter, p.384.
3 Interpres clinicus, p.293.
4 Neue Heilart der Kinderpocken. Ulm, 1769, p.68; and Specim., obs. No. 18.
5 Op. cit.
6 Nov. Act. Nat. cur., vol, I, obs. 22.
7 Nachricht Von dem Krankeninstitut zu Erlangen, 1783.
8 A new footnote is added here in the Sixth Edition, as follows:

This seems to be the reason for this beneficial remarkable fact namely that since the general distribution of Janner's Cow-pox vaccination, human small-pox never again appeared as epidemically or virulently as 40-45 years before when one city visited lost at least one-half and often three-quarters of its children by death of this miserable pestilence.

9 Willian, Ueber die Kuhpockenimpfung, aus dem Engl., mit Zusatzen G. P. Muhry, Gottingen, 1808.

10 Especially Clavier, Hurel and Desmormeaux, in the Bulletin des sciencs medicales, publie par les membres de l' Eure, 1808, also in the Journal de medicine continue, vol. xv, p.206.

11 Balhorn, in Hufeland's Journal, 10, ii.

12 Stevenson, in Duncan's Annals of Medicine, lustr. 2, vol. I, pt. 2, No. 9.

13 In Hufeland's Journal, xxiii.

14 On the Veneral Disease, p.4.

15 Cullen's Elements of Practical Medicine, pt. 2, I, 3, ch. vii.

16 Or at least that symptom was removed.

17 In Hufeland's Journal, xx, 3, p.50.

18 Rau, Ueber d. Werth des hom. Heidelb., 1824, p.85.

EXPLANATION

- Here Hahnemann gives example in nature where the d/s have been homoeopathically cured by other d/s having similar symptoms.
  E.g- Smallpox, is a dreaded d/s as it produces serious symptoms, it has removed & cured a number of maladies with similar symptoms.
- Smallpox produces violent opthalmia sometimes it even causes blindness, Dezotevx & Leroy cured a chronic opthalmia by the inoculation of smallpox.
- Smallpox causes deafness & dyspnoea, so it cured both these chronic diseases on reaching its peak, this was observed by, J. FR. CLoss
- Klein saw that swelling of the testicle is a frequent [common], symptom of smallpox, he observed that a person had a bruise due to which a large hard swelling of the left testicle occured, it was cured on inoculation of smallpox in that patient.
- Smallpox caused dysentery so it cures dysentery, this was observed by FR. WENDE
- Smallpox removes cow pox homoeopathically because of its similarity with cow -pox & greater strength than cow -pox.
- Small-pox the cow-pox homoeopathically diminish the smallpox & make it much milder as observed by MUHRY.
- Cow-pox has a peculiar symptom of swelling of the arm, it cured a swollen half-paralyzed arm.
- The measles causes eruption so when it comes in contact with a d/s with its chief symptoms the eruption, it can remove & cure it homoeopathically.
- Kortum observed that a chronic herpetic eruption was entirely & permanently [homoeopathically] cured by the breaking out of measles in patient.
- A person had excessively burning miliary rash on the face, neck and arms, for six years and it was aggravated by every change if weather. When the person contacted measles the rash assumed the form of a swelling on the surface of the skin. After the measles had run its course the exanthem was cured and did not return back.

§ 47

TEACH

Nothing could teach the physician in a plainer and more convincing manner than the above what kind of artificial morbific agent (medicine) he ought to choose in order to cure in a sure, rapid and permanent manner, conformably with the process that takes place in nature.

EXPLANATION

In all the above aphorism how clearly Hahnemann has taught the physician that what artificial morbific agent [medicine] he needs to choose so that cure is sure. The cure should be rapid, in permanent manner & with the process that takes place in nature.

- ✦ Nature cures a existing d/s only by producing similar & stronger d/s.
- ✦ This is the basic principle of Homoeopathic remedy.
- ✦ It chooses the most similar remedy which produces most of the totality of symptoms of patient to be cured, in a healthy person.

§ 48

ORDINARY SCHOOL OF MEDICINE

Neither in the course of nature, as we see from all the above examples, nor by the physician's art, can an existing affection or malady in any one instance be removed by a dissimilar morbific agent, be it ever so strong, but solely by one that is similar in symptoms and is somewhat stronger, according to eternal, irrevocable laws of nature, which have not hitherto been recognized.

EXPLANATION

- In nature also, we have already seen many examples [as explained in earlier aphorisms] that prove that a dissimilar morbific agent [medicine] can never cure a d/s.
- Even if the dissimilar morbific agent is very strong it can never cure a patient.
- Sick can only be cured by a malady that is similar in symptoms & somewhat stronger than the existing d/s

- But the ordinary school of medicine don't follow this law & they fail to cure in the most harmless way based on easily comprehensible principles.
- They don't follow the nature's law of cure.

§ 49

MINUTE OBSERVATION

We should have been able to meet with many more real, natural homoeopathic cures of this kind if, on the one hand, the attention of observers had been more directed to them, and, on the other hand, if nature had not been so deficient in helpful homoeopathic diseases.

EXPLANATION

- In this aphorism he says that during his time the attention of observers was not more directed to meet with many more real, natural homeopathic cures of this kind.
- They did not observe the natural Homeopathic cure & this is the reason, we don't have many real, natural homeopathic cures of this kind in note.
- The second reason for less note of natural homeopathic cures is that nature had been deficient in these helpful homeopathic d/s
- This means the cure by nature based on law of similia is not frequent.

§ 50

WE CANNOT DEPEND ON NATURE'S CURE

Mighty Nature herself has, as we see, at her command, as instruments for effecting homoeopathic cures, little besides the miasmatic diseases of constant character, (the itch) measles and smallpox1, morbific agents which2, as remedies, are either more dangerous to life and more to be dreaded than the disease they are to cure, they themselves require curing, in order to be eradicated in their turn – both circumstances that make their employment, as homoeopathic remedies, difficult, uncertain and dangerous. And how few diseases are there to which man is subject that find their similar remedy in smallpox, measles or itch! Hence, in the course of nature, very few maladies can be cured by these uncertain and hazardous homoeopathic remedies, and the cure by their instrumentality is also attended with danger and much difficulty, for this reason that the doses

of these morbific powers cannot be diminished according to circumstances, as doses of medicine can; but the patient afflicted with an analogous malady of long standing must be subjected to the entire dangerous and tedious disease, to the entire disease of smallpox, measles (or itch), which in its turn has to be cured. And yet, as is seen, we can point to some striking homoeopathic cures effected by this lucky concurrence, all so many incontrovertible proofs of the great, the sole therapeutic law of nature that obtains in them: Cure by symptoms similarity!

1 And the exanthematous contagious principle present in the cow-pox lymph.
2 Namely, small-pox and measles.

EXPLANATION

In above context he says again that nature herself can cure the miasmatic d/s of constant character like itch, measles & smallpox, morbific agents only.

- These agents are either more dangerous to life & more harmful & serious than the d/s they are to cure.
- They are of such type like the itch, that they themselves require their own treatment & eradication afterwards the original d/s is cured. The patient is afflicted with a similar malady of long standing entirely dangerous and tedious disease like smallpox, measles, itch etc which in turn has to be cured. In the course of Nature, very few maladies can be cured by these uncertain and hazardous Homoepathic remedies of Nature and the cure by their instrumentality is dangerous and much difficult.
- These above circumstances make their utilization as homeopathic remedies difficult, uncertain & dangerous
- So, we can not depend on nature's cure, it is more dangerous & uncertain.
- We can also see that the diseases which find their similar remedy in nature are very few.
- One more thing to be noted is that the doses of these morbific powers of nature cannot be diminished or controlled according to the situation whereas the doses of medicine can be controlled & is in the hands of careful physician.
- So we can see that we cannot depend on nature's cure based on cure by symptom similarity as it is not sure, not reliable & harmful too & itself requires cure.
- What we can utilise from this is, is how the cure should be directed based on the principle or therapeutic law of nature, " Cure by symptom similarity. "

§ 51

BENEFIT OF HOMOEOPATHIC AID OVER NATURE CURE

This therapeutic law is rendered obvious to all intelligent minds by these instances, and they are amply sufficient for this end. But, on the other hand, see what advantages man has over crude Nature in her happy-go-lucky operations. How many thousands more of homoeopathic morbific agents has not man at his disposal for the relief of his suffering fellow-creatures in the medicinal substances universally distributed throughout creation! In them he has producers of disease of all possible varieties of action, for all the innumerable, for all conceivable and inconceivable natural diseases, to which they can render homoeopathic aid – morbific agents (medicinal substances), whose power, when their remedial employment is completed, being overcome by the vital force, disappears spontaneously without requiring a second course of treatment for its extirpation, like the itch – artificial morbific agents, which the physician can attenuate, subdivide and potentize almost to an infinite extent, and the dose of which he can diminish to such a degree that they shall remain only slightly stronger than the similar natural disease they are employed to cure; so that in this incomparable method of cure, there is no necessity for any violent attack upon the organism for the eradication of even an inveterate disease of old standing; the cure by this method takes place by only a gentle, imperceptible and yet often rapid transition from the tormenting natural disease to the desired state of permanent health.

EXPLANATION

- In this aphorism he say that:-
- The therapeutic law " cure by symptom similarity "is now very clear to the intelligent minds by above facts.
- There are many examples to state it.
- We can also see that what advantage the homeopathic remedy have over crude nature's cure.
- Medicinal substances are universally present throughout the world.
- Man for the relief of the suffering sick creatures has more than thousands of homeopathic morbific agents.
- In these medicinal substances he has producers of variety of natural diseases to which they can give homeopathic aid[cure].
- These medicinal substances [morbific agents] after their remedies action is completed are removed by Vital force.
- After the remedial action of these medicine substances is completed, they are overcome by the vital-force & disappear spontaneously, they don't require a second course of treatment for their removal from body.
- We have seen that the natural cure by nature requires the removal of the second d/s which cured the original one but by using homeopathic aid we don't face this problem.
- The dose of homeopathic medicine can be controlled by the physician.
- The dose can be diminshed to such a degree that they remain only slightly stronger than the similar natural d/s for which they are employed to cure.
- By above employment of medicine there is no chance of any violent attack upon the human body, for eradication of even an deep-stated d/s of old duration.
- In this way the cure by this method takes place by gentle, rapid & harmless way, thus bringing the sick person back to health.

§ 52

THE PRINCIPAL METHODS OF CURE

There are but two principle methods of cure: the one based only on accurate observation of nature, on careful experimentation and pure experience, the homoeopathic (before we never designedly used) and a second which does not do this, the heteropathic or allopathic. Each opposes the other, and only he who does not know either can hold the delusion that they can ever approach each other or even become united, or to make himself so ridiculous as to practice at one time homoeopathically at another allopathically, according to the pleasure of the patient; a practice which may be called criminal treason against divine homoeopathy.

EXPLANATION

There are two principal methods of bringing cure.
I.   one is based on accurate observation of nature, on careful experiments & based on pure experience I.e- Homoepathic
II. Second one does not follow above the heteropathic or allopathic

Each of the methods opposes the other.

- We cannot practice both of them as they are totally different.
- Those who do not know either of them have a delusion that they can approach each other or becomes united. These people use homoepathy sometimes & allopathy the other times according to the pleasure of the patient. This type of practice of treating of sick maybe called criminal treason against divine homoeopathy.

§ 53

WHY HOMEOPATHY IS BEST?

The true mild cures take place only according to the homoeopathic method, which, as we have found (§§ 7-25) by experience and deduction, is unquestionably the proper one by which through art the quickest, most certain and most permanent cures are obtained since this healing art rests upon an eternal infallible law of nature.

The pure homoeopathic healing art is the only correct method, the one possible to human art, the straightest way to cure, as certain as that there is but one straight line between two given points.

EXPLANATION

As we have seen in aphorism 7 to 25 that the true mild cures occurs only by homoepathic method.

- ✦ We also know that this healing art is based upon an eternal infalliable law of nature, so without any doubt it is the proper one by which the quickest, most certain & most permanent cures are obtained.
- ✦ The pure homeopathic art of healing is the only correct method & the shortest & straightest way to cure of the sick.

§ 54

THE ALLOPATHIC METHOD

The allopathic method of treatment utilized many things against disease, but usually only improper ones (alloea) and ruled for ages in different forms called systems. Every one of these, following each other from time to time and differing greatly each from the other, honored itself with the name of Rational Medicine1.

Every builder of such a system cherished the haughty estimation of himself that he was able to penetrate into the inner nature of life of the healthy as well as of the sick and clearly to recognize it and accordingly gave the prescription which noxious matter2 should be banished from the sick man, and how to banish it in order to restore him to health, all this according to empty assumptions and arbitrary suppositions without honestly questioning nature and listening without prejudice to the voice of experience. Diseases were held to be conditions that reappeared pretty much in the same manner. Most systems gave, therefore, names to their imagined disease pictures and classified them, every system differently. To medicines were ascribed actions which were supposed to cure these abnormal conditions. (Hence the numerous text books on Materia Medica.3)

1 As if the establishment of a science, based only on observation of nature and pure experiment and experience idle speculation and scholastic vaporings could have a place.

2 Up to the most recent times what is curable in sickness was supposed to be material that had to be removed since no one could conceive of a dynamic effect (§ 11 note) of morbific agencies, such as medicines exercise upon the life of the animal organism.

3 To fill the measure of self infatuation to overflowing here were mixed (very learnedly) constantly more, indeed, many different medicines in so-called prescriptions to be administered in frequent and large doses and thereby the precious, easily-destroyed human life was endangered in the hands of these perverted ones. Especially so with seton, venesection, emetics, purgatives, plasters, fontanelles and cauterization.

EXPLANATION

The allopathic method of treatment uses many things against diseases called with the name of Rational Medicine but usually they are improper ones.

- Their mode of employment of medicine is according to empty assumptions and without listening to the voice of experience & nature.
- The builder of this system of treatment feels happy that he is able to penetrate into the inner nature of life of the healthly and also sick, based on it gives the prescription to banish the noxious matter from the sick man, in order to restore him to health.
- According to them d/s are conditions that reappear in some what same manner, they therefore, started giving names to imagined d/s pictures & also they classified them, every system differently.
  The medicines which they used were described actions which were thought to cure theses abnormal conditions.
- According to them what is to be cured in sick is a material thing that has to be removed since they could not conceive of a dynamic effect of morbific agents causing d/s in human body.
  Many different medicines were prescribed in frequent & large doses
- This endangered the precious human life in the hands of these physician who don't believe in law of cure based on similarity "

Footnote1:
As if the establishment of a science, based only on observation of nature and pure experiment and experience idle speculation and scholastic vaporings could have a place.

Footnote 2:
According to them what is to be cured in sick is a material thing that has to be removed since they could not conceive of a dynamic effect of morbific agents, such as medicines have upon the life of the animal organism.

Footnote 3:
Many different medicines and procedures like seton, venesection, emetics, purgatives, plasters, fontanelles and cauterization etc were prescribed to be administered in frequent and large doses. The precious human life was endangered in the hands of these physicians.

§ 55

TEMPORARY RELIEF

Soon, however, the public became convinced that the sufferings of the sick increased and heightened with the introduction of every one of these systems and methods of cure if

followed exactly. Long ago these allopathic physicians would have been left had it not been for the palliative relief obtained at times from empirically discovered remedies whose almost instantaneous flattering action is apparent to the patient and this to some extent served to keep up their credit.

EXPLANATION

In short time, the public was convinced that with their system the sufferings of the sick was not cured.

Instead of treating, the sufferings of the sick increased & kept on increasing with the introduction of every one of these systems & methods of cure.

This method of treatment would have been left long ago but it provided the palliative relief at times. The instantaneous relief action of these remedies is what the patient sees & praises.

But what this method does to the body we have already seen in aphorism 41.

§ 56

ISOPATHY & ALLOPATHY ARE NOT MODE OF TREATMENT

By means of this palliative (antipathic, enantiopathic) method, introduced according to Galen's teaching "Contraria contrariis" for seventeen centuries, the physicians hitherto could hope to win confidence while they deluded with almost instantaneous amelioration. But how fundamentally unhelpful and hurtful this method of treatment is (in diseases not running a rapid course) we shall see in what follows. It is certainly the only one of the modes of treatment adopted by the allopaths that had any manifest relation to a portion of the sufferings caused by the natural disease; but what kind of relation? Of a truth the very one (the exact contrary of the right one) that ought carefully to be avoided if we would not delude and make a mockery of the patient affected with a chronic disease1.

1 A third mode of employing medicines in diseases has been attempted to be created by means of Isopathy, as it is called – that is to say, a method of curing a given disease by the same contagious principle that produces it. But even granting this could be done, yet, after all, seeing that the virus is given to the patient highly potentized, and consequently, in an altered condition, the cure is effected only by opposing a simillimum to a simillimum.

To attempt to cure by means of the very same morbific potency (per Idem) contradicts all normal human understanding and hence all experience. Those who first brought Isopathy to notice, probably thought of the benefit which mankind received from cowpox vaccination by which the vaccinated individual is protected against future cowpox infection and as it were cured in advance. But both, cowpox and smallpox are only similar, in no way the same disease. In many respects they differ, namely in the more rapid course and mildness of cowpox and especially in this, that is never contagious to man by more nearness. Universal vaccination put an end to all epidemics of that deadly fearful smallpox to such an extent that the present generation does no longer possess a clear conception of the former frightful smallpox plague.

Moreover, in this way, undoubtedly, certain diseases peculiar to animals may give us remedies and thus happily enlarge our stock of homoeopathic remedies.

But to use a human morbific matter (a Psorin taken from the itch in man) as a remedy for the same itch or for evils arisen therefrom is –?

Nothing can result from this but trouble and aggravation of the disease.

EXPLANATION

According to Galen's teaching 'Contraria contraris" which was practised for seventeen centuries by this pallative [antipathic, enantipathic] method the physicians had hope to win the confidence of the people by the instantaneous amelioration by palliative treatment

But we see that how fundamentally unhelpful & hurtful is this method of treatment for the patients [in d/s which don't run a rapid course]

This mode of treatment only gives instant relief to the patient & suppresses his symptoms but the body is still diseased, it is not cured.

Footnote 1:

Hahnemann says:- A third mode of employing medicines in d/s is by 'ISOPATHY '.

In isopathy the given d/s is cured by the same contagious principle that causes the d/s.

- To bring cure by use of same morbific potency, was thought to be useful for mankind.
- They started believing in isopathy because on vaccination for cowpox the individual who is vaccinated is protected by smallpox infection in future
- But both cowpox & smallpox are similar but not same d/s
- Both differ from each other in many ways, cowpox has more rapid course & is mild & it is not spread to man by mere nearness
- By universal vaccination all epidemics of deadly smallpox d/s was prevented
  In this way, some d/s which are peculiar to animals may give us remedies for the human d/s which are similar to them.
- But do you think use of human matter can act as a remedy?

E.g- a psorin taken from the itch in man if used a remedy for the same human, itch will trouble the patient and cause aggravation of the disease but we know that remedy should be one which cure patient in the most harmless way without such aggravation and without causing discomfort.

§ 57

ALLOPATHIC METHOD

In order to carry into practice this antipathic method, the ordinary physician gives, for a single troublesome symptom from among the many other symptoms of the disease which he passes by unheeded, a medicine concerning which it is known that it produces the exact opposite of the morbid symptom sought to be subdued, from which, agreeably to the fifteen – centuries – old traditional rule of the antiquated medical school (contraria contrariis) he can expect the speediest (palliative) relief. He gives large doses of opium for pains of all sorts, because this drug soon benumbs the sensibility, and administers the same remedy for diarrhoeas, because it speedily puts a stop to the peristaltic motion of the intestinal canal and makes it insensible; and also for sleeplessness, because opium rapidly produces a stupefied, comatose sleep; he gives purgatives when the patient has suffered long from constipation and costiveness; he causes the burnt hand to be plunged into cold water, which, from its low degree of temperature, seems instantaneously to remove the burning pain, as if by magic; he puts the patient who complains of chilliness and deficiency of vital heat into warm baths, which warm him immediately; he makes him who is suffering from prolonged debility drink wine, whereby he is instantly enlivened and refreshed; and in like manner he employs other opposite (antipathic) remedial means, but he has very few besides those just mentioned, as it is only of very few substances that some peculiar (primary) action is known to the ordinary medical school.

EXPLANATION

1. As we all know the antipathic method gives medicine for a single troublesome symptom among all other symptoms of d/s
   - The antipathic physician gives medicine that produce exactly opposite action of the morbid symptom which he is trying to treat.
   - The patient gets immediate relief of symptoms & is happy that now he is treated but as we have already seen this does not cure the patient at all.

E.g- If the patient comes with pain of any kind, the ordinary physician gives large doses of opium, we know that opium denumbs the senses.

He gives same opium remedy for diarrhoea because it stops the peristaltic motion of intestine.
For sleeplessness also he gives opium because it rapidly produces a comatose sleep.

- Similarly for constipation purgative are given
- He dips burnt hand into cold water which removes the burning pain immediately from low degree of temperature of cold water,
- He gives wine to a person suffering from prolonged debility.

- Like above we gives other opposite [antipathic] remedial means to treat the sick.
- But very few substances with some peculiar [primary] action is known to the ordinary medical school.

§ 58

ALLOPATHY CONTINUED

If, in estimating the value of this mode of employing medicines, we should even pass over the circumstance that it is an extremely faulty symptomatic treatment (v. note to § 7), wherein the practitioner devotes his attention in a merely one-sided manner to a single symptom, consequently to only a small part of the whole, whereby relief for the totality of the disease, which is what the patient desires, cannot evidently be expected, – we must, on the other hand, demand of experience if, in one single case where such antipathic employment of medicine was made use of in a chronic or persisting affection, after the transient amelioration there did not ensue an increased aggravation of the symptom which was subdued at first in a palliative manner, an aggravation, indeed, of the whole disease? And every attentive observer will agree that, after such short antipathic amelioration, aggravation follows in every case without exception, although the ordinary physician is in the habit of giving his patient another explanation of this subsequent aggravation, and ascribes it to malignancy of the original disease, now for the first time showing itself, or to the occurrence of quite a new disease1.

1 Little as physicians have hitherto been in the habit of observing accurately, the aggravation that so certainly follows such palliative treatment could not altogether escape their notice. A striking example of this is to be found in J. H. Schulze's Diss. qua corporis humani momentanearum alterationum specimina quoedam expenduntur, Hale, 1741, § 28. Willis bears testimony to something similar (Pharm. rat., § 7, cap. I, p.298): "Opiata dolores atroscissimos plerumque sedant atque indolentiam – procurant, camque – aliquamdiu et pro stato quodam tempore continuant, quo spatio elapso dolores mox recrusescunt et brevi ad sol itam ferociam augentur." And also at page 295: "Exactis opii viribus illico redeunt tormina, nec atrocitatem suam remittunt, nisi dum ab eodem pharmaco rursus incantuntur." In like manner J. Hunter (On the Venereal Disease, p.13) says that wine and cordials given to the weak increase the action without giving real strength, and the powers of the body are afterwards sunk proportionally as they have been raised, by which nothing can be gained, but a great deal may be lost.

EXPLANATION

1. In this aphorism Hahnemann says that, this symptomatic treatment is extremely faulty [wrong] because it gives attention to a single symptom, to only a small part of the whole d/s
2. The practitioner gives his attention in one-sided manner to a single symptom.

3. As the totality of d/s is not cured the patient is not cured.
4. Every attentive observer finds that after short amelioration by antipathic treatment the aggravation occurs in every case without exception.
5. We have also seen that the physician gives his patient another explanation of this subsequent aggravation & says that it is due to malignancy of the original d/s or due to occurrence of a new d/s.

Footnote 1:
J. Hunter says that if wine & cordials are given to the weak it increase the action without giving real strength & afterwards the power of the body are sunk 'proportionally 'as they have been raised. This way a great deal may be lost in body.

§ 59

EXAMPLE OF DISADVANTAGE

Important symptoms of persistent diseases have never yet been treated with such palliative, antagonistic remedies, without the opposite state, a relapse – indeed, a palpable aggravation of the malady – occurring a few hours afterwards. For a persistent tendency to sleepiness during the day the physician prescribed coffee, whose primary action is to enliven; and when it had exhausted its action the day – somnolence increased; – for frequent waking at night he gave in the evening, without heeding the other symptoms of the disease, opium, which by virtue of its primary action produced the same night (stupefied, dull) sleep, but the subsequent nights were still more sleepless than before; – to chronic diarrhoeas he opposed, without regarding the other morbid signs, the same opium, whose primary action is to constipate the bowels, and after a transient stoppage of the diarrhoea it subsequently became all the worse; – violent and frequently recurring pains of all kinds he could suppress with opium for but a short time; they then always returned in greater, often intolerable severity, or some much worse affection came in their stead. For nocturnal cough of long standing the ordinary physician knew no better than to administer opium, whose primary action is to suppress every irritation; the cough would then perhaps cease the first night, but during the subsequent nights it would be still more severe, and if it were again and again suppressed by this palliative in increased doses, fever and nocturnal perspiration were added to the disease; – weakness of the bladder, with consequent retention of urine, was sought to be conquered by the antipathic work of cantharides to stimulate the urinary passages whereby evacuation of the urine was certainly at first effected but thereafter the bladder becomes less capable of stimulation and less able to contract, and paralysis of the bladder is imminent; – with large doses of purgative drugs and laxative salts, which excite the bowels to frequent evacuation, it was sought to remove a chronic tendency to constipation, but in the secondary action the bowels became still more confined; – the ordinary physician seeks to remove chronic debility by the administration of wine, which, however, stimulates only in its primary action, and hence the forces sink all the lower in the secondary its primary action, and hence the forces sink all the lower in the secondary action; – by bitter substances and heating condiments he tries to strengthen and warm the chronically weak and cold stomach, but in the secondary action of these palliatives, which are stimulating in their primary action only, the stomach becomes yet more inactive; – long standing deficiency of vital heat and chilly disposition ought surely to yield to prescriptions of warm baths, but still more weak, cold, and chilly do the patients subsequently become; – severely burnt parts feel instantaneous alleviation from the application of cold water, but the burning pain afterwards increases to an incredible degree, and the inflammation spreads and rises to a still greater height;1 – by means of the sternutatory remedies that provoke a secretion of mucus, coryza with stoppage of the nose of long standing is sought to be removed, but it escapes observation that the disease is aggravated all the more by these antagonistic remedies (in their secondary action), and the nose becomes still more stopped; – by electricity and galvanism, with in their primary action greatly stimulate muscular action, chronically weak and almost paralytic limbs were soon excited to more active movements, but the consequence (the secondary action) was complete deadening of all muscular irritability and complete paralysis; – by venesections it was attempted to remove chronic determination of blood to the head, but they were always followed by greater congestion; – ordinary medical practitioners know nothing better with which to treat the paralytic torpor of the corporeal and mental organs, conjoined with unconsciousness, which prevails in many kinds of typhus, than with large doses of valerian, because this is one of the most powerful medicinal agents for causing animation and increasing the motor faculty; in their ignorance, however, they knew not that this action is only a primary action, and that the organism, after that is passed, most certainly falls back, in the secondary (antagonistic) action, into still greater stupor and immobility, that is to say, into paralysis of the mental and corporeal organs (and death); they did not see, that the very diseases they supplied most plentifully with valerian, which is in such cases an oppositely acting, antipathic remedy, most infallibly terminated fatally. The old school physician rejoices2 that he is able to reduce for several hours the velocity of the small rapid pulse in cachectic patients with the very first dose of uncombined purple foxglove (which in its primary action makes the pulse slower); its rapidity, however, soon returns; repeated, and now increased doses effect an ever smaller diminution of its rapidity, and at length none at all – indeed – in the secondary action the pulse becomes uncountable; sleep, appetite and strength depart, and a speedy death is invariably the result, or else insanity ensues. How often, in one word, the disease is aggravated, or something even worse is effected by the secondary action of such antagonistic (antipathic) remedies, the old school with its false theories does not perceive, but experience teaches it in a terrible manner.

1 Vide Introduction.
2 Vide Hufeland, in his pamphlet, Die Homoopathie, p.20.

EXPLANATION

1. In this aphorism he says that the important symptoms of the persistent d/s are never treated with such antagonistic remedies which only palliate.
2. A palpable aggravation of the malady occurs a few hours afterwards

E.g- A person with persistent tendency to sleepiness during the day is prescribed coffee by the physician, its primary action is to awake [enliver] & when this primary action is over the day -sleepiness increased more. Rather than relief of symptoms its intensity increased
, opium by its primary action produced the same night sleep but the subsequent nights were more sleepless than before.

E.g-Opium given for chronic diarrhoea without taking into account other morbid signs, by its primary action cause constipation of the bowels& after a short period of diarrhoea it subsequenty become worse.

E.g- A patient with recuring pains of all kind is given opium, it suppress pain for a short time, then it returned in greater & often intolerable severity or some much more affection came.

E.g- For a person with long-standing nocturnal cough, ordinary physician gives opium whose primary action is to suppress every irritation, the cough would stop the first night but the coming nights would be more severe & if this cough is again & again suppressed by this palliative drug in increased doses, fever & nocturnal perspiration were also added to cough.

E.g- For constipation large doses of purgative drugs & laxative salts were given which by this palliative action excites the bowels to frequent evacuation but in secondary action the bowels became still more constipated.

E.g- The severly burnt parts feel instant relief on applying cold water but the burning pain increases afterwards to great degree & inflammation spreads.

E.g- Coryza with stoppage of nose is given remedies that cause secretion of mucus but in their secondary action the d/s is aggravated & nose becomes more 'stopped'.

E.g-For a case of chronic weak, electricity & galvanism was used which in their primary action stimulates muscular action & active movements but the result was complete deadening of all muscular irritability & complete paralysis.

Old school with its false theories does not perceive that by this treatment the d/s is not cured but aggravated or sometimes. even worse occurs by the secondary action of such antipathic remedies.

But the ordinary physician feels happy that he is able to reduce the symptoms for several hours & does not see the results after.

§ 60

DISADVANTAGE OF INCREASING POTENCY

If these ill-effects are produced, as may very naturally be expected from the antipathic employment of medicines, the ordinary physician imagines he can get over the difficulty by giving, at each renewed aggravation, a stronger dose of the remedy, whereby an equally transient suppression1 is effected; and as there then is a still greater necessity for giving ever – increasing quantities of the palliative there ensues either another more serious disease or frequently even danger to life and death itself, but never a cure of a disease of considerable or of long standing.

1 All usual palliatives given for the suffering of the sick have (as is seen here) as after-effects an increase of the same suffering and the older physicians had to repeat them in ever stronger doses in order to achieve a similar modification, which however, was never permanent and never sufficient to prevent an increased recurrence of the ailment. But Brousseau, who twenty-five years before contended against the senseless mixing of different drugs in prescription and thereby ending its reign in France, (for which mankind is grateful to him) introduced his so-called physiological system (without taking note of the homoeopathic method then already established), a method of treatment, while effectively lessening and permanently preventing the return of all the sufferings, was applicable to all diseases of mankind; a thing that the palliatives then in use were not capable of affecting.

Being able to heal disease with mild innocent remedies and thus establish health, Brousseau found the easier way to quiet the sufferings of patients more and more at the cost of their life and at last to extinguish life wholly – a method of treatment that, alas, seemed sufficient to his contemporaries. In the degree that the patient retains his strength will his ailments be apparent and the more intensely will he feel his pains. He moans and groans and cries out and calls for help more and more vociferously so that the physician cannot come any too soon to give relief. Brousseau needed only to depress the vital force, to lessen it more and more and behold, the more frequently the patient was bled, the more leeches and cupping glasses sucked out the vital fluid (for the innocent irreplaceable blood was according to him responsible for almost all ailments). In the same proportion the patient lost strength to feel pain or to express his aggravated condition by violent complaint and gestures. The patient appears more quiet in proportion as he grows weaker, the bystanders rejoice in his apparent improvement, ready to return to the same measures on the renewal of his sufferings – be they spasms, suffocation, fears or pain, for they had so beautifully quieted him before and gave promise of further ease. In disease of long duration and when the patient retained some strength, he was deprived of food, put on a "hunger diet," in order to depress life so much more successfully and inhibit the restless states. The debilitated patient feels unable to protest against further similar measures of blood-letting leeches, vesication, warm baths and so forth to refuse their employment. That death must follow such frequently repeated reduction and exhaustion of the vital energy is not noticed by the patient, already robbed of all consciousness, and the relatives, blinded by the improvements even of the last sufferings of the patient by means of blood letting and warm baths, cannot understand and are surprised when the patient quietly slips away.

"But God knows the patient on his bed of sickness was not treated with violence, for the prick of a small lancet is not really painful and the gum Arabic solution (Eau de Gourme, almost the only medicine that Brousseau used) was mild in taste and without apparent action – the bite of the leeches insignificant and the blood letting by the physician done quietly while the luke warm baths could only soothe, hence the disease from the very start must have been fatal, so that the patient, notwithstanding all efforts of the physician, had to leave the earth." In this way the relatives, and especially the heirs of the dear departed, consoled themselves.

The physicians in Europe and elsewhere accepted this convenient treatment of all disease according to a single rule, since it saved them from all further thinking (the most laborious of all work under the sun). They only had to take care "to assuage the pangs of conscience and console themselves that they were not the originators of this system and this method of treatment, that all the other thousands of Brousseauists did the same and that possibly everything would cease with death anyway as was taught by their master." In this way many thousand physicians were miserably misled to shed (with cold heart) the warm blood of their patients that were capable of cure and thereby rob millions of men gradually of their life, according to Brousseau's method, more than fell on Napoleon's battlefields. Was it perhaps necessary by the disposition of God for that system of Brousseau which destroyed medically the life of curable patients to precede homoeopathy in order to open the eyes of the world to the only true science and art of medicine, homoeopathy, in which curable patients find health and new life when this most difficult of all arts is practised by an indefatigable discriminating physician in a pure and conscientious manner?

EXPLANATION

When the ordinary physician gives antipathic remedy to the patient, the patient gets instant relief. After the primary action of the remedy is over, ill-effects are produced.

- Those ill-effects are due to secondary action of the remedy.
- When the patient comes back with these ill-effects, the ordinary physician imagines that he can remove this ill-effect by giving a stronger dose of remedy each time.
- This process goes on due to which either another more serious d/s or frequently incurable d/s, even danger to life & death occurs.
- But there is never a cure of a d/s of considerable or of long standing, in short the patient is not cured.

Footnote 1:
In this footnote, an another method of treatment which was introduced by 'BROSSEAU "is explained.
Brousseau, 25 years before stood against this senseless use of mixing different drugs in prescriptions to patients in France & introduced his so-called physiological system

- He didn't take note of the homoepathic method of treatment.
- His method of treatment permanently prevented the return of all the suffering & was applicable to all the d/s of mankind
- Brousseau found easier way to quiet the suffering of the patients at the cost of the life of the patients & ultimately this treatment lead to death
- Brousseau depressed the vital force by his method
- according to him the blood was responsible for almost all ailments & so he used more leeches & cupping glasses to suck out the vital fluid [blood]
- this way the patient lost strength to feel pain or express his aggravation by violent complaints because he didn't now have any power left.
  The patient now appears more quiet as he grows weaker & his relatives feel happy that he is improving & the patient is not able to complain now,
- if he complains of spasm, fears or pain the relatives take him back to the same physician.

In d/s of long duration & when patient had some strength, he was given restricted diet"hunger diet". The patient becomes so weak that he is unable to protest against measures of physician like blood -letting leeches, vesication, warm baths etc.

This way repeated reduction & exhaustion of vital energy occurs & the patient quietly dies away.

The relatives see that during treatment no violence was done & physician tried all efforts but patient died. This way the relatives console themselves.

The physician in europe & elsewhere also accepted this convenient treatment of all d/s where all d/s were treated according to a single rule, since it saved them from all further thinking.

* Brosseau destroyed medically the life of curable patients.

Now it became necessary to follow homoepathy to open eyes of the world that only true science & art of medicine is homoepathy.

By the homoeopathic treatment all curable patients find health & new life when this art is practised in a pure & conscientious manner

§ 61

ORDINARY PHYSICIAN

Had physicians been capable of reflecting on the sad results of the antagonistic employment of medicines, they had long since discovered the grand truth, THAT THE TRUE RADICAL HEALING ART MUST BE FOUND IN THE EXACT OPPOSITE OF SUCH AN ANTIPATHIC TREATMENT OF THE SYMPTOMS OF DISEASE; they would have become convinced, that as a medicinal action antagonistic to the symptoms of the disease (an antipathically employed medicine) is followed by only transient relief, and after that is passed, by invariable aggravation, the converse of that procedure, the homoeopathic employment of medicines according to similarity of symptoms, must effect a permanent and perfect cure, if at the same time the opposite of their large doses, the most minute doses, are exhibited. But neither the obvious aggravation that ensued from their antipathic treatment, nor the fact that no physician ever effected a permanent cure of disease of considerable or of long standing unless some homoeopathic medicinal agent was accidentally a chief ingredient in his prescription, nor yet the circumstances that all the rapid and perfect cures that nature ever performed (§ 46), were always effected by the supervention upon the old disease of one of a similar character, ever taught them, during such a long series of centuries, this truth, the knowledge of which can alone conduce to the benefit of the sick.

EXPLANATION

Physicians never thought seriously on the sad results of the antagonistic employment of medicines.

- ✦ If they would have thought seriously they would have found that the true radical healing art must be explored in exactly opposite of antipathic treatment of the symptoms of d/s by homoeopathic employment of medicines according to the similarity of symptoms.

- The antipathic or antagonistic action of medicine is followed by only short relief & aggravation thereafter
- Whereas Homeopathic action of medicine based on similarity of symptoms gives permanent & perfect cure
- The allopathic system uses large doses but in Homoeopathy much minute doses are used.
- But the ordinary physician neither learned from the aggravation that occured by their antipathic treatment, nor from the fact that no physician ever affected a permanent cure of d/s of long standing, nor they observed nature in her mode of treatment [aphorism 46].
- They were far behind the truth, the knowledge of healing the sick.

§ 62

HAHNEMANN WAS FIRST TO OBSERVE HEALING ART

But on what this pernicious result of the palliative, antipathic treatment and the efficacy of the reverse, the homoeopathic treatment, depend, is explained by the following facts, deduced from manifold observations, which no one before me perceived, though they are so very palpable and so very evident, and are of such infinite importance to the healing art.

EXPLANATION

In this aphorism Hahnemann says that he was the first physician to observe the very evident & important art of healing.

How palliative, antipathic treatment is harmful & the Homeopathic treatment the healing art is explained by the following facts in coming aphorism.

- Hahnemann deduced all this from many observations he made, which no one before him could observe & make note of.

§ 63

PRIMARY ACTION & SECONDARY ACTION

Every agent that acts upon the vitality, every medicine, deranges more or less the vital force, and causes a certain alteration in the health of the individual for a longer or a shorter period. This is termed primary action. Although a product of the medicinal and vital powers conjointly, it

is principally due to the former power. To its action our vital force endeavors to oppose its own energy. This resistant action is a property, is indeed an automatic action of our life-preserving power, which goes by the name of secondary action or counteraction.

EXPLANATION

Every agent & every medicine both, more or less derange the vital force & act upon the vitality.

- This causes a certain change in the health of the individual for a shorter or a longer period. This is called 'Primary action'.
- This primary action is mainly due to the medicinal power.

As we know every action has a reaction

- So to its action our vital force oppose its own energy, This resistent action is automatic action of our life-preserving power called secondary action or counteraction.

§ 64

COUNTERACTION & CURATIVE ACTION

During the primary action of the artificial morbific agents (medicines) on our healthy body, as seen in the following examples, our vital force seems to conduct itself merely in a passive (receptive) manners, and appears, so to say, compelled to permit the impressions of the artificial power acting from without to take place in it and thereby after its state of health; it then, however, appears to rouse itself again, as it were, and to develop (A) the exact opposite condition of health (counteraction, secondary action) to this effect (primary action) produced upon it, if there be such an opposite, and that in as great a degree as was the effect (primary action) of the artificial morbific agent on it, and proportionate to its own energy; – or (B) if there be not in nature a state exactly the opposite of the primary action, it appears to endeavor to indifferentiate itself, that is, to make its superior power available in the extinction of the change wrought in it from without (by the medicine), in the place of which it substitutes its normal state (secondary action, curative action).

EXPLANATION

When the artificial morbific agents [medicines] are given to the healthy person, the primary action of medicines acts on the vital force.

The vital force permits the impressions of the artificial power & it alters the state of health of body, this is the primary action of medicine on the vital force.

Now every action has a reaction.

A] The vital force in reaction produces the exact opposite condition of health called counteraction/ secondary action in reaction to the primary action.

This occurs if there is an opposite & as great action, as was the primary action of medicine on it & proportionate to its own energy [Counteraction or secondary action]

B] If it is not exactly the opposite of the primary action the vital force makes its superior power to extinct the change brought upon the vital force by medicine & brings its normal state [secondary action, curative action]

In both above cases by counteraction or by curative action the vital force brings body back to normal state by opposing the change brought to the vital force by the medicinal agent[Primary action].

§ 65

EXAMPLES OF COUNTERACTION

Examples of (A) are familiar to all. A hand bathed in hot water is at first much warmer than the other hand that has not been so treated (primary action); but when it is withdrawn from the hot water and again thoroughly dried, it becomes in a short time cold, and at length much colder than the other (secondary action). A person heated by violent exercise (primary action) is afterwards affected with chilliness and shivering (secondary action). To one who was yesterday heated by drinking much wine (primary action), today every breath of air feels too cold (counteraction of the organism, secondary action). An arm that has been kept long in very cold water is at first much paler and colder (primary action) than the other; but removed from the cold water and dried, it subsequently becomes not only warmer than the other, but even hot, red and inflamed (secondary action, reaction of the vital force). Excessive vivacity follows the use of strong coffee (primary action), but sluggishness and drowsiness remain for a long time afterwards (reaction, secondary action), if this be not always again removed for a short time by imbibing fresh supplies of coffee (palliative). After the profound stupefied sleep caused by opium (primary action), the following night will be all the more sleepless (reaction, secondary action). After the constipation produced by opium (primary action), diarrhoea ensues (secondary action); and after purgation with medicines that irritate the bowels, constipation of several days' duration ensues (secondary action). And in like manner it always happens, after the primary action of a medicine that produces in large doses a great change in the health of a healthy person, that its exact opposite, when, as has been observed, there is actually such a thing, is produced in the secondary action by our vital force.

EXPLANATION

- ✦ He says that examples of [A] (see Aphorism 64)to occur in body are known to all of us.
- ✦ Some of them are:--

E.g. The left hand is bathed in hot water, it becomes warmer than the right one [primary action], but when the left hand is removed from the hot water & dried, in short time it becomes colder than the other [secondary action]

E.g. A person doing violent exercise is heated [primary action] but after sometime he feels chilly & shivers [secondary action].

E.g. A person had wine yesterday is heated [primary action], but today air feels too cold to him [Counter-action, secondary action]

E.g. An arm if kept in very cold water for long becomes pales & colder [primary action] but when it is removed from cold water & dried it becomes hot, red & inflamed [secondary action reaction of the vital force].

E.g. Excessive use of strong coffee brings alertness [Primary action] but afterwards drowsiness occurs [reaction, secondary reaction]

E.g. Opium produces constipation [primary action], but afterwards diarrhoea occurs [secondary action]

Thus we see that after the primary action of a medicine great change in the health of a healthy person occur exactly opposite in nature due to secondary action by our vital force.

§ 66

TWO TYPES OF ACTION

An obvious antagonistic secondary action, however, is, as may readily be conceived, not to be noticed from the action of quite minute homoeopathic doses of the deranging agents on the healthy body. A small dose of every one of them certainly produces a primary action that is perceptible to a sufficiently attentive; but the living organism employs against it only so much reaction (secondary action) as is necessary for the restoration of the normal condition.

EXPLANATION

- This antagonistic secondary action may not be noticed from the minute Homeopathic doses used on the healthy body.
- A small dose of the Homeopathic medicine produces a primary action [Observed only by a attentive observer]but the living organism produces against it only that much reaction [Secondary action] as it is necessary for restoration of the normal condition.
- It means the secondary action is very minute due to minute Homeopathic dose & the person is cured back to health.

§ 67

ALLOPATHIC PALLIATION REQUIRED IN SOME CASES

These incontrovertible truths, which spontaneously offer themselves to our notice and experience, explain to us the beneficial action that takes place under homoeopathic treatment; while, on the other hand, they demonstrate the perversity of the antipathic and palliative treatment of diseases with antagonistically acting medicines.1

1 Only in the most urgent cases, where danger to life and imminent death allow no time for the action of a homoeopathic remedy – not hours, sometimes not even quarter-hours, and scarcely minutes – in sudden accidents occurring to previously healthy individuals – for example, in asphyxia and suspended animation from lightning, from suffocation, freezing, drowning, etc. – is it admissible and judicious, at all events as a preliminary measure to stimulate the irritability and sensibility (the physical life) with a palliative, as for instance, with gentle electrical shocks, with clysters of strong coffee, with a stimulating odor, gradual application of heat, etc. When this stimulation is effected, the play of the vital organs again goes on in its former healthy manner, for there is here no disease* to be removed, but merely an obstruction and suppression of the healthy vital force. To this category belong various antidotes to sudden poisoning: alkalies from mineral acids, hepar sulphuris for metallic poisons, coffee and camphora (and ipecacuanha) for poisoning by opium, etc.

It does not follow that a homoeopathic medicine has been ill selected for a case of disease because some of the medicinal symptoms are only antipathic to some of the less important and minor symptoms of the disease; if only the others, the stronger well-marked (characteristic), and peculiar symptoms of the disease are covered and matched by the same medicine with similarity of symptoms – that is to say, overpowered, destroyed and extinguished; the few opposite symptoms also disappear of themselves after the expiry of the term of action of the medicament, without retarding the cure in the least.

* And yet the new sect that mixes the two systems appeals (though in vain) to this observation, in order that they may have an excuse for encountering everywhere such exceptions to the general rule in diseases, and to justify their convenient employment of allopathic palliatives, and of other injurious allopathic trash besides, solely for the sake of sparing themselves the trouble of seeking for the suitable homoeopathic remedy for each case of disease – and thus conveniently appear as homoeopathic physicians, without being such. But their performances are on a par with the system they pursue; they are corrupting.

EXPLANATION

- In nature and by experience these undeniable truths explain us the beneficial action of homeopathic treatment.
- On the other hand, they also demonstrate the unpleasant antipathic & palliative treatment of d/s by antagonistically acting medicines.

Footnote 1:
- In most urgent cases, where there is danger to life & imminent death risk. It does not allow time for action of a homeopathic remedy -we have time of minutes or hours or less than hours.

E.g. In cases of asphyxia, lightning, suffocation, freezing, drowning etc, it becomes necessary to stimulate the sensibility [the physical life]with a palliative treatment like- gentle electrical shocks, strong coffee, stimulating odour, application of heat etc as we have no time for the action of a homoeoapthic remedy.

In these cases there is no d/s to be removed but only an obstruction & suppression of the healthy vital force, by these stimulation the vital organs again goes on in its former healthy manner [as it is not diseased or deranged]

E.g- Antidotes to sudden poisonings

- ✦ Alkali for mineral acids
- ✦ Coffee & camphor for opium poisoning.

But some Homeoapthic physicians mix the two systems based on above observation & employ allopathic palliative & other allopathic methods to avoid trouble of selecting the suitable Homoepathic remedy for each case of d/s. They are not true Homeopathic physician.

Those palliative methods are only applicable in most urgent cases, where no disease is to be removed.

§ 68

ADVANTAGE OF HOMEOPATHY

In homoeopathic cures they show us that from the uncommonly small doses of medicine (§§ 275 – 287) required in this method of treatment, which are just sufficient, by the similarity of their symptoms, to overpower and remove from the sensation of the life principle the similar natural disease there certainly remains, after the destruction of the latter, at first a certain amount of medicinal disease alone in the organism, but, on account of the extraordinary minuteness of the dose, it is so transient, so slight, and disappears so rapidly of its own accord, that the vital force has no need to employ, against this small artificial derangement of its health, any more considerable reaction than will suffice to elevate its present state of health up to the healthy point – that is, than will suffice to effect complete recovery, for which after the extinction of the previous morbid derangement but little effort is required (§ 64, B).

EXPLANATION

In Homeopathic cure [aphorism 275-287] small doses of medicine is required, these medicines by the similarity of their symptoms, in minute doses overpower & remove the similar natural d/s

- After the similar natural d/s is removed, now a certain amount of medicinal d/s is left in the organism.
- On account of the extraordinary minuteness of the dose this medicinal d/s is so short-lived, so slight & it disappears rapidly of its own.
- The vital force has no need to employ any more reaction to elevate it's present State of health up to the healthy point I.e-Complete recovery occurs, for which, after removal of the previous morbid derangement little effort is required [aphorism 64, B].

§ 69

DISADVANTAGE OF ANTIPATHY

In the antipathic (palliative) mode of treatment, however precisely the reverse of this takes place. The medicinal symptom which the physician opposes to the disease symptom (for example, the insensibility and stupefaction caused by opium in its primary action to acute pain) is certainly not alien, not allopathic of the latter; there is a manifest relation of the medicinal symptom to the disease symptom, but it is the reverse of what should be; it is here intended that the annihilation of the disease symptom shall be effected by an opposite medicinal symptom, which is nevertheless impossible. No doubt the antipathically chosen medicine touches precisely the same diseased point in the organism as the homoeopathic medicine chosen on account of the similar affection it produces; but the former covers the opposite symptom of the disease only as an opposite, and makes it unobservable to our life principle for a short time only, so that in the first period of the action of the antagonistic palliative the vital force perceives nothing disagreeable from either if the two (neither from the disease symptom nor from the medicinal symptom), as they seem both to have mutually removed and dynamically neutralized one another as it were (for example, the stupefying power of opium does this to the pain). In the first minutes the vital force feels quite well, and perceives neither the stupefaction of the opium nor the pain of the disease. But as the antagonistic medicinal symptom cannot (as in the homoeopathic treatment) occupy the place of the morbid derangement present in the organism in the sensation of the life principle as a similar, stronger (artificial) disease, and cannot, therefore, like a homoeopathic medicine, affect the vital force with a similar artificial disease, so as to be able to step into the place of the original natural morbid derangement, the palliative medicine must, as a thing totally differing from, and the opposite of the disease derangement, leave the latter uneradicated; it renders it, as before said, by a semblance of dynamic neutralization,1 at first unfelt by the vital force, but, like every medicinal disease, it is soon spontaneously extinguished, and not only leaves the disease behind, just as it was, but compels the vital force (as it must, like all palliatives, be given in large doses in order to effect the apparent removal) to produce an opposite condition (§§ 63,64) to this palliative medicine, the reverse of the medicinal action, consequently the analogue of the still present, undestroyed, natural morbid derangement, which is necessarily strengthened and increased2 by this addition (reaction against the palliative) produced by the vital force. The disease symptom (this single part of the disease) consequently becomes worse after the term of the action of the palliative has expired; worse in proportion to the magnitude of the dose of the palliative. Accordingly (to keep to the same example) the larger the dose of opium given to allay the pain, so much the more does the pain increase beyond its original intensity as soon as the opium has exhausted its action.3

1 In the living human being no permanent neutralization of contrary or antagonistic sensations can take place, as happens with substances of opposite qualities in the chemical laboratory, where, for instance, sulphuric acid and potash unite to form a perfectly different substance, a neutral salt, which is now no longer either acid or alkali, and is not decomposed even by heat. Such amalgamations and thorough combinations to form something permanently neutral and indifferent do not, as has been said, ever take place with respect to synamic impressions of an antagonistic nature in our sensific apparatus. Only a semblance of neutralization and mutual removal occurs in such cases at first, but the antagonistic sensations do not permanently remove one another. The tears of the mourner will be dried for but a short time by a laughable play; the jokes are, however, soon forgotten, and his tears then flow still more abundantly than before.

2 Plain as this proposition is, it has been misunderstood, and in opposition to it some have asserted "that the palliative in its secondary action, would then be similar to the disease present, must be capable of curing just as well as a homoeopathic medicine does by its primary action." But they did not reflect that the secondary action is not a product of the medicine, but invariably of the antagonistically acting vital force of the organism; that therefore this secondary action resulting from the vital force on the employment of a palliative is a state similar to the symptoms of the disease which the palliative left uneradicated, and which the reaction of the vital force against the palliative consequently increased still more.

3 As when in a dark dungeon, where the prisoner could with difficulty recognize objects close to him, alcohol is suddenly lighted, everything is instantly illuminated in a most consolatory manner to the unhappy wretch; but when it is extinguished, the brighter the flame was previously the blacker is the night which now envelopes him, and renders everything about him much more difficult to be seen than before.

EXPLANATION

In the antipathic (palliative) mode of treatment the reverse of this takes place. The medicinal symptom which the physician opposes to the disease symptom are reverse of what should be.

e.g. the insensibility and stupefaction caused by opium in its primary action to acute pain. Opium is given to reduce the pain.

It is expected that the annihilation of the disease symptom shall be effected by an opposite medicinal symptom, which is never possible.

Let us understand this with an example. When the stupefying power of opium is given for the symptom of pain. In the first minutes the vital force feels quite well and it neither perceives the stupefaction of the opium nor the pain of the disease. But as the antagonistic medicinal symptom cannot occupy the place of the morbid derangement present in the organism in the sensation of the life principle as a similar, stronger (artificial) disease, and cannot affect the vital force with a similar artificial disease and cannot step into the place of the original natural morbid derangement and leaves the disease uneradicated. It renders it, by the semblance of dynamic neutralization, at first unfelt by the vital force. Like every medicinal disease, it is soon spontaneously extinguished and leaves the disease behind just as it was but compels the vital force to produce an opposite condition (aphorism 63,64) to this palliative medicine, the reverse of the medicinal action, analogous to the undestroyed natural morbid derangement which is increased by this addition (reaction against the palliative) produced by the vital force.

The disease symptom consequently becomes worse after the term of the action of the palliative has expired. The extent of worse action occurs in proportion to the magnitude of the dose of the palliative given.

Accordingly the larger the dose of opium given to allay the pain, so much the more does the pain increase beyond its original intensity as soon as the opium action is exhausted.

Footnote 1:
In the living human being no permanent neutralization of antagonistic sensations can take place. This happens only with substances of opposite qualities in the chemical laboratory e.g. sulphuric acid and potash unite to form a perfectly different substance, a neutral salt, which is now no longer acidic or basic and is not decomposed even by heat.

Such combinations to form something permanently neutral and indifferent do not take place with respect to dynamic impressions of an antagonistic nature in our body.

Only a semblance of neutralization and mutual removal occurs in such cases at first, but the antagonistic sensations do not permanently remove one another. e.g. the tears of the mourner will be dried for a short time by a laughable play or jokes but as soon as the jokes are forgotten his tears then flow still more abundantly than before.

Footnote 2:
It has been misunderstood that the palliative in its secondary action, which would be similar to the disease present, must be capable of curing like a homoeopathic medicine does by its primary action.

But they did not reflect that the secondary action is not a product of the medicine, but product of the antagonistically acting vital force of the organism. Therefore this secondary action resulting from the vital force due to employment of a palliative is a state similar to the disease symptoms, which the palliative left uneradicated and increased too.

Footnote 3:
In a dark prison, where the prisoner could recognise objects with difficulty. If alcohol is suddenly lighted, everything is instantly illuminated but when it is extinguished, the brighter the flame was, the blacker is the darkness and makes everything around him more difficult to be seen than before.

§ 70

SUMMERY

From what has been already adduced we cannot fail to draw the following inferences:

That everything of a really morbid character and which ought to be cured that the physician can discover in diseases consists solely of the sufferings of the patient, and the sensible alterations in his health, in a word, solely of the totality of the symptoms, by means of which the disease demands the medicine requisite for its relief; while, on the other hand, every internal cause attributed to it, every occult quality or imaginary material morbific principle, is nothing but an idle dream;

That this derangement of the state of health, which we term disease, can only be converted into health by another revolution effected in the state of health by means of medicines, whose sole curative power, consequently, can only consist in altering man's state of health – that is to say, in a peculiar excitation of morbid symptoms, and is learned with most distinctness and purity by testing them on the healthy body;

That, according to all experience, a natural disease can never be cured by medicines that possess the power of producing in the healthy individual an alien morbid state (dissimilar morbid symptoms) differing from that of the disease to be cured (never, therefore, by an allopathic mode of treatment), and that even in nature no cure ever takes place in which an inherent disease is removed, annihilated and cured by the addition of another disease dissimilar to it, be the new one ever so strong;

That, moreover, all experience proves that, by means of medicines which have a tendency to produce in the healthy individual an artificial morbid symptom, antagonistic to the single symptom of disease sought to be cured, the cure of a long-standing affection will never be effected, but merely a very transientalleviation, always follows by its aggravation; and that, in a word, this antipathic and merely palliative treatment in long-standing diseases of a serious character is absolutely inefficacious;

That, however, the third and only other possible mode of treatment (the homoeopathic), in which there is employed for the totality of the symptoms of a natural disease a medicine capable of producing the most similar symptoms possible in the healthy individual, given in suitable dose, is the only efficacious remedial method whereby diseases, which are purely dynamic deranging irritations of the vital force, are overpowered, and being thus easily, perfectly and permanently extinguished, must necessarily cease to exist. This is brought about by means of the stronger similar deranging irritation of the homoeopathic medicine in the sensation of the life principle. – and for this mode of procedure we have the example of unfettered Nature herself, when to an old disease there is added a new one similar to the first, whereby the new one is rapidly and forever annihilated and cured.

EXPLANATION

In this aphorism he has drawn the following inferences:-

A] When a sick person comes to the physician, the sole importance is to give relief to the sufferings of the patient & the sensible alterations in his health.
In short, to give relief solely of the totality of the symptoms, through which d/s demands medicine for its relief.
- On the other hand, trying to find out or explain every imaginary material morbific principle is nothing but a dream & of no use to sick.

B] This derangement of the state of health is termed disease. It can be converted to health by means of medicines, whose sole curative power is altering man's state of health.

C] As we have seen in nature also no cure occurs by addition of dissimilar d/s to original d/s be the new dissimilar d/s be ever so strong.
According to all experience, a natural d/s can never be cured by medicines that have power of producing dissimilar morbid symptoms[In the healthy individual] differing from that of the d/s to be cured, therefore allopathic mode of treatment cannot bring cure.

D] The anti- pathic & only palliative treatment in long -standing d/s of a serious character has no use & can never cure it.
- By Use of medicines producing an artificial morbid symptom [in healthy individual], antagonistic [opposite]to the single symptom of d/s to be cured, the cure of long -standing d/s will never occur. In this case only short relief occurs followed by d/s aggravation.

E] The third & the only possible mode of treatment is the homeopathic. Here a medicine which produces the most similar symptoms possible in the healthy individual is employed for the totality of the symptoms of a natural d/s in suitable dose is the only remedial method, where d/s, which are dynamic derangement of vital force, are overpowered & are permanently & easily removed from the body.
For this mode of procedure we have example of nature herself, where an old d/s is rapidly cured when a new similar d/s is added to the first.

§ 71

3 POINTS TO NECESSARY TO CURING

As it is now no longer a matter of doubt that the diseases of mankind consist merely of groups of certain symptoms, and may be annihilated and transformed into health by medicinal substances, but only by such as are capable of artificially producing similar morbid symptoms (and such is the process in all genuine cures), hence the operation of curing is comprised in the three following points:

I. How is the physician to ascertain what is necessary to be known in order to cure the disease?

II. How is he to gain a knowledge of the instruments adapted for the cure of the natural disease, the pathogenetic powers of the medicines?

III. What is the most suitable method of employing these artificial morbific agents (medicines) for the cure of natural disease?

EXPALNATION

Thus it is very clear now that the d/s of mankind consist of groups of certain symptoms.

The d/s maybe annihilated & transformed into health by medicinal substances capable of producing similar morbid symptom in healthy individual.

- ✦ Hence the operation of curing consists of 3 points:-
    1. How physician ascertain that what is necessary he should know in order to cure the d/s?
    2. How he will gain knowledge of pathogenetic powers of medicines.
    3. What is the most suitable method of employing these medicines for the cure of natural d/s?

§ 72

ACUTE & CHRONIC D/S

With respect to the first point, the following will serve as a general preliminary view. The disease to which man is liable are either rapid morbid processes of the abnormally deranged vital force, which have a tendency to finish their course more or less quickly, but always in a moderate time – these are termed acute diseases; – or they are diseases of such a character that, with small, often imperceptible beginnings, dynamically derange the living organism, each in its own peculiar manner, and cause it gradually to deviate from the healthy condition, in such a way that the automatic life energy, called vital force, whose office is to preserve the health, only opposes to them at the commencement and during their progress imperfect, unsuitable, useless resistance, but is unable of itself to extinguish them, but must helplessly suffer (them to spread and) itself to be ever more and more abnormally deranged, until at length the organism is destroyed; these are termed chronic diseases. They are caused by infection with a chronic miasm.

EXPLANATION

- For the first point, the following will serve as a general view.
- Acute d/s: Acute d/s are the d/s, an abnormally deranged vital force, which have tendency to finish their course more or less quickly but always in a moderate time.
- Chronic d/s: The d/s with small, often imperceptible beginnings, which dynamically derange the living organism and cause it gradually to deviate from the healthy condition, Here the vital force

opposes them imperfectly at the beginnings & during their progress but is unable to extinguish them by itself. The person suffers helplessly & vital force becomes more & more abnormally deranged. Finally at length, the organism is destroyed, these are termed chronic d/s.
They are caused by dynamic infection with a chronic miasm.

§ 73

ACUTE D/S

As regards acute diseases, they are either of such a kind as attack human beings individually, the exciting cause being injurious influences to which they were particularly exposed. Excesses in food, or an insufficient supply of it, severe physical impression, chills, over heatings, dissipation, strains, etc., or physical irritations, mental emotions, and the like, are exciting causes of such acute febrile affections; in reality, however, they are generally only a transient explosion of latent psora, which spontaneously returns to its dormant state if the acute diseases were not of too violent a character and were soon quelled. Or they are of such a kind as attack several persons at the same time, here and there (sporadically), by means of meteoric or telluric influences and injurious agents, the susceptibility for being morbidly affected by which is possessed by only a few persons at one time. Allied to these are those diseases in which many persons are attacked with very similar sufferings from the same cause (epidemically); these diseases generally become infectious (contagious) when they prevail among thickly congregated masses of human beings. Thence arise fevers1, in each instance of a peculiar nature, and, because the cases of disease have an identical origin, they set up in all those they affect an identical morbid process, which when left to itself terminates in a moderate period of time in death or recovery. The calamities of war, inundations and famine are not infrequently their exciting causes and producers – sometimes they are peculiar acute miasms which recur in the same manner (hence known by some traditional name), which either attack persons but once in a lifetime, as the smallpox, measles, whooping-cough, the ancient, smooth, bright red scarlet fever2 of Sydenham, the mumps, etc., or such as recur frequently in pretty much the same manner, the plague of the Levant, the yellow fever of the sea-coast, the Asiatic cholera, etc.

1 The homoeopathic physician, who does not entertain the foregone conclusion devised by the ordinary school (who have fixed upon a few names of such fevers, besides which mighty nature dare not produce any others, so as to admit of their treating these disease according to some fixed method), does not acknowledge the names goal fever, bilious fever, typhus fever, putrid fever, nervous fever or mucous fever, but treats them each according to their several peculiarities.

2 Subsequently to the year 1801 a kind of pupura miliaris (roodvonk), which came from the West, was by physicians confounded with the scarlet fever, notwithstanding that they exhibited totally different symptoms, that the latter found its prophylatic and curative remedy in belladonna, the former in aconite, and that the former was generally merely sporadic, while the latter was invariable

epidemic. Of late years it seems as if the two occasionally joined to form an eruptive fever of a peculiar kind, for which neither the one nor the other remedy, alone, will be found to be exactly homoeopathic.

EXPLANATION

- Acute d/s, attack human beings individually or attacks several persons.
- The exciting cause is injurious influences like excess in food or an insufficient supply of it, severe physical impressions, chills, overheating, dissipation, strains etc or physical irritations, mental emotions etc.
- In reality, they are only a transient explosion of latent psora which, if acute d/s are not too violent, returns to its dormant state.
- They attack several persons at the same time, here & there [spordically], the cause is meteoric or telluric influences & injurious agents.
  The susceptibility for being affected is possessed by only a few persons at one time.
- Those d/s in which many persons are attacked with very similar sufferings from the same cause is called epidemic d/s
- These d/s generally become infections [contagious] when it occurs in thickly populated areas.
- Then fevers of a peculiar nature [we don't categorize fever as ordinary school does eg.-typhus fever, typhoid fever, bilious fever etc]arise, As the cases of d/s have an identical origin, they setup identical morbid process in all those they affect.
  If it is left to itself, no medicine is given, it terminates in a moderate period of time in death or recovery.
- Calamities of war, inundations & famine are frequently their exciting causes & producers -sometimes peculiar acute miasms, which recur in the same manner.
  They either attack person once in a lifetime, as smallpox, measles, whooping cough, red scarlet fever of sydenham, mumps etc. Or recur in the pretty same manner e. g- Plague of the levant, yellow fever of sea-coast, the asiatic cholera etc.

Footnote 1:
The homoeopathic physician does not follow these conclusions of ordinary school who have given fixed names of such fevers, like Gaol fever, typhus fever, typhus fever, putrid fever, nervous fever or mucous fever but treats them each According to their peculiarities.

Footnote 2:
In year 1801, a kind of purpura miliaris [roodvonk], was confused by physician with scarlet fever, but curative remedy of scarlet fever was belladonna & of purpura miliaris was aconite, scarlet fever was epidemic & other merely sporadic.

- ✦ Later it seemed as if two joined to form an eruptive fever of a peculiar kind for which neither belladonna nor aconite was the homoeapthic remedy.

§ 74

CHRONIC D/S

Among chronic diseases we must still, alas!, reckon those so commonly met with, artificially produced in allopathic treatment by the prolonged use of violent heroic medicines in large and increasing doses, by the abuse of calomel, corrosive sublimate, mercurial ointment, nitrate of silver, iodine and its ointments, opium, valerian, cinchona bark and quinine, foxglove, prussic acid, sulphur and sulphuric acid, perennial purgatives1, venesections, shedding streams of blood, leeches, issues, setons, etc., whereby the vital energy is sometimes weakened to an unmerciful extent, sometimes, if it do not succumb, gradually abnormally deranged (by each substance in a peculiar manner) in such a way that, in order to maintain life against these inimical and destructive attacks, it must produce a revolution in the organism, and either deprive some part of its irritability and sensibility, or exalt these to an excessive degree, cause dilatation or contraction, relaxation or induration or even total destruction of certain parts, and develop faulty organic alterations here and there in the interior or the exterior (cripple the body internally or externally), in order to preserve the organism from complete destruction of the life by the ever – renewed, hostile assaults of such destructive forces.3

1 The only possible case of plethora shows itself with the healthy woman, several days before her monthly period, with a feeling of a certain fullness of womb and breasts, but without inflammation.

2 Among all imaginable methods for the relief of sickness, no greater allopathic, irrational or inappropriate one can be thought of than this Brousseauic, debilitating treatment by means of venesection and hunger diet, which for many years has spread over a large part of the earth. No intelligent man can see in it anything medical, or medically helpful, whereas real medicines, even if chosen blindly and administered to a patient, may at times prove of benefit in a given case of sickness because they may accidentally have been homoeopathic to the case. But from venesection, healthy common sense can expect nothing more than certain lessening and shortening of life. It is a sorrowful and wholly groundless fallacy that most and indeed all diseases depend on local inflammation. Even for true local inflammation, the most certain and quickest cure is found in medicines capable of taking away dynamically the arterial irritation upon which the inflammation is based and this without the least loss of fluids and strength. Local venesections, even from the affected part, only tend to increase renewed inflammation of these parts. And precisely so it is generally inappropriate, aye, murderous to take away many pounds of blood from the veins in inflammatory fevers, when a few appropriate medicines would dispel this irritated arterial state, driving the hitherto quiet blood together with the disease in a few hours without the least loss of fluids and strength. Such great loss of blood is evidently irreplaceable for the remaining continuance of life, since the organs intended by the Creator for bloodmaking have thereby become so weakened that while they may manufacture blood in the same quantity but not again of the same good quality. And how impossible is it for this imagined plethora to have been produced in such remarkable rapidity and so to drain it off by frequent venesections

when yet an hour before the pulse of this heated patient (before the fever and chill stage) was so quiet. No man, no sick person has ever too much blood or too much strength. On the contrary, every sick man lacks strength, otherwise his vital energy would have prevented the development of the disease. Thus it is irrational and cruel to add to this weakened patient, a greater, indeed the most serious source of debility that can be imagined. It is a murderous malpractice irrational and cruel based on a wholly groundless and absurd theory instead of taking away his disease which is ever dynamic and only to be removed by dynamic potencies.

EXPLANATION

Among the chronic d/s we must recall those commonly caused by allopathic treatment by use of violent medicines in large & increasing doses for prolonged time.

- These allopathic medicines artifically produce a chronic d/s in human, e.g- Abuse of calomel, corrosive bark & quinine, sulphur, opium, nitrate of silver, iodine & its ointment, opium, cinchona bark & quinine, sulphur & sulphuric acid, purgatives, venesections, shedding streams of blood, leeches, issues, setons etc.
- By these methods the vital energy is weakened to great extent, gradually, it is abnormally deranged in such a way that in order to maintain life against these destructive attacks, it brings changes in the body.
- It produces a revolution in the organism & either some part of the body is deprived of its irritability & sensibility or, raises these to an excessive degree cause dilation or contraction in body organs, relaxation or induration or even total destruction of certain parts & develop organic changes in the interior or the exterior.
- This vital energy does in order to preserve the organism from complete destruction of life caused by these assaults of such destructive forces.

Footnote 1:
Plethora shows itself in a healthy woman, several days before her monthly period, with a feeling of fullness of womb and breasts, but without inflammation.

Footnote 2:
He explains the unmerciful treatment done by physician of that time.

- The Brousseau's mode of treatment is the most irrational & inappropriate method of treatment. Allopathic treatment is better than this Brousseauic.
  Brousseau's treatment is a debilitating & hunger diet [see aph-60]
- It is never medicinally helpful. The real medicines even if they are chosen blindly may prove beneficial in a given case of sickness because they may accidentally have been homoeopathic to the case.
- But from methods by Brousseau, like venesection we can only expect shortening of life. Local venesections, even from the affected part, only tends to increase renewed inflammation of these parts.

- It is inappropriate, murderous act to remove pounds of blood from veins in cases of inflammatory fevers.
- Such organs of blood making have become, so weak that may produce blood in the same quantity but not of same good quality.
- Every sick man lacks strength, otherwise his vital energy would have prevented the d/s development in the body, thus it is irrational & cruel to add to this weakened patient a source of debility, it is a murderous malpractice irrational & cruel.
- D/s should be removed only by dynamic potencies[as homoeopathy does]

§ 75

INCURABLE

These inroads on human health effected by the allopathic non-healing art (more particularly in recent times) are of all chronic diseases the most deplorable, the most incurable; and I regret to add that it is apparently impossible to discover or to hit upon any remedies for their cure when they have reached any considerable height.

EXPLANATION

- Of all the chronic d/s, these effects on human health caused by the Allopathic non-healing art is the most incurable one,
- It becomes impossible to discover or hit any remedies for their cure when they have reached the height in human body.

§ 76

VITAL-FORCE DAMAGED

Only for natural diseases has the beneficent Deity granted us, in Homoeopathy, the means of affording relief; but those devastations and maimings of the human organism exteriorly and interiorly, effected by years, frequently, of the unsparing exercise of a false art,1 with its hurtful drugs and treatment, must be remedied by the vital force itself (appropriate aid being given for the eradication of any chronic miasm that may happen to be lurking in the background), if it has not already been too much weakened by such mischievous acts, and can devote several years

to this huge operation undisturbed. A human healing art, for the restoration to the normal state of those innumerable abnormal conditions so often produced by the allopathic non-healing art, there is not and cannot be.

1 If the patient succumbs, the practiser of such a treatment is in the habit of pointing out to the sorrowing relatives, at the post-mortem examination, these internal organic disfigurements, which are due to his pseudo-art, but which he artfully maintains to be the original incurable disease (see my book, Die Alloopathie, ein Wort deh Warnung an Kranke jeder Art, Leipzig, bei Baumgartner [translated in Lesser Writings]). Those deceitful records, the illustrated works on pathological anatomy, exhibit the products of such lamentable bungling. Deceased people from the country and those from the poor of cities who have died without such bungling with hurtful measures are not opened up through pathological anatomy as a rule. Such corruption and deformities would not be found in their corpses. From this fact can be judged the value of the evidence drawn from these beautiful illustrations as well as of the honesty of these authors and book makers.

EXPLANATION

- For natural d/s [which do not occur due to wrong treatment], the god has given us Homeopathy as the relief or cure.
  But the destruction & permanent damage caused to human body interiorly and exteriorly by false art for years with hurtful drugs & treatment now must be remedied by the vital force itself, though appropriate aid is eradication of any chronic miasm that may be present in the background.
- Now vital force will be able to do so only it has not been too much weakened by such acts & takes several years if not disturbed.
- For those all abnormal conditions which are produced by the allopathic non-healing art there is no human healing art.

Footnote 1:
If the patient dies, the practisers of such a treatment points out to the sorrowing relatives, at the Post-mortem examination that these internal organic disfigurement, which really are due to his pseudo-art, but he artfully claims it to be the original incurable disease.

This way such corruption and deformities goes un- noticed

§ 77

FALSE CHRONIC D/S

Those diseases are inappropriately named chronic, which persons incur who expose themselves continually to avoidable noxious influences, who are in the habit of indulging in injurious liquors or aliments, are addicted to dissipation of many kinds which undermine the health, who

undergo prolonged abstinence from things that are necessary for the support of life, who reside in unhealthy localities, especially marshy districts, who are housed in cellars or other confined dwellings, who are deprived of exercise or of open air, who ruin their health by overexertion of body or mind, who live in a constant state of worry, etc. These states of ill-health, which persons bring upon themselves, disappear spontaneously, provided no chronic miasm lurks in the body, under an improved mode of living, and they cannot be called chronic diseases.

EXPLANATION

Sometimes those d/s which occur due to exposure to noxious influences which can be avoided, they cannot be called chronic d/s.

E.g. A person who has habit of taking injurious liquors or ailments or who undergo prolonged abstinence from things that are necessary for the support of life.

- ✦ Who reside in unhealthy areas especially marshy districts
- ✦ Who are deprived of confined dwellings.
- ✦ Who ruin their health by over exertion of body or mind or Who live in constant worry etc.

These states of ill-health, which persons bring on themselves, it disappear spontaneously [provided no chronic miasm is present in the body], if mode of living is improved, so they cannot be called Chronic d/s.

§ 78

TRUE NATURAL, CHRONIC D/S

The true natural chronic diseases are those that arise from a chronic miasm, which when left to themselves, and unchecked by the employment of those remedies that are specific for them, always go on increasing and growing worse, notwithstanding the best mental and corporeal regimen, and torment the patient to the end of his life with ever aggravated sufferings. These, excepting those produced by medical malpractice (§ 74), are the most numerous and greatest scourges of the human race; for the most robust constitution, the best regulated mode of living and the most vigorous energy of the vital force are insufficient for their eradication.1

1 During the flourishing years of youth and with the commencement of regular menstruation joined to a mode of life beneficial to soul, heart and body, they remain unrecognized for years. Those afflicted appeal in perfect health to their relatives and acquaintances and the disease that was received by infection or inheritance seems to have wholly disappeared. But in later years, after adverse events and conditions of life, they are sure to appear anew and develop the more rapidly and assume a more serious character in proportion as the vital principle has become disturbed by debilitating passions, worry and care, but especially when disordered by inappropriate medicinal treatment.

EXPLANATION

- Those d/s that arise from a chronic miasm are called true natural chronic d/s.
- These d/s without employment of specific remedy, always go on increasing & grow worse.
- Even the best mental & corporeal regimen cannot help.
- It leads patient to the end of his life with aggravated sufferings.
- These, except those produced by malpractice of medicine [aph-74 allopathic medicine use], are the most numerous & greatest disaster of human because even the best mode of living and the most vigorous energy of the vital force are insufficient for their removal or eradication.

Footnote 1:
During youth years & the menarche [starting of menses] with a mode of life beneficial to soul, heart & body, these remain unrecognized for years.

- Those afflicted appear healthy to their relatives & the d/s that was received by infection or inheritance, it looks that it has disappeared totally.

But in later years, in adverse conditions of life & adverse events, they appear a new & develop more rapidly & are more serious as the vital principle has become disturbed by debilitating motions, worry & care & especially when it is disordered by inappropriate medicinal treatment.

§ 79

KNOWLEDGE OF SYPHILIS, SYCOSIS

Hitherto syphilis alone has been to some extent known as such a chronic miasmatic disease, which when uncured ceases only with the termination of life. Sycosis (the condylomatous disease), equally ineradicable by the vital force without proper medicinal treatment, was not recognized as a chronic miasmatic disease of a peculiar character, which it nevertheless undoubtedly is, and physicians imagined they had cured it when they had destroyed the growths upon the skin, but the persisting dyscrasia occasioned by it escaped their observation.

EXPLANATION

Until then syphilis alone was known as such a chronic miasmatic d/s.

- Syphilis if uncured ends only with the termination of life.
- Sycosis [the condylomatous d/s] is also equally ineradicable without proper medicinal treatment, but it was not recognized till then as a chronic miasmatic d/s.
- The physicians thought that they had cured it by destroying the growths upon the skin but abnormal disordered state still persisted in the body but it escaped their observation.

§ 80

PSORA

Incalculably greater and more important than the two chronic miasms just named, however, is the chronic miasm of psora, which, while those two reveal their specific internal dyscrasia, the one by the venereal chancre, the other by the cauliflower-like growths, does also, after the completion of the internal infection of the whole organism, announce by a peculiar cutaneous eruption, sometimes consisting only of a few vesicles accompanied by intolerable voluptuous tickling itching (and a peculiar odor), the monstrous internal chronic miasm – the psora, the only real fundamental cause and producer of all the other numerous, I may say innumerable, forms of disease1, which, under the names of nervous debility, hysteria, hypochondriasis, mania, melancholia, imbecility, madness, epilepsy and convulsions of all sorts, softening of the bones (rachitis), scoliosis and cyphosis, caries, cancer, fungus nematodes, neoplasms, gout, haemorrhoids, jaundice, cyanosis, dropsy, amenorrhoea, haemorrhage from the stomach, nose, lungs, bladder and womb, of asthma and ulceration of the lungs, of impotence and barrenness, of megrim, deafness, cataract, amaurosis, urinary calculus, paralysis, defects of the senses and pains of thousands of kinds, etc., figure in systematic works on pathology as peculiar, independent diseases.

1 I spent twelve years in investigating the source of this incredibly large number of chronic affections, in ascertaining and collecting certain proofs of this great truth, which had remained unknown to all former or contemporary observers, and in discovering at the same time the principal (antipsoric) remedies, which collectively are nearly a match for this thousand-headed monster of disease in all its different developments and forms. I have published my observations on this subject in the book entitled The Chronic Diseases (4 vols., Dresden, Arnold. [2nd edit., Dusseldorf, Schaub.]) before I had obtained this knowledge I could only treat the whole number of chronic diseases as isolated, individual maladies, with those medicinal substances whose pure effects had been tested on healthy persons up to that period, so that every case of chronic disease was treated by my disciples according to the group of symptoms it presented, just like an idiopathic disease, and it was often so for cured that sick mankind rejoiced at the extensive remedial treasures already amassed by the new healing art. How much greater cause is there now for rejoicing that the desired goal has been so much more nearly attained, inasmuch as the recently discovered and far more specific homoeopathic remedies for chronic affections arising from psora (properly termed antipsoric remedies) and the special instructions for their preparation and employment have been published; and from among them the true physician can now select for his curative agents those whose medicinal symptoms correspond in the most similar (homoeopathic) manner to the chronic disease he has to cure; and thus, by the employment of (antipsoric) medicines more suitable for this miasm, he is enabled to render more essential service and almost invariably to effect a perfect cure.

EXPLANATION

- In this aphorism he has talked about greater & more important than the two chronic miasms, the psora

As the other two miasms, syphilis reveal its specific internal dyscrasila by venereal chancre &sycosis by the cauliflower- like growth, the psora also does reveal itself after the complete internal infection of the whole organism.

The psora reveals itself by peculiar cutaneous eruption, sometimes which consist of a few vesicles with intolerable voluptuons tickling itching & a peculiar odour.

The psora is the only real fundamental cause & producer of all the other numerous forms of d/s, under the names like nervous debility, hysteria, hypochondriasis, mania, melan cholia, inbecility, madness, epilepsy & convulsion, softening of the bones [rachitis], scoliosis & cyphosis, caries, cancer, neoplasms, gout, haemorrhoids, jaundice, cyanosis, dropsy, amenorrhoea, haemorrhage from the stomach, nose, lungs, bladder & womb, asthma& ulceration of the lungs, impotence & barrenness, megrim, deafness, cataract, amaurosis, urinary calculus, paralysis, defects of the senses & pains of thousands of kinds etc.

Footnote:

He says that. 'I spent twelve years to investigate the source of this large numbers of chronic affections, in collecting certain proofs of this great truth, which was unknown to all former observers.

He at the same time discovered the principal [antipsoric] remedies for this monster of d/s. He has published his observations on this subject in the book 'THE CHRONIC DISEASES'

[4 Volumes, dresden, arnold[2nd edition, dusseldorf, schaub]

- He taught how to treat a number of chronic d/s with those medicinal substances whose pure effects had been tested on healthy persons upto that period.
  So every case of chronic d/s was treated by his disciples according to the group of symptoms it presented & it was cured. The sick mankind rejoiced at the extensive remedial new healing art.
- By now many antipsoric remedies have been discovered & the special instructions for their preparation & employment have been published.
- Now the true physician can select among those remedies his curative agents whose medicinal symptoms correspond in the most similar [Homoeopathic] manner to the chronic d/s he has to cure.
- By the employment of antipsoric medicine, he gives more essential service towards a perfect cure.

§ 81

DEVELOPMENT OF PSORA

The fact that this extremely ancient infecting agent has gradually passed, in some hundreds of generations, through many millions of human organisms and has thus attained an incredible

development, renders it in some measure conceivable how it can now display such innumerable morbid forms in the great family of mankind, particularly when we consider what a number of circumstances[1] contribute to the production of these great varieties of chronic diseases (secondary symptoms of psora), besides the indescribable diversity of men in respect of their congenital corporeal constitutions, so that it is no wonder if such a variety of injurious agencies, acting from within and from without and sometimes continually, on such a variety of organisms permeated with the psoric miasm, should produce an innumerable variety of defects, injuries, derangements and sufferings, which have hitherto been treated of in the old pathological works[2], under a number of special names, as diseases of an independent character.

1 Some of these causes that exercise a modifying influence on the transformation of psora into chronic diseases manifestly depend sometimes on the climate and the peculiar physical character of the place of abode, sometimes on the very great varieties in the physical and mental training of youth, both of which may have been neglected, delayed or carried to excess, or on their abuse in the business or conditions of life, in the matter of diet and regimen, passions, manners, habits and customs of various kinds.

2 How many improper ambiguous names do not these works contain, under each of which are included excessively different morbid conditions, which often resemble each other in one single symptom only, as ague, jaundice, dropsy, consumption, leucorrhoea, haemorrhoids, rheumatism, apoplexy, convulsions, hysteria, hypochondriasis, melancholia, mania, quinsy, palsy, etc., which are represented as diseases of a fixed and unvarying character, and are treated, on account of their name, according to a determinate plan! How can the bestowal of such a name justify an identical medical treatment? And if the treatment is not always to be the same, why make use of an identical name which postulates an identity of treatment? "Nihil sane in artem medicam pestiferum magis unquam irrepsit malum, quam generalia quaedam medicinam," says Huxham, a man as clear-sighted as he was estimable on account of his conscientiousness (Op. phys. med., tom. I.). And in like manner Frittze laments (Annalen, I, p.80) "that essentially different diseases are designated by the same name." Even those epidemic diseases, which undoubtedly may be propagated in every separate epidemic by a peculiar contagious principle which remains unknown to us, are designated, in the old school of medicine by particular names, just as if they were well-known fixed diseases that invariably recurred under the same form, as hospital fever, goal fever, camp fever, putrid fever, bilious fever, nervous fever, mucous fever, although each epidemic of such roving fevers exhibits itself at every occurrence as another, a new disease, such as it has never before appeared in exactly the same form, differing very much, in every instance, in its course, as well as in many of its most striking symptoms and its whole appearance. Each is so for dissimilar to all previous epidemics, whatever names they may bear, that it would be dereliction of all logical accuracy in our ideas of things were we to give to these maladies, that differ so much among themselves, one of those names we meet with in pathological writings, and treat them all medicinally in conformity with this misused name. The candid Sydenham alone perceived this, when he (Obs. med., cap. ii, De morb, epid.) insists upon the necessity of not considering any epidemic disease as having occurred before and treating it in the same way as another, since all that occur successively, be they ever so numerous, differ from one another: "Nihil quicquam (opinor,) animum universae qua patet medicinae pomoeria perlustrantem, tanta admiratione percellet, quam discolor illa et sui plane dissimilis morborum Epidemicorum facies; non tam qua varias ejusdem anni tempestates, quam qua discrepantes divewrsorum ab invicem annorum constitutiones referunt, ab iisque dependent. Quae

tam aperta praedictorum morborum diversitas tum propriis ac sibi peculiaribus symptomatis, tum etiam medendi ratione, quam hi ab illis disparem prorsus sibi vendicant, satis illucescit. Ex quibus constat morbus hosce, ut ut externa quadantenus specie, er symptomatis aliquot utrisque pariter super venientibus, convenire paulo incautioribus videantur, re tamen ipsa (si bene adverteris animum), alienae admondum esse indolis, et distare ut aera lupinis."

From all this it is clear that these useless and misused names of diseases ought to have no influence on the practice of the true physician, who knows that he has to judge of and to cure diseases, not according to the similarity of the name of a single one of their symptoms, but according to the totality of the signs of the individual state of each particular patient, whose affection it is his duty carefully to investigate, but never to give a hypothetical guess at it.

If, however, it is deemed necessary sometimes to make use of names of diseases, in order, when talking about a patient to ordinary persons, to render ourselves intelligible in few words, we ought only to employ them as collective names, and tell them, eg., the patient has a kind of St. Vitus's dance, a kind of dropsy, a kind of typhus, a kind of ague; but (in order to do away once and for all with the mistaken notions these names give rise to) we should never say he has the St. Vitus's dance, the typhus, the dropsy, the ague, as there are certainly no disease of these and similar names of fixed unvarying character.

EXPLANATION

- This extremely ancient infecting agent psora has passed gradually from generation to generations through millions of human organisms & developed.
- A number of circumstances contribute to the production of these great varieties of chronic d/s [secondary symptoms of psora], along with congenital corporeal constitutions of individuals.
- The injurious agencies which from within & from without & sometimes continually, produces an innumerable variety of defects, injuries, Derangements and sufferings, which till then were treated under a number of special names, as d/s of an independent character.

Footnote 1:
Some of the causes that act as a modifying influence in transforming psora into chronic d/s, depend sometimes on climate & peculiar physical character of place, physical & mental conditions of youth, physical & mental abuse in business or conditions of life, diet & regimen, passions, manners, habit & customs of various kinds.

Footnote 2:
Here hahnemann has discussed, about the works of that times of physicians.

- These works contain many improper ambiguous names, under which different morbid conditions are included, which often resemble each other in one single symptom only e.g- ague, jaundice, dropsy, consumption, leucorrhoea, haemorrhoids, rheumatism, apoplexy, convulsion, hysteria, hypochrondriasis, mania melancholia, quinsy, palsy etc. They are represented as d/s of a fixed character & are treated based on their name, according to a determinate plan.

Few questions arise:-

1. How can application of such a name justify that they require identical medical treatment?
2. If the treatment is not always same, then why make use of an identical name?

Like Huxham, Fritze laments said that 'different d/s are designated by the same name."

- ✦ Even those epidemic d/s, which are propagated in every separate epidemic by a peculiar contagious principle which is unknown to us, they were well-known fixed d/s that recurred under the same form, as hospital fever, gaol fever, camp fever, putrid fever.bilious fever, nervous fever, mucous fever. But the truth is that such fevers exhibits them at every occurance as another, a new d/s, such as it has never before appeared in exactly the same form.
  These fever differ in its course, striking symptoms & its whole appearance.
  Each one is very far dissimilar to all previous epidemics.
- ✦ Sydenham also observed this & said not to consider any epidemic d/s that it is same as before one & stop treating them in the same way because they differ from one another.
- ✦ From all this it is clear that these useless names of d/s should have no influence on the practice of the true physician because he has to cure d/s according to the similarity of totality of the symptoms & signs of each particular patient. It should not be according to the similarity of the name of a single one of their symptoms.
- ✦ If, however, it becomes neccessary to make use of names of diseases, when talking about a patient to ordinary persons we can use as collective names as e.g- the patient has a kind of St. Vitus's dance, a kind of dropsy, a kind of typhus, a kind of ague. We should never say he has the St. Vitus's dance, the typhus, the dropsy, the ague.

§ 82

INDIVIDUALIZATION

Although, by the discovery of that great source of chronic diseases, as also by the discovery of the specific homoeopathic remedies for the psora, medicine has advanced some steps nearer to a knowledge of the nature of the majority of diseases it has to cure, yet, for settling the indication in each case of chronic (psoric) disease he is called on to cure, the duty of a careful apprehension of its ascertainable symptoms and characteristics is as indispensable for the homoeopathic physician as it was before that discovery, as no real cure of this or of other diseases can take place without a strict particular treatment (individualization) of each case of disease – only that in this investigation some difference is to be made when the affection is an acute and rapidly developed disease, and when it is a chronic one; seeing that, in acute disease, the chief symptoms strike us and become evident to the senses more quickly, and hence much less time is requisite for tracing the picture of the disease and much fewer questions are required to be asked1, as almost

everything is self-evident, than in a chronic disease which has been gradually progressing for several years, in which the symptoms are much more difficult to be ascertained.

1 Hence the following directions for investigating the symptoms are only partially applicable for acute diseases.

EXPLANATION

- By the discovery of great source of chronic d/s & discovery of the specific homoeopathic remedies for the psora, medicine has now advanced nearer to a knowledge of the nature of the majority of diseases it has to cure. Yet for each case of chronic (psoric) disease the duty of a careful physician is to consider all the disease symptoms & characteristics, because no real cure of d/s can occur without a strict individualization of each case of d/s.
- In acute cases, the chief symptoms strike us & become evident to senses more quickly. Hence less time is required to get the picture of the d/s & much fewer questions are required to be asked. This is because almost everything is self-evident, hence the following directions for investigating the symptoms are only partially applicable for acute d/s.

In chronic case which has been gradually progressing for several years, here the symptoms are much more difficult to be ascertained.

Footnote 1:
Therefore the following directions for investigating the symptoms are only partially applicable for acute diseases

§ 83

TRUE PHYSICIAN-FREE FROM PREJUDICE, SOUND SENSE & ATTENTIVE

This individualizing examination of a case of disease, for which I shall only give in this place general directions, of which the practitioner will bear in mind only what is applicable for each individual case, demands of the physician nothing but freedom from prejudice and sound senses, attention in observing and fidelity in tracing the picture of the disease.

EXPLANATION

- Here Hahnemann says that in individualizing examination of a case of d/s, I shall only give general directions.
- In each individual case, the physician should be 'free from PREJUDICE & should have 'sound senses', attention in observing [faithfulness] in tracing the picture of the d/s.

§ 84

RECORDING OF SYMPTOMS

The patient details the history of his sufferings; those about him tell what they heard him complain of, how he has behaved and what they have noticed in him; the physician sees, hears, and remarks by his other senses what there is of an altered or unusual character about him. He writes down accurately all that the patient and his friends have told him in the very expressions used by them. Keeping silence himself he allows them to say all they have to say, and refrains from interrupting them1 unless they wander off to other matters. The physician advises them at the beginning of the examination to speak slowly, in order that he may take down in writing the important parts of what the speakers say.

1 Every interruption breaks the train of thought of the narrators, and all they would have said at first does not again occur to them in precisely the same manner after that.

EXPLANATION

- The patient gives details of his sufferings. He relatives tell physician what they have heard the patient complain of, how was his behaviour & what they noticed in him.
- The physician sees, hears & by his senses notices the unusual character about the patient.
- The physician writes down all that the patient & his friends told him in the same words used by them, accurately.
- He allows them to say all they have to say & should not interrupt them in between because it breaks the train of thought.
- He can interrupt only when they wander off to other matters.
- The physician advises them to speak slowly so that he may take notes of important parts of what speakers say.

Footnote 1:
He allows them to say all they have to say & should not interrupt them in between because it breaks the train of thought.

§ 85

NEW SYMPTOMS ON FRESH LINE

He begins a fresh line with every new circumstance mentioned by the patient or his friends, so that the symptoms shall be all ranged separately one below the other. He can thus add to any

one, that may at first have been related in too vague a manner, but subsequently more explicitly explained.

EXPLANATION

- The physician starts a fresh line with every new circumstance told by the patient or his friends.
- This way symptoms are all arranged separately one below the other.
- He can thus add to any one which at first may have been related in too vague manner but later more explicitly explained.

§ 86

OBSERVATIONS

When the narrators have finished what they would say of their own accord, the physician then reverts to each particular symptom and elicits more precise information respecting it in the following manner; he reads over the symptoms as they were related to him one by one, and about each of them he inquires for further particulars, e.g., at what period did this symptom occur? Was it previous to taking the medicine he had hitherto been using? While taking the medicine? Or only some days after leaving off the medicine? What kind of pain, what sensation exactly, was it that occurred on this spot? Where was the precise spot? Did the pain occur in fits and by itself, at various times? Or was it continued, without intermission? How long did it last? At what time of the day or night, and in what position of the body was it worst, or ceased entirely? What was the exact nature of this or that event or circumstance mentioned – described in plain words?

EXPLANATION

- When the patients & his relatives have finished saying what they have to say.
- Now the physician goes back to each symptom & finds out more precise information required by asking questions.
- It is done in following manner:-

    1. He reads the symptoms one by one
    2. Then is inquires further details about each of them.

    E.g- At what period did this symptom occur?, was it before taking medicine he has been using till now? Or While the use of medicine? Or some days after leaving off the medicine??

- What type of pain, sensation exactly & which spot?
- Where was the precise spot?
- Did pain occur in fits or by itself, at various times?
- Was it continued, without intermission?
- How long did it last?
- At what time of the day or night?
- In which position was pain worst or stopped completely?
- What was the exact nature of his or that event mentioned -described in plain words?
- So you need to get full details regarding symptoms.

§ 87

DETAILS OF SYMPTOMS

And thus the physician obtains more precise information respecting each particular detail, but without ever framing his questions so as to suggest the answer to the patient1, so that he shall only have to answer yes or no; else he will be misled to answer in the affirmative or negative something untrue, half true, or not strictly correct, either from indolence or in order to please his interrogator, from which a false picture of the disease and an unsuitable mode of treatment must result.

1 For instance the physician should not ask, Was not this or that circumstance present? He should never be guilty of making such suggestions, which tend to seduce the patient into giving a false answer and a false account of his symptoms.

EXPLANATION

- Thus the physician obtains more precise information & each particular detail.
- But you should not frame questions that suggest the answer to the patient -in yes or no. Never do this
- Otherwise he will be missed to answer in the affirmative or negative something that is not true or half true or not strictly correct because the patient from indolence or in order to please his physician can give false information.

Footnote 1:
For instance the physician should not ask, Was not this or that circumstance present? He should never be guilty of making such suggestions, which tend to seduce the patient into giving a false answer and a false account of his symptoms.

§ 88

GENERAL EXPRESSION

If in these voluntary details nothing has been mentioned respecting several parts or functions of the body or his metal state, the physician asks what more can be told in regard to these parts and these functions, or the state of his disposition or mind1, but in doing this he only makes use of general expressions, in order that his informants may be obliged to enter into special details concerning them.

1 For example what was the character of his stools? How does he pass his water? How is it with his day and night sleep? What is the state of his disposition, his humor, his memory? How about the thirst? What sort of taste has he in his mouth? What kinds of food and drink are most relished? What are most repugnant to him? Has each its full natural taste, or some other unusual taste? How does he feel after eating or drinking? Has he anything to tell about the head, the limbs or the abdomen?

EXPLANATION

- If when giving details the patient has not mentioned several facts or functions of the body or his mental state, the physician asks what he want to ask regarding these parts & these functions or state of his disposition or mind.
- But while doing this he should use general expressions, so that the physician or his relatives maybe obliged to give special details concerning them.

Footnote 1:-
- E.g. What is the character of his stools?
- How does he pass his water?
- How is it with his day & night sleep?
- What is the state of his disposition, his humour his memory?
- How about the thirst?
- What sort of taste has he in his mouth?
- What kinds of food and drink are most relished?
- are most repugnant to him?
- Has each food its full natural taste, or some other unusual taste?
- How does he feel after eating or drinking?
- Has he anything to tell about the head, the limbs or the abdomen?etc.

§ 89

SPECIAL

When the patient (for it is on him we have chiefly to rely for a description of his sensations, except in the case of feigned diseases) has by these details, given of his own accord and in answer to inquiries, furnished the requisite information and traced a tolerably perfect picture of the disease, the physician is at liberty and obliged (if he feels he has not yet gained all the information he needs) to ask more precise, more special questions.1

1 For example, how often are his bowels moved? What is the exact character of the stools? Did the whitish evacuation consist of mucus or faeces? Had he or had he not pains during the evacuation? What was their exact character, and where were they seated? What did the patient vomit? Is the bad taste in the mouth putrid, or bitter, or sour, or what? before or after eating, or during the repast? At what period of the day was it worst? What is the taste of what is eructated? Does the urine only become turbid on standing, or is it turbid when first discharged? What is its color when first emitted? Of what color is the sediment? How does he behave during sleep? Does he whine, moan, talk or cry out in his sleep? Does he start during sleep? Does he snore during inspiration, or during expiration? Does he lie only on his back, or on which side? Does he cover himself well up, or can he not bear the clothes on him? Does he easily awake, or does he sleep too soundly? How often does this or that symptom occur? What is the cause that produces it each time it occurs? does it come on whilst sitting, lying, standing, or when in motion? only when fasting, or in the morning, or only in the evening, or only after a meal, or when does it usually appear? When did the rigor come on? was it merely a chilly sensation, or was he actually cold at the same time? if so, in what parts? or while feeling chilly, was he actually warm to the touch? was it merely a sensation of cold, without shivering? was he hot without redness of the face? what parts of him were hot to the touch? or did he complain of heat without being hot to the touch? How long did the chilliness last? how long the hot stage? When did the thirst come on – during the cold stage? during the heat? or previous to it? or subsequent to it? How great was the thirst, and what was the beverage desired? When did the sweat come on – at the beginning or the end of the heat? or how many hours after the heat? when asleep or when awake? How great was the sweat? was it warm or cold? on what parts? how did it smell? What does he complain of before or during the cold stage? what during the hot stage? what after it? what during or after the sweating stage?

(Added to the Sixth Edition)

In women, note the character of menstruation and other discharges, etc.

EXPLANATION

- When the patient has given the details, we have to rely on him for description of his sensations, except in the case of fake d/s [not true d/s]

- Even after we have asked questions to him & he has answered them. The physician, if he feels he has not gained all the information he needs, he can ask more precise & more special questions.

Footnote 1:
EXAMPLE
- How often are his bowels moved?
- What is the exact character of the stools?
- Did the whitish evacuation consist of mucus or faeces?
- Had he or had he not pains during the evacuation?
- What was their exact character, and where were they seated?
- What did the patient vomit?
- Is the bad taste in the mouth putrid, or bitter, or sour, or what?
- before or after eating, or during the repast?
- At what period of the day was it worst?
- What is the taste of what is eructated?
- Does the urine only become turbid on standing, or is it turbid when first discharged?
- What is its color when first emitted?
- Of what color is the sediment?
- How does he behave during sleep?
- Does he whine, moan, talk or cry out in his sleep?
- Does he start during sleep?
- Does he snore during inspiration, or during expiration?
- Does he lie only on his back, or on which side?
- Does he cover himself well up, or can he not bear the clothes on him?
- Does he easily awake, or does he sleep too soundly?
- How often does this or that symptom occur?
- What is the cause that produces it each time it occurs?
- Does it come on whilst sitting, lying, standing, or when in motion?
- Only when fasting, or in the morning, or only in the evening, or only after a meal, or when does it usually appear?
- When did the rigor come on?
- Was it merely a chilly sensation, or was he actually cold at the same time?
- If so, in what parts? or while feeling chilly, was he actually warm to the touch?
- Was it merely a sensation of cold, without shivering?
- Was he hot without redness of the face?
- What parts of him were hot to the touch? or did he complain of heat without being hot to the touch?
- How long did the chilliness last?
- How long the hot stage?
- When did the thirst come on – during the cold stage? during the heat? or previous to it? or subsequent to it?
- How great was the thirst, and what was the beverage desired?

- When did the sweat come on – at the beginning or the end of the heat? or how many hours after the heat?
- When asleep or when awake?
- How great was the sweat? was it warm or cold? on what parts? how did it smell?
- What does he complain of before or during the cold stage? what during the hot stage? what after it? what during or after the sweating stage?
- In women, note the character of menstruation and other discharges, etc

§ 90

PHYSICIAN OBSERVATION CASE & PATIENT

When the physician has finished writing down these particulars, he then makes a note of what he himself observes in the patient1, and ascertains how much of that was peculiar to the patient in his healthy state.

1 For example, how the patient behaved during the visit – whether he was morose, quarrelsome, hasty, lachrymose, anxious, despairing or sad, or hopeful, calm etc. Whether he was in a drowsy state or in any way dull of comprehension; whether he spoke hoarsely, or in a low tone, or incoherently, or how other wise did he talk? what was the color of his face and eyes, and of his skin generally? what degree of liveliness and power was there in his expression and eyes? what was the state of his tongue, his breathing, the smell from his mouth, and his hearing? were his pupils dilated or contracted? how rapidly and to what extent did they alter in the dark and in the light? what was the character of the pulse? what was the condition of the abdomen? how moist or hot, how cold or dry to the touch, was the skin of this or that part or generally? whether he lay with head thrown back, with mouth half or wholly open, with the arms placed above the head, on his back, or in what other position? what effort did he make to raise himself? and anything else in him that may strike the physician as being remarkable.

EXPLANATION

- When the physician has finished writing down all these particulars, now he makes a note of what all he himself observes in the patient.
- He now ascertains how much of all what patient has told, is peculiar to the patient in his healthy state.

Footnote 1:
- How was the behaviour of the patient during the visit -whether he was morose, quarrelsome, hasty, anxious, despairing or sad, or hopeful, calm etc
- whether he was in a drowsy state or dull of comprehension.

- whether he spoke hoarsely, or in a low tone, or incoherently, or how other wise did he talk? what was the color of his face and eyes, and of his skin generally?
- what degree of liveliness and power was there in his expression and eyes?
- what was the state of his tongue, his breathing, the smell from his mouth, and his hearing? were his pupils dilated or contracted?
- how rapidly and to what extent did they alter in the dark and in the light?
- what was the character of the pulse? what was the condition of the abdomen?
- how moist or hot, how cold or dry to the touch, was the skin of this or that part or generally? whether he lay with head thrown back, with mouth half or wholly open, with the arms placed above the head, on his back, or in what other position? what effort did he make to raise himself?
- Physician can ask anything else in him that the physician may found remarkable or useful.
- So that the proper totality of symptoms is prepared & based on it the most suitable remedy can be given for cure of the sick.

§ 91

HISTORY & RECORDING

The symptoms and feelings of the patient during a previous course of medicine do not furnish the pure picture of the disease; but on the other hand, those symptoms and ailments which he suffered from before the use of the medicines, or after they had been discontinued for several days, give the true fundamental idea of the original form of the disease, and these especially the physician must take note of. When the disease is of a chronic character, and the patient has been taking medicine up to the time he is seen, the physician may with advantage leave him some days quite without medicine, or in the meantime administer something of an unmedicinal nature and defer to a subsequent period the more precise scrutiny of the morbid symptoms, in order to be able to grasp in their purity the permanent uncontaminated symptoms of the old affection and to form a faithful picture of the disease.

EXPLANATION

- The physician should take note of whether the symptoms & feelings of the patient are during a course of medicine he was taking because this would not furnish the pure picture of the d/s.
- The symptoms & ailments which he suffered from before the use of the medicines, or after they had been discontinued for several days, should be noted. It gives the true fundamental idea of the original form of the d/s. So physician should note this thing while taking a case.

- In case of a d/s of chronic character in which the patient has been taking medicine upto the time he is seen, the physician should leave the patient for some days without medicine or administer an unmedicinal substances for a subsequent period and then take a the case as a fresh one.
- This is important in order to group the permanent uncontaminated symptoms of the old affections and form a faithful picture of the d/s, so that the proper remedy can be chosen.

§ 92

RECORDING-ACUTE SYMPTOM

But if it be a disease of a rapid course, and if its serious character admit of no delay, the physician must content himself with observing the morbid condition, altered though it may be by medicines, if he cannot ascertain what symptoms were present before the employment of the medicines, – in order that he may at least form a just apprehension of the complete picture of the disease in its actual condition, that is to say, of the conjoint malady formed by the medicinal and original diseases, which from the use of inappropriate drugs is generally more serious and dangerous than was the original disease, and hence demands prompt and efficient aid; and by thus tracing out the complete picture of the disease he will be enabled to combat it with a suitable homoeopathic remedy, so that the patient shall not fall a sacrifice to the injurious drugs he was swallowed.

EXPLANATION

If the d/s is of a rapid course & if its of a serious character that no delay can be made, the physician must observe the morbid condition[Although it may be by the medicines he is taking for the d/s]

- He may form a just apprehension of the complete picture of the d/s in its actual condition -The conjoint malady = Medicinal symptom + Original symptoms.
- Usually in these cases the original d/s has been made generally more serious & dangerous from the use of inappropriate drugs.
- Hence it demands fast & efficient aid.
- The physician thus by tracing out the complete picture of the d/s will be able to fight it with a suitable Homeopathic remedy, so that the life of the patient can be saved & not sacrificed to the injurious drugs he has swallowed.

§ 93

PRIVATELY?

If the disease has been brought on a short time or, in the case of a chronic affection, a considerable time previously, by some obvious cause, then the patient – or his friends when questioned privately – will mention it either spontaneously or when carefully interrogated.1

1 Any causes of a disgraceful character, which the patient or his friends do not like to confess, at least not voluntarily, the physician must endeavor to elicit by skilfully framing his questions, or by private information. To these belong poisoning or attempted suicide, onanism, indulgence in ordinary or unnatural debauchery, excess in wine, cordials, punch and other ardent beverages, or coffee, – over-indulgence in eating generally, or in some particular food of a hurtful character, – infection with venereal disease or itch, unfortunate love, jealousy, domestic infelicity, worry, grief on account of some family misfortune, ill-usage, balked revenge, injured pride, embarrassment of a pecuniary nature, superstitious fear, – hunger, – or an imperfection in the private parts, a rupture, a prolapse, and so forth.

EXPLANATION

- If the d/s has been brought on a short time or in case of a chronic d/s a considerable time before.
- The patient or his relatives should be questioned privately & they will now mention the history of intake of injurious agents because many times in these cases the patient or his friends don't like to confess, voluntarily so it is the duty of the physician to elicit it by skilfully framing his questions or by private information.

Footnote 1:
Example:-
These may belong to cases by poisoning or attempted suicide, onanism[Ejaculating outside the vagina during intercourse]

Ordinary or unnatural addictions, excess in wine, cordials [Alcoholic beverages], punch etc or coffee.

- Over -indulgence in eating or intake of hurtful food.
- Infection with veneral d/s or itch.
- Unfortunate love, jealously, worry, grief, illusuage, balked revenge, injured pride, superstitious fear
- Hunger
- Imperfection in the private parts, rupture, a prolapse & so forth.

§ 94

INVESTIGATION OF MAINTAINING CAUSE

While inquiring into the state of chronic disease, the particular circumstances of the patient with regard to his ordinary occupations, his usual mode of living and diet, his domestic situation, and so forth, must be well considered and scrutinized, to ascertain what there is in them that may tend to produce or to maintain disease, in order that by their removal the recovery may by prompted.1

1 In chronic diseases of females it is specially necessary to pay attention to pregnancy, sterility, sexual desire, accouchements, miscarriages, suckling, and the state of the menstrual discharge. With respect to the last-named more particularly, we should not neglect to ascertain if it recurs at too short intervals, or is delayed beyond the proper time, how many days it lasts, whether its flow is continuous or interrupted, what is its general quality, how dark is its color, whether there is leucorrhoea before its appearance or after its termination, but especially by what bodily or mental ailments, what sensations and pains, it is preceded, accompanied or followed; if there is leucorrhoea, what is its nature, what sensations attend its flow, in what quantity it is, and what are the conditions and occasions under which it occurs?

EXPLANATION

- In cases of chronic d/s while inquiring the patient, the physician should also ask questions regarding particular circumstance of the patient.
    - Like his ordinary occupations, his usual mode of living & diet, his domestic situation etc.
    - These are useful in order to find out that what is there which is producing or maintaining the d/s.
    - If this is found out, their removal may help in promoting the recovery faster.

Footnote:-
In chronic d/s of females, pay attention to pregnancy, sterility, sexual desire, miscarriage, suckling, accouchements [delivery] & the state of menstrual discharge.

- We should ask whether menses recur at too short intervals or delayed beyond the proper time, duration, whether flow is continuous or interrupted, quantity, colour, whether there is leucorrhoea before its appearance or after its termination, by what bodily or mental ailments.

What sensations & pains, it is preceded accompanied or followed.

§ 95

RECORDING OF LONG SUFFERING

In chronic disease the investigation of the signs of disease above mentioned, and of all others, must be pursued as carefully and circumstantially as possible, and the most minute peculiarities must be attended to, partly because in these diseases they are the most characteristic and least resemble those of acute diseases, and if a cure is to be affected they cannot be too accurately noted; partly because the patients become so used to their long sufferings that they pay little or no heed to the lesser accessory symptoms, which are often very pregnant with meaning (characteristic) – often very useful in determining the choice of the remedy – and regard them almost as a necessary part of their condition, almost as health, the real feeling of which they have well-nigh forgotten in the sometimes fifteen or twenty years of suffering, and they can scarcely bring themselves to believe that these accessory symptoms, these greater or less deviations from the healthy state, can have any connection with their principal malady.

EXPLANATION

- In chronic d/s the case-taking is a bit tedious task.
- In chronic d/s because the patients become so used to their long sufferings that they pay little or no heed[importance], to the lesser accessory symptoms, they may have forgotten the symptoms due to long 15 or 20 years of suffering. They think that these accessory symptoms can have no connection with their, main malady [d/s condition]
- Therefore in chronic d/s detailed history should be taken proper investigation of the signs of d/s as mentioned in above aphorism & all others must be carefully pursued.

Because in these d/s these accessory symptoms are the most characteristic often very useful in determining the choice of the remedy & so the most minute peculiarities must be attended to in these cases.

§ 96

RECORDING OF HYPOCHONDRIC CASE

Besides this, patients themselves differ so much in their dispositions, that some, especially the so-called hypochondriacs and other persons of great sensitiveness and impatient of suffering,

portray their symptoms in too vivid colors and, in order to induce the physician to give them relief, describe their ailments in exaggerated expression.1

1 A pure fabrication of symptoms and sufferings will never be met with in hypochondriacs, even in the most impatient of them – a comparison of the sufferings they complain of at various times when the physician gives them nothing at all, or something quite unmedical, proves this plainly; – but we must deduct something from their exaggeration, at all events ascribe the strong character of their expressions to their expressions when talking of their ailments becomes of itself an important symptom in the list of features of which the portrait of the disease is composed. The case is different with insane persons and rascally feigners of disease.

EXPLANATION

- One can find a totally different picture, in cases of so-called hypochondriacs & other persons with great sensitivity & impatient of suffering.
- These people portray their symptoms in exaggerated manner, so as to induce the physicians to give them relief.

Footnote 1:
A pure deliberate act of deviating from the actual symptoms & sufferings will not be seen in hypochondriacs, even in the most impatient patient.

- When the physician gives them nothing at all or something which is quite unmedicinal the comparison of the sufferings they complain then proves this plainly.
- In cases with very exaggeration of their expressions when telling their ailments /sufferings becomes an important symptom and is included in establishing the portrait of the d/s.
- The case is different with insane persons & feigners.

§ 97

RECORDING OF INDOLENT CASE

Other individuals of an opposite character, however, partly from indolence, partly from false modesty, partly from a kind of mildness of disposition or weakness of mind, refrain from mentioning a number of their symptoms, describe them in vague terms, or allege some of them to be of no consequence.

EXPLANATION

- Sometimes individuals of an opposite character are also encountered.
- They refrain or hesitate from mentioning a number of their symptoms, describe them in vague terms or think that some of them may not be useful, so do not mention them.

- Partey from lethargy, partly from false modesty, party from mildness of disposition or weakness of mind they refrain from telling some symptoms.
- This may lead to false formation of potrait of d/s.

§ 98

RECORD ONLY PATIENT LANGUAGE

Now, as certainly as we should listen particularly to the patient's description of his sufferings and sensations, and attach credence especially to his own expressions wherewith he endeavors to make us understand his ailments – because in the mouths of his friends and attendants they are usually altered and erroneously stated, – so certainly, on the other hand, in all diseases, but especially in the chronic ones, the investigation of the true, complete picture and its peculiarities demands especial circumspection, tact, knowledge of human nature, caution in conducting the inquiry and patience in an eminent degree.

EXPLANATION

- Here he says that we should listen mainly to the patient's descriptive about his sufferings & sensations & attach credence, especially to his own expressions because in the mouths of friends & attendants they are usually altered.
- In all d/s, but especially the chronic ones, the investigation of the true, complete picture requires especial, tact, knowledge of human nature, proper conducting of inquiry & patience.

§ 99

RECORDING ACUTE CASE IS EASY

On the whole, the investigation of acute diseases, or of such as have existed but a short time, is much the easiest for the physician, because all the phenomena and deviations from the health that has been put recently lost are still fresh in the memory of the patient and his friends, still continue to be novel and striking. The physician certainly requires to know everything in such cases also; but he has much less to inquire into; they are for the most part spontaneously detailed to him.

EXPLANATION

1. On the whole, the investigation of acute d/s or of such d/s that existed for a short time, is much easy for physician because all the deviations from the health are recent one & fresh in the memory of the patient & his friends.
2. The patient & his friends can easily recall the symptoms as they are fresh ones.
3. In such cases also, the physician requires to know everything about the case.
4. Here he requires less to inquire into as the patient himself spontaneously gives details to him.

§ 100

INVESTIGATION OF THE EPIDEMIC D/S

In investigating the totality of the symptoms of epidemic and sporadic diseases it is quite immaterial whether or not something similar has ever appeared in the world before under the same or any other name. The novelty or peculiarity of a disease of that kind makes no difference either in the mode of examining or of treating it, as the physician must any way regard to pure picture of every prevailing disease as if it were something new and unknown, and investigate it thoroughly for itself, if he desire to practice medicine in a real and radical manner, never substituting conjecture for actual observation, never taking for granted that the case of disease before him is already wholly or partially known, but always carefully examining it in all its phases; and this mode of procedure is all the more requisite in such cases, as a careful examination will show that every prevailing disease is in many respects a phenomenon of a unique character, differing vastly from all previous epidemics, to which certain names have been falsely applied – with the exception of those epidemics resulting from a contagious principle that always remains the same, such as smallpox, measles, etc.

EXPLANATION

- In investigating the totality of the symptoms of epidemic and sporadic d/s we need to be careful.
- Every prevailing d/s is unique in character & differ from all previous epidemics, to which certain names have been falsely applied.
- Here one thing needs to be noted that there is one exception that is in those epidemics which result from a contagious principle that always remains the same, such as small-pox, measles etc.
- Other than above; it is quite immaterial whether something similar has ever appeared in the world before under the same, or any other name. This will not effect our process of investigation.
- The mode of examination or treating the d/s will be as if it were something new & unknown & investigate it thoroughly.

- If a physician wants to practice medicine in a real manner, he should never think that case of d/s before him is already wholly or partially known to him.
- He should carefully examine it in all its phases as every new d/s differs from all previous ones.

§ 101

INVESTIGATION

It may easily happen that in the first case of an epidemic disease that presents itself to the physician's notice he does not at once obtain a knowledge of its complete picture, as it is only by a close observation of several cases of every such collective disease that he can become conversant with the totality of its signs and symptoms. The carefully observing physician can, however, from the examination of even the first and second patients, often arrive so nearly at a knowledge of the true state as to have in his mind a characteristic portrait of it, and even to succeed in finding a suitable, homoeopathically adapted remedy for it.

EXPLANATION

- It may happen that in an epidemic d/s the physician in the first case [patient] may not at once obtain a knowledge of the complete picture of d/s.
- It requires a close observation of several cases of every such collective d/s of an epidemic, now he can become familiar with the totality of its signs & symptoms.
  But a carefully observing physician can arrive so nearly at a knowledge of the true state of d/s from the examination of even the first & second patients.
  He makes a characteristic portrait of it in his mind & find a suitable, homoeopathically adapted remedy for it.
- Such physician is an unprejudiced physician who takes each case as a fresh one totally different from any epidemic ever occured before.

§ 102

PORTRAIT OF D/S

In the course of writing down the symptoms of several cases of this kind the sketch of the disease picture becomes ever more and more complete, not more spun out and verbose, but more significant (more characteristic), and including more of the peculiarities of this collective disease; on the one hand, the general symptoms (e.g., loss of appetite, sleeplessness, etc.) become precisely defined as to their peculiarities; and on the other, the more marked and special symptoms which are peculiar to but few diseases and of rarer occurrence, at least in the same combination, become prominent and constitute what is characteristic of this malady.1 All those affected with the disease prevailing at a given time have certainly contracted it from one and the same source and hence are suffering from the same disease; but the whole extent of such an epidemic disease and the totality of its symptoms (the knowledge whereof, which is essential for enabling us to choose the most suitable homoeopathic remedy for this array of symptoms, is obtained by a complete survey of the morbid picture) cannot be learned from one single patient, but is only to be perfectly deduced (abstracted) and ascertained from the sufferings of several patients of different constitutions.

1 The physician who has already, in the first cases, been able to choose a remedy approximating to the homoeopathic specific, will, from the subsequence cases, be enabled either to verify the suitableness of the medicine chosen, or to discover a more appropriate, the most appropriate homoeopathic remedy.

EXPLANATION

- In such cases of epidemic d/s, all those affected with the d/s at given time have certainly contracted it from one & the same source & hence are suffering from the same d/s.
- The whole extent of such an epidemic d/s & totality of its symptoms, which is essential to choose the most suitable homeopathic remedy, is obtained by a complete survey of the morbid picture.
- It means it cannot be learned from one single patient but is only perfectly deduced from the observation of the sufferings of several patients of different constitutions.
- While writing down the symptoms of several cases of this kind, the complete picture becomes more & more clear.
- The general symptoms e.g- Loss of appetite, sleeplessness etc & the more marked & special symptoms which are peculiar to few d/s & of rarer occurrence in patient become prominent & constitute the characteristic of this malady.

Footnote:
The physician who has in the first case, been able to choose a remedy. He will be able to verify the medicine chosen or discover a more appropriate remedy by examining the subsequent [other] cases.

§ 103

INVESTIGATION OF PSORA

In the same manner as has here been taught relative to the epidemic disease, which are generally of an acute character, the miasmatic chronic maladies, which, as I have shown, always remain the same in their essential nature, especially the psora, must be investigated, as to the whole sphere of their symptoms, in a much more minute manner than has ever been done before, for in them also one patient only exhibits a portion of their symptoms, a second, a third, and so on, present some other symptoms, which also are but a (dissevered, as it were), portion of the totality of the symptoms which constitute the entire extent of this malady, so that the whole array of the symptoms belonging to such a miasmatic, chronic disease, and especially to the psora, can only be ascertained from the observation of very many single patients affected with such a chronic disease, and without a complete survey and collective picture of these symptoms the medicines capable of curing the whole malady homoeopathically (to wit, the antipsorics) cannot be discovered; and these medicines are, at the same time, the true remedies of the several patients suffering from such chronic affections.

EXPLANATION

- As we have learned in case of epidemic d/s, in the same manner the miasmatic chronic maladies, especially the psora, must be investigated.
- Here the whole sphere of their symptoms must be observed in much more minute manner.
- This is because one patient only exhibits a portion of their symptoms.
- A second patient, a third & so on, present some other symptoms which are also a portion of the totality of the symptoms which constitute the entire extent of this malady.
- So in order to find all the symptoms of such a miasmatic, chronic d/s & especially the psora, we have to observe very many single patients effected with such a chronic d/s.
- In such a way by complete survery & collective picture of these symptoms the best suitable Homeopathic remedy can be discovered.
- These medicines are the true remedies of the several patients suffering from such chronic d/s.

§ 104

SPECIALLY MARK

When the totality of the symptoms that specially mark and distinguish the case of disease or, in other words, when the picture of the disease, whatever be its kind, is once accurately sketched,1 the most difficult part of the task is accomplished. The physician has then the picture of the disease, especially if it be a chronic one, always before him to guide him in his treatment; he can investigate it in all its parts and can pick out the characteristic symptoms, in order to oppose to these, that is to say, to the whole malady itself, a very similar artificial morbific force, in the shape of a homoeopathically chosen medicinal substance, selected from the lists of symptoms of all the medicines whose pure effects have been ascertained. And when, during the treatment, he wishes to ascertain what has been the effect of the medicine, and what change has taken place in the patient's state, at this fresh examination of the patient he only needs to strike out of the list

of the symptoms noted down at the first visit those that have become ameliorated, to mark what still remain, and add any new symptoms that may have supervened.

1 The old school physician gave himself very little trouble in this matter in his mode of treatment. He would not listen to any minute detail of all the circumstances of his case by the patient; indeed, he frequently cut him short in his relation of his sufferings, in order that he might not be delayed in the rapid writing of his prescription, composed of a variety of ingredients unknown to him in their true effects. No allopathic physician, as has been said, sought to learn all the circumstances of the patient's case, and still less did he make a note in writing of them. On seeing the patient again several days afterwards he recollected nothing concerning the few details he had heard at the first visit (having in the meantime seen so many other patients laboring under different affections); he had allowed everything to go in at one ear and out at the other. At subsequent visits he only asked a few general questions, went through the ceremony of feeling the pulse at the wrist, looked at the tongue, and at the same moment wrote another prescription, on equally irrational principles, or ordered the first one to be continued (in considerable quantities several times a day), and, with a graceful bow, he hurried off to the fiftieth or sixtieth patient he had to visit, in this thoughtless way, in the course of that forenoon. The profession which of all others requires actually the most reflection, a conscientious, careful examination of the state of each individual patient and a special treatment founded thereon, was conducted in this manner by persons who called themselves physicians, rational practitioners. The result, as might naturally be expected, was almost invariably bad; and yet patients had to go to them for advise, partly because there were none better to be had, partly for fashion's sake.

EXPLANATION

- When the totality of the symptoms of the case of d/s is made, hence the picture of the d/s is accurately sketched, the most difficult part of the task is completed.
- Now the physician has the picture of the d/s especially if it is chronic d/s. This guides him in his treatment, he can investigate it & pick out the characteristic symptoms & choose a very similar artificial morbific force, the homoeopathically chosen medicinal substance.
- The most similar homoeopathic remedy is then selected from the lists of symptoms of all the medicines who have been proved.
- If during the treatment, he wants to ascertain the effects of the medicine given & he want to know the changes that has taken place in the patients state. He examines the patient as fresh case & strike out the symptoms, noted down at the first visit, which have become ameliorated [treated] & mark out symptoms which remain now & if any new symptoms have appeared add them to the left symptoms & now based on the old symptoms left + new symptoms a new totality of symptoms is examined.

Footnote:
The old school physician don't take pain of detailed history of each symptom, as we take in homeopathy.

- ✦ He does not listen to any minute details of all the circumstances of his case told by the patients.
- ✦ He cuts the patient short & does not delay in the rapid writing of his prescription, consisting of a variety of ingredients unknown to him in their true effects.

- On seeing the patient again after several days of first visit, he only ask a few general questions, feels the pulse at the wrist, looks the tongue & at the same irrational principles writes another prescription or orders the first one to be continued.
- The result is what we except, that is almost invariably bad & then also patients go to them for advice because there were none better to be according to them, also due to fashion's sake[because all others also go].

§ 105

INVESTIGATION OF PATHOGENETIC POWER OF MEDICINE

The second point of the business of a true physician related to acquiring a knowledge of the instruments intended for the cure of the natural diseases, investigating the pathogenetic power of the medicines, in order, when called on to cure, to be able to select from among them one, from the list of whose symptoms an artificial disease may be constructed, as similar as possible to the totality of the principal symptoms of the natural disease sought to be cured.

EXPLANATION

- After proper case taking and proper evaluation of the totality of symptoms, now the second most important work of a true physician is to have a proper knowledge of the instruments which cure the natural d/s.
- He should be able to investigate the pathogenetic power of the medicines.
- He should be able to select a remedy as similar as possible to the totality of the principal symptoms of the natural d/s, which needs to be cured.
- He should be able to select from among the listen of medicines whose symptoms are most similar to the case to be cured.

§ 106

KNOWLEDGE OF MEDICINE

The whole pathogenetic effect of the several medicines must be known; that is to say, all the morbid symptoms and alterations in the health that each of them is specially capable of developing in the healthy individual must first have been observed as far as possible, before we can hope to be able to find among them, and to select, suitable homoeopathic remedies for most of the natural disease.

EXPLANATION

- According to Hahnemann, the physician should know the whole pathogenic effects of the several medicines.
- He should have knowledge, what symptoms & alterations in the health does each medicine develop in the healthy individual [d/s individual cannot prove a remedy]
- Then only a physician will be able to select the suitable homeopathic remedies for most of the natural d/s among the remedies known to us.

§ 107

DRUG PROVING ON SICK

If, in order to ascertain this, medicines be given to sick persons only, even though they be administered singly and alone, then little or nothing precise is seen of their true effects, as those peculiar alterations of the health to be expected from the medicine are mixed up with the symptoms of the disease and can seldom be distinctly observed.

EXPLANATION

- If we want to know the pathogenetic power of the medicines, we have to prove them on the healthy individual.
- Healthy individual will give true effects & alterations of the health produced by the medicine.
- If the drug proving be given to sick persons, even though we give the medicine, singly & alone it will not give true effects.
- This is because the peculiar alterations of the health due the medicine are mixed up with the symptoms of the d/s of the sick person.
- So, we get a mixed or false picture of medicine if proved on a sick person as he himself is suffering from a d/s which has its peculiar symptoms.

§ 108

DRUG PROVING HEALTHY-INDIVIDUAL

There is, therefore, no other possible way in which the peculiar effects of medicines on the health of individuals can be accurately ascertained – there is no sure, no more natural way of accomplishing this object, than to administer the several medicines experimentally, in moderate doses, to healthy persons, in order to ascertain what changes, symptoms and signs of their influence each individually produces on the health of the body and of the mind; that is to say, what disease elements they are able and tend to produce1, since, as has been demonstrated (§§ 24-27), all the curative power of medicines lies in this power they possess of changing the state of man's health, and is revealed by observation of the latter.

1 Not one single physician, as far as I know, during the previous two thousand five hundred years, thought of this so natural, so absolutely necessary and only genuine mode of testing medicines for their pure and peculiar effects in deranging the health of man, in order to learn what morbid state each medicine is capable of curing, except the great and immoral Albrecht von Haller. He alone, besides myself, saw the necessity of this (vide the Preface to the Pharmacopoeia Helvet, Basil, 1771, fol., p.12); Nempe primum in corpore sano medela tentanda est, sine peregrina ulla miscela; odoreque et sapore ejus exploratis, exigua illiu dosis ingerenda et ad ommes, quae inde contingunt, affectiones, quis pulsus, qui calor, quae respiratia, quaenam excretiones, attendum. Inde ad ductum phaenomenorum, in sano obviorum, transeas ad experimenta in corpore aegroro," etc. But no one, not a single physician, attended to or followed up this invaluable hint.

EXPLANATION

- He says that if we want to know the peculiar effects of medicines on the health of individuals we need to test & prove them on healthy humans.
- We administer the several medicines, experimentally in moderate doses, to healthy person, then we observe what all changes, symptoms & signs of their influence each individually produces on the health of the body & of the mind.
- We now find out, what d/s elements they are able & tend to produce.
- Earlier also we have read that [aphr-24-27], all the curative power of medicines lies in the power they possess of changing the state of man's health & is revealed by observation of the latter.

Example- a medicine 'A' produces a group of symptoms when given to a healthy person.

Now when a sick person with similar group of symptoms comes for cure we give the medicine 'A' which cures the sick.

So in Homeopathy cure occurs based on similarity of the symptoms.

Footnote:
Hahnemann says that during the last 2500 years, not even one single physician thought this so natural & only genuine mode testing medicines.

- ✦ This mode of testing medicine to get the pure & peculiar effects they produce in the health of man help us to learn the morbid state each medicine is capable of curing.
- ✦ He says that only 'Albrecht von haller' along with me saw the necessity of this, except him no one, not a single physician attended or followed this invaluable hint.

§ 109

HAHNEMANN PATH

I was the first that opened up this path, which I have pursued with a perseverance that could only arise and be kept up by a perfect conviction of the great truth, fraught with such blessings to humanity, that it is only by the homoeopathic employment of medicines1 that the certain cure of human maladies is possible.2

1 It is impossible that there can be another true, best method of curing dynamic diseases (i.e., all diseases not strictly surgical) besides homoeopathy, just as it is impossible to draw more than one straight line betwixt two given points. He who imagines that there are other modes of curing diseases besides it could not have appreciated homoeopathy fundamentally nor practised it with sufficient care, nor could he ever have seen or read cases of properly performed homoeopathic cures; nor, on the other hand, could he have discerned the baselessness of all allopathic modes of treating diseases and their bad or even dreadful effects, if, with such lax indifference, he places the only true healing art on an equality with those hurtful methods of treatment, or alleges the latter to be auxiliaries to homoeopathy which it could not do without! My true, conscientious followers, the pure homoeopathists, with their successful, almost never-failing treatment, might teach these persons better.

2 The first fruits of these labors, as perfect as they could be at that time, I recorded in the Fragmenta de viribus medicamentorum positivis, sive in sano corpore humano observatis, pts. I, ii, Lipsiae, 8, 1805, ap. J. A. Barth; the more mature fruits in the Reine Arzneimittellebre, I Th., dritte Ausg.; II Th., dritte Ausg., 1833; III Th., zweite Ausg., 1825; IV Th., zw. Ausg., 1827 (English translation, Materia Medica Pura, vols I and ii); and in the second, third, and fourth parts of Die chronischen Krankheiten, 1828, 1830, Dresden bei Arnold (2nd edit., with a fifth part, Dusseldorf bei Schaub, 1835, 1839).

EXPLANATION

- Hahnemann says that he was the first one that opened up this path.
- He was the one who gave humanity such blessing, the cure of human maladies.
- It is only by the homoeopathic employment of medicines that the certain cure of human maladies is possible, Hahnemann was the first physician to discover it.

Footnote:

It is not possible that there can be any another true, best method of curing dynamic d/s I.e- all d/s not strictly surgical other than homoeopathy.

- Like we can never draw more than one straight line b/w two given points.
- Similarly there is no other pathy or method of curing dynamic d/s other than homoeopathy.
- The person who imagines that there are other modes of curing d/s means that he has, not been able to appreciate homeopathy & not practised it with sufficient care. He has also not seen or read cases of properly performed homoeopathic cures, nor, on the other hand he could observe the baselessness of all allopathic modes of treating d/s & their bad, even dreadful effects, otherwise he would have not placed the only true healing art on an equality with those hurtful methods of treatment.
- Hahnemann says, ' My true followers, the pure, homeopathists, with their successful almost never- failing treatment, might teach these persons better."

§ 110

ALLOPATHY EFFECT OF DRUG

I saw, moreover, that the morbid lesions which previous authors had observed to result from medicinal substances when taken into the stomach of healthy persons, either in large doses given by mistake or in order to produce death in themselves or others, or under other circumstances, accorded very much with my own observations when experimenting with the same substances on myself and other healthy individuals. These authors give details of what occurred as histories of poisoning and as proofs of the pernicious effects of these powerful substances, chiefly in order to warn others from their use; partly also for the sake of exalting their own skill, when, under the use of the remedies they employed to combat these dangerous accidents, health gradually returned; but partly also, when the persons so affected died under their treatment, in order to seek their own justification in the dangerous character of these substances, which they then termed poisons. None of these observers ever dreamed that the symptoms they recorded merely as proofs of the noxious and poisonous character of these substances were sure revelations of the power of these drugs to extinguish curatively similar symptoms occurring in natural disease, that these their pathogenetic phenomena were intimations of their homoeopathic curative action, and that the only possible way to ascertain their medicinal powers is to observe those changes of health medicines are capable of producing in the healthy organism; for the pure, peculiar powers of medicines available for the cure of disease are to be learned neither by any ingenious a priori speculations, nor by the smell, taste or appearance of the drugs, nor by their chemical analysis, nor yet by the employment of several of them at one time in a mixture (prescription) in diseases; it was never suspected that these histories of medicinal diseases would one day furnish the first rudiments of the true, pure materia medica, which from the earliest times until now has consisted solely of false conjectures and fictions of the imagination – that is to say, did not exist at all.1

1 See what I have said on this subject in the "Examination of the Sources of the Ordinary Materia Medica," prefixed to the third part of my Reine Arzneimittellebre (translated in the Materia Medica Pura, vol. ii).

EXPLANATION

- Here Hahnemann says that, he saw authors had observed when the medicinal substances were taken into the stomach of healthy persons in large doses given by mistake or in order to produce death in themselves or others produced morbid lesion.
- He also observed the action of these medicinal substances on himself & other healthy individuals.
- These authors have given details of what happened as histories of poisoning & pernicious effects of these powerful substances mainly to warn others from their use.
- None of these observers ever dreamed that the symptoms they recorded only as proofs of the noxious & poisonous character of these substances were actually the proof of the power of these drugs to remove similar symptoms occurring in natural d/s, curatively.
- Their pathogenetic phenomena were indicator of their homeopathic curative action.
- The way to confirm their medicinal powers is to observe those changes medicines produce in the healthy organism.
- The pure, peculiar powers of medicines available for the cure of d/s can only be learned by their action on healthy human, not by just guessing nor by the smell, taste or appearance of the drugs, nor by their chemical analysis, nor by employment of several of them at one time in a mixture [prescription] in d/s.
- No one ever thought those histories of medicinal d/s would one day give us the seed of the true, pure materia medica[which was until then thought to be imaginary]

Footnote:
Hahnemann —{ what I have said on this subject in the "Examination of the Sources of the Ordinary Materia Medica," prefixed to the third part of my Reine Arzneimittellebre (translated in the Materia Medica Pura, vol. ii).}

§ 111

AGREEMENT WITH POISON DRUG EFFECT

The agreement of my observations on the pure effects of medicines with these older ones – although they were recorded without reference to any therapeutic object, – and the very concordance of these accounts with others of the same kind by different authors must easily convince us that medicinal substances act in the morbid changes they produce in the healthy human body according to fixed, eternal laws of nature, and by virtue of these are enabled to produce certain, reliable disease symptoms each according to its own peculiar character.

EXPLANATION

- Based on his observations on the pure effects of medicines & similarly with these older observation, though these older ones were recorded without any therapeutic object.
- Based on observations of the same kind by different authors points us that medicinal substances act in human body & produce morbid changes in the healthy human body according to fixed, external laws of nature.
- By the virtue of these, medicines are able to produce certain, reliable d/s symptoms according to their own peculiar character.

§ 112

PRIMARY & SECONDARY ACTION OF DRUG

In those older prescriptions of the often dangerous effects of medicines ingested in excessively large doses we notice certain states that were produced, not at the commencement, but towards the termination of these sad events, and which were of an exactly opposite nature to those that first appeared. These symptoms, the very reverse of the primary action (§ 63) or proper action of the medicines on the vital force are the reaction of the vital force of the organism, its secondary action (§§ 62-67), of which, however, there is seldom or hardly ever the least trace from experiments with moderate doses on healthy bodies, and from small doses none whatever. In the homoeopathic curative operation the living organism reacts from these only so much as is requisite to raise the health again to the normal healthy state (§ 67).

EXPLANATION

- During the older prescriptions done by physician of old school they used to prescribe medicines in excessively large doses producing dangerous effects.
- They produced certain states towards the termination which were of an exactly opposite nature [secondary action] to those that first appeared [primary action].
- These symptoms are the reaction of the vital force of the organism, its secondary action [aph 62-67], to the primary action[aph- 63], of the medicines on the vital force.
- In the homeopathic curative operation the living organism reacts from these medicines to the level as is requistie to raise the health again to the normal healthy state[aph-67].

§ 113

EXCEPTIONS NARCOTIC MEDICINE

The only exceptions to this are the narcotic medicines. As they, in their primary action, take away sometimes the sensibility and sensation, sometimes the irritability, it frequently happens that in their secondary action, even from moderate experimental doses on healthy bodies, an increased sensibility (and a greater irritability) is observable.

EXPLANATION

- In this aphorism Hahnemann says that the only exceptions to above are the narcotic medicines.
- As the narcotic medicines, in their primary action, sometimes take away the sensibility & sensation, sometimes even the irritability so that in their secondary action an increased sensibility & a greater irritability is observed even from moderate experimental doses on healthy bodies.
- Here with narcotic medicines we see both the primary & secondary actions.
- Whereas with other medicines we get only the primary actions.

§ 114

PRIMARY ACTION IN NARCOTIC DOSES

With the exception of these narcotic substances, in experiments with moderate doses of medicine on healthy bodies, we observe only their primary action, i.e., those symptoms wherewith the medicine deranges the health of the human being and develops in him a morbid state of longer or shorter duration.

EXPLANATION

- In experiments with moderate doses of medicine on healthy bodies, we observe only their primary action, except these narcotic substances.
- We see only the primary action.
- So, we can say that when medicine in moderate doses are proved on healthy bodies, we observe only their primary action, the symptoms they produce, I.e- those symptoms wherewith the medicine deranges the health of the human -being & develops a morbid state of longer or shorter duration.

§ 115

ALTERNATING ACTION

Among these symptoms, there occur in the case of some medicines not a few which are partially, or under certain conditions, directly opposite to other symptoms that have previously or subsequently appeared, but which are not therefore to be regarded as actual secondary action or the mere reaction of the vital force, but which only represent the alternating state of the various paroxysms of the primary action; they are termed alternating actions.

EXPLANATION

- Here Hahnemann describes the alternating actions of the medicine.
- In the case of some medicines, we get symptoms which are partially opposite or under certain condition, directly opposite to other symptoms, obtained previously in other healthy person, which represents the alternating state of the various paroxysms of the primary action. They are termed as alternating actions.
- Do not confuse these alternating actions with actual secondary action or mere reaction of the vital force.

§ 116

PROVE DRUGS IN DIFFERENT PERSON'S

Some symptoms are produced by the medicines more frequently – that is to say, in many individuals, others more rarely or in few persons, some only in very few healthy bodies.

EXPLANATION

- While drug proving of medicines on healthy individuals, some symptoms are produced by the medicines more frequently.
    - I] These symptoms are produced in many individuals.
    - II] Other symptoms more rarely or in few persons only.
    - III] Some symptoms are produced only in very few healthy bodies.

§ 117

IDIOSYNCRASIES

To the latter category belong the so-called idiosyncrasies, by which are meant peculiar corporeal constitutions which, although otherwise healthy, possess a disposition to be brought into a more or less morbid state by certain things which seem to produce no impression and no change in many other individuals.1 But this inability to make an impression on every one is only apparent. For as two things are required for the production of these as well as all other morbid alterations in the health of man – to wit., the inherent power of the influencing substance, and the capability of the vital force that animates the organism to be influenced by it – the obvious derangements of health in the so-called idiosyncrasies cannot be laid to the account of these peculiar constitutions alone, but they must also be ascribed to these things that produce them, in which must lie the power of making the same impressions on all human bodies, yet in such a manner that but a small number of healthy constitutions have a tendency to allow themselves to be brought into such an obvious morbid condition by them. That these agents do actually make this impression on every healthy body is shown by this, that when employed as remedies they render effectual homoeopathic service2 to all sick persons for morbid symptoms similar to those they seem to be only capable of producing in so-called idiosyncratic individuals.

1 Some few persons are apt to faint from the smell of roses and to fall into many other morbid, and sometimes dangerous states from partaking of mussels, crabs or the roe of the barbel, from touching the leaves of some kinds of sumach, etc.

2 Thus the Princess Maria Porphyroghnita restored her brother, the Emperor Alexius, who suffered from faintings, by sprinkling him with rose water in the presence of his aunt Eudoxia (Hist. byz. Alexias, lib. xv, p. 503, ed. Posser); and Horstius (Oper., iii, p.59) saw great benefit from rose vinegar in cases of syncope.

EXPLANATION

To the third category of aph- 116 belong the so-called IDIOSYNCRASIES.

This is termed idiosyncrasy. These people are otherwise healthy.

Two things are required for production of these as well as all other morbid alterations in health of man-

- A]   The inherent power of the influencing substance.
- B]   Capability of the vital force [which animates the organism to be influenced by it]
- C]   The derangements of health in the so-called Idiosyncrasies are due to peculiar constitutions & the things that produce them.

These things that produce indiosyncrasies, have the power of making the same impressions on all human beings, yet small number of healthy constitutions have the tendency to allow themselves to produce morbid condition due to them.

- ✦ When these agents are employed as remedies they render Homeopathic cure to all sick persons with these morbid symptoms similar to those produced in idiosyncratic individuals.

Footnote:
Let us understand this with an example as mentioned in the footnote of this aphorism.

- ✦ A person faints from the smell of roses & gets many other morbid & dangerous states from taking mussels crab etc or from touching the leaves of sumach etc, while other produce no change.
- ✦ Princess Maria's brother was fainted she sprinkled some rose water on him & he was restored. Horsitus saw great benefit from rose vinegar in cases of syncope.

§ 118

PECULIAR ACTION

Every medicine exhibits peculiar actions on the human frame, which are not produced in exactly the same manner by any other medicinal substance of a different kind.1

1 This fact was also perceived by the estimable A. v. Haller, who says (Preface to his Hist. stirp. helv.): "Latet immensa virium diversitas in iis ipsis plantis, quarum facies externas dudum novimus, animas quasi et quodcunque caelestius habent, nondum perspeximus."

EXPLANATION

- Every medicine exhibits peculiar actions the human body.
- No two medicine of a different kind can produce actions exactly in the same manner.

Footnote:
This fact was also perceived by the A. V. Haller, who says in his own italian words ("Latet immensa virium diversitas in iis ipsis plantis, quarum facies externas dudum novimus, animas quasi et quodcunque caelestius habent, nondum perspeximus.)

§ 119

INDIVIDUALIZATION OF DRUG

As certainly as every species of plant differs in its external form, mode of life and growth, in its taste and smell from every other species and genus of plant, as certainly as every mineral and salt differs from all others, in its external as well as its internal physical and chemical properties (which alone should have sufficed to prevent any confounding of one with another), so certainly do they all differ and diverge among themselves in their pathogenetic – consequently also in their therapeutic – effects.1 Each of these substances produces alterations in the health of human beings in a peculiar, different, yet determinate manner, so as to preclude the possibility of confounding one with another.2

1 Anyone who has a thorough knowledge of, and can appreciate the remarkable difference of, effects on the health of man of every single substance from those of every other, will readily perceive that among them there can be, in a medical point of view, no equivalent remedies whatever, no surrogates. Only those who do not know the pure, positive effects of the different medicines can be so foolish as to try to persuade us that one can serve in the stead of the other, and can in the same disease prove just as serviceable as the other. Thus do ignorant children confound the most essential different things, because they scarcely know their external appearances, far less their real value, their true importance and their very dissimilar inherent properties.

2 If this be pure truth, as it undoubtedly is, then no physician who would not be regarded as devoid of reason, and who would not act contrary to the dictates of his conscience, the sole arbiter of real worth, can employ in the treatment of diseases any medicinal substance but one with whose real significance he is thoroughly and perfectly conversant, i.e., whose positive action on the health of healthy individuals he has so accurately tested that he knows for certain that it is capable of producing a very similar morbid state, more similar than any other medicine with which he is perfectly acquainted, to that presented by the case of disease he intends to cure by means of it; for, as has been shown above, neither man, nor mighty Nature herself, can effect a perfect, rapid and permanent cure otherwise than with a homoeopathic remedy. Henceforth no true physician can abstain from making such experiment, in order to obtain this most necessary and only knowledge of the medicines that are essential to cure, this knowledge which has hitherto been neglected by the physicians in all ages. In all former ages – posterity will scarcely believe it – physicians have hitherto contented themselves with blindly prescribing for diseases medicines whose value was unknown, and which had never been tested relative to their highly important, very various, pure dynamic action on the health of man; and, moreover, they mingled several of these unknown medicines that differed so vastly among each other in one formula, and left it to chance to determine what effects should thereby be produced on the patient. This is just as if a madman should force his way into the workshop of an artisan, seize upon handfuls of very different tools, with the uses of all of which he is quite unacquainted, in order, as he imagines, to work at the objects of art he sees around him. I need hardly remark that these would be destroyed, I may say utterly ruined, by his senseless operations.

EXPLANATION

- Every species of plant differs in its external form, mode of life & growth, in its taste & smell from every other species & genus of plant.
- Also every mineral & salt differs from all others, in its external as well as its internal physical & chemical properties.
- So, certainly they all differ & diverge among themselves in their pathogenetic & therapeutic effects
- Each of these substances produces alterations in the health of human beings in a peculiar, different & determinate manner, so this prevents the possibility of confusing one with another.

Footnote:

Anyone who has a thorough knowledge of & can observe the difference of effects of every single substance from those of every other, on the health of man, he will see that, from medical point of view, that there is no equivalent remedies, no surrogates.

- Only those who do not know the pure, positive effects of different medicines can be so foolish & say that one medicine can serve in place of the other in a given d/s, other medicine can be used in place of this.
  Physician employs one medicinal substance whose real significance, whose positive action on the health of healthy individuals he has so accurately tested that he knows for certain that it is capable of producing a very similar morbid state, more similar than any other medicine with which he is perfectly familiar.
- Neither man, nor mightly nature herself, can bring a perfect, rapid & permanent cure than with a homeopathic remedy.
- True physician should not abstain from making such experiment, in order to obtain this most necessary & only knowledge of the medicines that are essential to cure.
- In all former times- physicians have blindly prescribed medicines. Those medicines whose value was unknown & which had never been tested for pure dynamic action on the health of man.
- They also mixed several of these unknown medicines that differ from each other vastly.
- They left it to chance to determine what effects should be produced on the patient.
- This is a senseless operation, destroying the precious life of human.

§ 120

CAREFUL DRUG-PROVING

Therefore medicines, on which depend man's life and death, disease and health, must be thoroughly and most carefully distinguished from one another, and for this purpose tested by

careful, pure experiments on the healthy body for the purpose of ascertaining their powers and real effects, in order to obtain an accurate knowledge of them, and to enable us to avoid any mistake in their employment in diseases, for it is only by correct selection of them that the greatest of all earthly blessings, the health of the body and of the mind, can be rapidly and permanently restored.

EXPLANATION

- The medicines should be tested by careful, pure experiments on the healthy body to ascertain their powers & real effects, so that accurate knowledge of medicines can be obtained because on those medicines depends the man's life & death, d/s & health.
- Proper knowledge of medicines enable us to avoid any mistake in their use. By the correct selection of medicines the health of the body & of the mind, can be rapidly & permanently restored.

§ 121

DRUG DOSES FOR PROVING

In proving medicines to ascertain their effects on the healthy body, it must be borne in mind that the strong, heroic substances, as they are termed, are liable even in small doses to produce changes in the health even of robust persons. Those of milder power must be given for these experiments in more considerable quantities; in order to observe the action of the very weakest, however, the subjects of experiment should be persons free from disease, and who are delicate, irritable and sensitive.

EXPLANATION

- While proving the medicines to ascertain their effects on the healthy body, it must be noted that the strong, heroic substances even in small doses, produces changes in the health even of robust persons.
- The substances of milder power must be given in more considerable quantities, in order to observe the action of the very weakest substances.
- The subjects of experiment should be persons free from d/s & who are delicate, irritable & sensitive.

§ 122

PROVE SINGLE DRUG

In these experiments – on which depends the exactitude of the whole medical art, and the weal of all future generations of mankind – no other medicines should be employed except such as are perfectly well known, and of whose purity, genuineness and energy we are thoroughly assured.

EXPLANATION

- In these experiments, medicines used should be perfectly well known & their purity, genuineness & energy should be thoroughly assured.
- Because on them depends the accuracy of the whole medical art & which is the best for future generation of the mankind.

§ 123

METHOD OF PREPARATION

Each of these medicines must be taken in a perfectly simple, unadulterated form; the indigenous plants in the form of freshly expressed juice, mixed with a little alcohol to prevent it spoiling; exotic vegetable substances, however, in the form of powder, or tincture prepared with alcohol when they were in the fresh state and afterwards mingled with a certain proportion of water; salts and gums, however, should be dissolved in water just before being taken. If the plant can only be procured in its dry state, and if its powers are naturally weak, in that case there may be used for the experiment an infusion of it, made by cutting the herb into small pieces and pouring boiling water on it, so as to extract its medicinal parts; immediately after its preparation it must be swallowed while still warm, as all expressed vegetable juices and all aqueous infusions of herbs, without the addition of spirit, pass rapidly into fermentation and decomposition, whereby all their medicinal properties are lost.

EXPLANATION

- Each of these medicines must be taken in a perfectly simple, unadulterated form, like
- Indigenous plants in the form of freshly expressed juice, which is mixed with a little alcohol to prevent it from, spoiling.

- Exotic vegetables in fresh state are taken in the form of powder or tincture prepared with alcohol & afterwards mixed with a certain proportion of water.
- Salts & gums should be dissolved in water just before taking.
- If the plant is available only in dry state & if its powers are naturally weak, cut the herb into small pieces & pour boiling water on it, so that the medicinal parts can be extracted.

It must be swallowed immediately after its preparation while it is warm, I.e- its infusion is used.

§ 124

SINGLE DRUG PROVING

For these experiments every medicinal substance must be employed quite alone and perfectly pure, without the admixture of any foreign substance, and without taking anything else of a medicinal nature the same day, nor yet on the subsequent days, nor during all the time we wish to observe the effects of the medicine.

EXPLANATION

- While drug -proving, every medicinal substance must be employed alone & perfectly pure, without admixing foreign substance.
- During experiment the healthy person on which proving is being performed should not take anything else of a medicinal nature same day, on subsequent days till we wish to observe the effects of the medicine.

§ 125

DIET

During all the time the experiment lasts the diet must be strictly regulated; it should be as much as possible destitute of spices, of a purely nutritious and simple character, green vegetables,1 roots and all salads and herb soups (which, even when most carefully prepared, possess some disturbing medicinal qualities) should be avoided. The drinks are to be those usually partaken of, as little stimulating as possible.2

1 Young green peas, green French beans ('boiled potatoes' in the Sixth Edition) and in all cases carrots are allowable, as the least medicinal vegetables.

2 The subject of experiment must either be not in the habit of taking pure wine, brandy, coffee or tea, or he must have totally abstained for a considerable time previously from the use of these injurious beverages, some of which are stimulating, others medicinal.

EXPLANATION

- During the experiment till we wish to observe the effects of the medicine, the diet of the person must be strictly regulated.
- It should be devoid of [does not include]spices, green vegetables, roots & all salads & herb soups.
- The diet should be purely nutritious & of simple character.
- The drinks should be as little stimulatory as possible.

Footnote:
- Diet can include green vegetables, young green peas, green french beans, boiled potatoes, carrot are allowed as they are the least medicial vegetables.
- Drinks like pure wine, brandy, coffee.tea are not allowed. The person should not have a habit of taking these or must have totally stopped their consumption for a considerable time. Some of these are stimulating, others are medicinal.

§ 126

QUALITIES OF PROVER

The person who is proving the medicine must be pre-eminently trustworthy and conscientious and during the whole time of the experiment avoid all over-exertion of mind and body, all sorts of dissipation and disturbing passions; he should have no urgent business to distract his attention; he must devote himself to careful self-observation and not be disturbed while so engaged; his body must be in what is for him a good state of health, and he must possess a sufficient amount of intelligence to be able to express and describe his sensations in accurate terms.

EXPLANATION

- The person who is proving the medicine must be trust -worthy and attentive.
- During the whole time of the experiment he should avoid all over-exertion of mind & body, all disturbing work.
- He should have no urgent business that can distract his attention.
- His body must be in a good state of health & he must possess a sufficient amount of intelligence so that he will be able to express & describe jis sensations in accurate words.

§ 127

DRUG PROVING ON BOTH SEXES

The medicines must be tested on both males and females, in order also to reveal the alterations of the health they produce in the sexual sphere.

EXPLANATION

- The medicines must be tested on both males & females.
- It is tested on both sexes in order to reveal the alteration of the health they produce in the sexual sphere.

§ 128

PROVE ONLY DYNAMIC DRUG

The most recent observations have shown that medicinal substances, when taken in their crude state by the experimenter for the purpose of testing their peculiar effects, do not exhibit nearly the full amount of the powers that lie hidden in them which they do when they are taken for the same object in high dilutions potentized by proper trituration and succussion, by which simple operations the powers which in their crude state lay hidden, and, as it were, dormant, are developed and roused into activity to an incredible extent. In this manner we now find it best to investigate the medicinal powers even of such substances as are deemed weak, and the plan we adopt is to give to the experimenter, on an empty stomach, daily from four to six very small globules of the thirtieth potency of such a substance, moistened with a little water or dissolved in more or less water and thoroughly mixed, and let him continue this for several days.

EXPLANATION

- The medicinal substances, when taken in their crude state by experimenter to test their effects, they found that the crude substances do not show the powers hidden in them.
- When the same substances is taken in high dilutions, potentized by proper trituration & succussion the hidden dormant powers roused into activity to an incredible extent.
- So now even such weak substances are given to experimenter after dilutions.

E.g. we give 4-6 very small globules of 30th potency, moistened with a little water or dissolved in more or less water & mixed thoroughly on an empty stomach for several days.

§ 129

MINIMUM DOSE

If the effects that result from such a dose are but slight, a few more globules may be taken daily, until they become more distinct and stronger and the alterations of the health more conspicuous; for all persons are not effected by a medicine in an equally great degree; on the contrary, there is a vast variety in this respect, so that sometimes an apparently weak individual may by scarcely at all affected by moderate doses of a medicine known to be of a powerful character, while he is strongly enough acted on by others of a much weaker kind. And, on the other hand, there are very robust persons who experience very considerable morbid symptoms from an apparently mild medicine, and only slighter symptoms from stronger drugs. Now, as this cannot be known beforehand, it is advisable to commence in every instance with a small dose of the drug and, where suitable and requisite, to increase the dose more and more from day to day.

EXPLANATION

- Different persons react to the given dose of drug differently.
- Sometimes an apparently weak individual may be scarcely [to a little degree] effected by moderate doses of medicine of powerful character.
  While he is strongly acted on by medicine of weaker character.
  Similarly a very robust [strong] person may experience very considerable morbid symptoms from a mild medicine & experiences only slight symptoms from stronger drugs.
- Now as this cannot be known to us, so it is advisable to start with a small dose of the drug & when suitable & required, increase the dose more & more from day to day.
- If the effects from such a dose are slight a few more globules may be taken daily until they become more distinct & stronger & alterations of the health becomes more conspicuous.

§ 130

FIRST DOSE

If, at the very commencement, the first dose administered shall have been sufficiently strong, this advantage is gained, that the experimenter learns the order of succession of the symptoms and can note down accurately the period at which each occurs, which is very useful in leading to a knowledge of the genius of the medicine, for then the order of the primary actions, as also that of the alternating actions, is observed in the most unambiguous manner. A very moderate dose, even, often suffices for the experiment, provided only the experimenter is endowed with sufficiently delicate sensitiveness, and is very attentive to his sensations. The duration of the action of a drug can only be ascertained by a comparison of several experiments.

EXPLANATION

If, at the starting the first dose administered has been sufficiently strong, the experimenter learns the order of succession of the symptoms & can note down the period at which each occurs,

This is very useful in getting information of the genius of the medicine. Genius means the innate nature of medicine, which is peculiar to anything & constitutes its identity, its nature, disposition, peculiar character etc.

It distinguishes it form all other medicines. Now the order of the primary actions & of the alternating, is observed in completely clear manner.

- Even a very moderate dose is yielding if the experimenter is sensitive & is very attentive to his sensations.
- The duration of the action of a drug can be confirmed by the comparison of several experiments.

§ 131

INCREASING THE DOSE

If, however, in order to ascertain anything at all, the same medicine must be given to the same person to test for several successive days in ever increasing doses, we thereby learn, no doubt, the various morbid states this medicine is capable of producing in a general manner, but we do not ascertain their order of succession; and the subsequent dose often removes, curatively, some one or other of the symptoms caused by the previous dose, or develops in its stead an opposite state; such symptoms should be enclosed in brackets, to mark their ambiguity, until subsequent purer experiments show whether they are the reaction of the organism and secondary action or an alternating action of this medicine.

EXPLANATION

- If we want to confirm anything, the same medicine must be given to the same person for several successive days in ever -increasing doses.
- We learn the various morbid states produced by medicine in a general manner but not about their order of succession.

- The subsequent dose often removes some symptoms caused by previous dose, curatively or develops an opposite state.
- Such symptoms should be in -closed in brackets until subsequent purer experiments show us that whether they are the reaction of the organism & secondary action or an alternating action of this medicine.

§ 132

DRUG PROVING OF WEAK MEDICINAL SUBSTANCES

But when the object is, without reference to the sequential order of the phenomena and the duration of the action of the drug, only to ascertain the symptoms themselves, especially those of a weak medicinal substance, in that case the preferable course to pursue is to give it for several successive days, increasing the dose every day. In this manner the action of an unknown medicine, even of the mildest nature, will be revealed, especially if tested on sensitive persons.

EXPLANATION

- If we want to ascertain the symptoms of the medicine especially those of a weak medicinal substances, we need to give it for several successive days.
- The dose of medicine is increased everyday.
- In this manner the action of an unknown medicine even of the mildest nature will be revealed, especially if tested on sensitive persons.

§ 133

FIRST OBSERVED

On experiencing any particular sensation from the medicine, it is useful, indeed necessary, in order to determine the exact character of the symptom, to assume various positions while it lasts, and to observe whether, by moving the part affected, by walking in the room or the open air, by standing, sitting or lying the symptom is increased, diminished or removed, and whether it returns on again assuming the position in which it was first observed, – whether it is altered by eating or drinking, or by any other condition, or by speaking, coughing, sneezing or any other action of the body, and at the same time to note at what time of the day or night it usually occurs in the most marked manner, whereby what is peculiar to and characteristic of each symptom will become apparent.

EXPLANATION

- In order to determine the exact character of the symptom, it is necessary to observe the symptom in various positions.
- Let us take an example, we got a symptom of Headache. Now we will determine the exact character of headache by the medicine.
- We will observe by moving the part affected, by walking in room or open air, by standing, sitting or lying the symptom of headache is increased, diminished or removed.
- Now we will again assume the position in which headache was first observed, to see if it returns or not.
- Now we observe if it is altered by eating or drinking or by any other condition, or by speaking, coughing, sneezing or any other action of the body.
- We also note at what time day or night it usually occurs in the most marked manner.
- This way what is peculiar to & characteristic of each symptom will become apparent.

§ 134

DRUG PROVING ON MULTIPLE PERSON

All external influences, and more especially medicines, possess the property of producing in the health of the living organism a particular kind of alteration peculiar to themselves; but all the symptoms peculiar to a medicine do not appear in one person, nor all at once, nor in the same experiment, but some occur in one person chiefly at one time, others again during a second or third trail; in another person some other symptoms appear, but in such a manner that probably some of the phenomena are observed in the fourth, eighth or tenth person which had already appeared in the second, sixth or ninth person, and so forth; moreover, they may not recur at the same hour.

EXPLANATION

- All external influences & medicine have the property of producing a particular kind of alteration peculiar to themselves, in the health of the living organism,
- But all the symptoms of a medicine do not appear in one person, nor all at once, nor in the same experiment.
- Some occur in one person chiefly at one time, others during a second or third trial.

- In another person some other symptoms appear in a manner observed in the 4th, 8th or 10th person which had already appeared in the 2nd, 6th, or 9th person & so on.
- Moreover the symptoms may not recur at the same hour.

§ 135

SURVEILLANCE DURING PROVING

The whole of the elements of disease a medicine is capable of producing can only be brought to anything like completeness by numerous observations on suitable persons of both sexes and of various constitutions. We can only be assured that a medicine has been thoroughly proved in regard to the morbid states it can produce – that is to say, in regard to its pure powers of altering the health of man – when subsequent experimenters can notice little of a novel character from its action, and almost always only the same symptoms as had been already observed by others.

EXPLANATION

- After numerous observations on suitable persons of both sexes & of various constitution we can get the whole elements of d/s, a medicine is capable of producing.
- We can get assured that a medicine has been thoroughly proved when subsequent experimenters can produce the same symptoms almost always observed by others.
- Like this the pure powers of medicine in altering the health of man is proved.

§ 136

ALL SYMPTOMS OF DRUG CAN'T BE NOTED ON ONE PERSON

Although, as has been said, a medicine, on being proved on healthy subjects, cannot develop in one person all the alterations of health it is capable of causing, but can only do this when given to many different individuals, varying in their corporeal and mental constitution, yet the tendency to excite all these symptoms in every human being exists in it (§ 117), according to an eternal and immutable law of nature, by virtue of which all its effects, even those that are but rarely developed in the healthy person, are brought into operation in the case of every individual if administered to him when he is in a morbid state presenting similar symptoms; it then, even in

the smallest dose, being homoeopathically selected, silently produces in the patient an artificial state closely resembling the natural disease, which rapidly and permanently (homoeopathically) frees and cures him of his original malady.

EXPLANATION

- A medicine, when it is proved on healthy subjects does not develop all the symptoms in one person.
- It develops all the alterations of health when given to many different individuals who differ in their corporeal & mental constitution.
- The tendency to excite all the symptoms in every human being exists in every medicine [aph-117].
- When a medicine is administered to a person [patient] (when he is in a morbid state presenting similar symptoms), then {a patient presenting with similar symptoms of medicine}, then all its effects, are brought into operation in the case of every individual.
- Even those symptoms which are rarely developed in the healthy person are brought into operation in every individual who is suffering from similar symptoms as of medicine [I.e-in the patient].
- The medicine even in the smallest dose, when selected homeopathically, silently produces an artificial state resembling the natural d/s, which rapidly & permanently cures the sick patient from original malady.

§ 137

MODERATE DOSE

The more moderate, within certain limits, the doses of the medicine used for such experiments are – provided we endeavor to facilitate the observation by the selection of a person who is a lover of truth, temperate in all respects, of delicate feelings, and who can direct the most minute attention to his sensation – so much the more distinctly are the primary effects developed, and only these, which are most worth knowing, occur without any admixture of secondary effects or reactions of the vital force. When, however, excessively large doses are used there occur at the same time not only a number of secondary effects among the symptoms, but the primary effects developed, and only these, which are most worth knowing, occur without any admixture of secondary effects or reactions of the vital force. When, however, excessively large doses are used there occur at the same time not only a number of secondary effects among the symptoms, but the primary effects also come on in such hurried confusion and with such impetuosity that nothing can be accurately observed; let alone the danger attending them, which no one who has any regard for his fellow-creatures, and who looks on the meanest of mankind as his brother, will deem an indifferent manner.

EXPLANATION

- Within certain limits, the more moderate the doses of medicine used for such experiment the more distinctly the primary effects develop & occur without any admixture of secondary effects or reactions of the vital force.
- Above can be achieved only if the person selelcted is a lover of truth, temperate [mind]in all respects, he has delicate feelings & can direct the most minute attention to his sensations.

§ 138

ALTERATION IN HEALTH DURING DRUG PROVING

All the sufferings, accidents and changes of the health of the experimenter during the action of a medicine (provided the above condition [§§ 124-127] essential to a good and pure experiment are complied with) are solely derived from this medicine, and must be regarded and registered as belonging peculiarly to this medicine, as symptoms of this medicine, even though the experimenter had observed, a considerable time previously, the spontaneous occurrence of similar phenomena in himself. The reappearance of these during the trial of the medicine only shows that this individual is, by virtue of his peculiar constitution, particularly disposed to have such symptoms excited in him. In this case they are the effect of the medicine; the symptoms do not arise spontaneously while the medicine that has been taken is exercising an influence over the health of the whole system, but are produced by the medicine.

EXPLANATION

- When a medicine is given to the experimenter during the action of a medicine, all the changes in the health, all the sufferings & accidents are due to this medicine.
- These sufferings must be registered as belonging to this medicine,
- For this, above [aph-124-127] all conditions mentioned in these aphorism should be followed.
- The experimenter may have observed similar phenoma in himself some time previously, but the reappearance of these symptom during the trial of the medicine means that in this case they are the effect of the medicine.
- In this case they are the effects of the medicine, the symptoms do not arise spontaneously they are produced by the medicine.

§ 139

BE CAREFUL WHILE WRITING THE SYMPTOMS

When the physician does not make the trial of the medicine on himself, but gives it to another person, the latter must note down distinctly the sensations, sufferings, accidents and changes of health he experiences at the time of their occurrence, mentioning the time after the ingestion of the drug when each symptom arose and, if it lasts long, the period of its duration. The physician looks over the report in the presence of the experimenter immediately after the experiment is concluded, or if the trial lasts several days he does this every day, in order, while everything is still fresh in his memory, to question him about the exact nature of every one of these circumstances, and to write down the more precise details so elicited, or to make such alterations as the experimenter may suggest.1

1 He who makes known to the medical world the results of such experiments becomes thereby responsible for the trustworthiness of the person experimented on and his statements, and justly so, as the weal of suffering humanity is here at stake.

EXPLANATION

- When the medicine is tested on another person & the physician does not make the trial of the medicine on himself.
- In these cases all the sensations, sufferings, accidents & changes of health he experiences should be noted down distinctly.
- The time of occurrence of each symptom after the ingestion of the drug & if the symptom lasts long, the period of its duration must be noted down.
- The physician looks over the report in the presence of the experimenter immediately after the experiment is completed.
- If the trial lasts several days he does this every day, when everything is still fresh in his memory, he questions him about the exact nature of every symptom & sensation & writes it down in details.

Footnote:
The person who makes us know the results of such experiments is responsible for the results of such experiments and the truthfulness of sensations rely on him.

§ 140

ILLITERATE PROVER

If the person cannot write, the physician must be informed by him every day of what has occurred to him, and how it took place. What is noted down as authentic information on this point, however, must be chiefly the voluntary narration of the person who makes the experiment, nothing conjectural and as little as possible derived from answers to leading questions should be admitted; everything must be ascertained with the same caution as I have counselled above (§§ 84-99) for the investigation of the phenomena and for tracing the picture of natural diseases.

EXPLANATION

- For the investigation of the phenomena & for tracing the picture of natural d/s following things should be noted.
- If the person cannot write, he should inform the physician what has occurred to him & how it look place every day.
- While noting down the information given, it should be voluntary narration of the person who makes the experiment.
- Try not to get answers to leading questions.
- Follow caution as told in [aph-84-99], for the investigation of the phenomena & for tracing the picture of natural d/s.

§ 141

IDEAL PROVER-PHYSICIAN HIMSELF

But the best provings of the pure effects of simple medicines in altering the human health, and of the artificial diseases and symptoms they are capable of developing in the healthy individual, are those which the healthy, unprejudiced and sensitive physician institutes on himself with all the caution and care here enjoined. He knows with the greatest certainty the things he has experienced in his own person.1

   1 Those trials made by the physician on himself have for him other and inestimable advantages. In the first place, the great truth that the medicinal virtue of all drugs, whereon depends their curative power, lies in the changes of health he has himself undergone from the medicines he has proved, and the morbid states he has himself experienced from them, becomes for him an incontrovertible

fact. Again by such noteworthy observations on himself he will be brought to understand his own sensations, his mode of thinking and his disposition (the foundation of all true wisdom "), and he will be also trained to be, what every physician ought to be, a good observer. All our observations on others are not nearly so interesting as those made on ourselves. The observer of others must always dread lest the experimenter did not feel exactly what he said, or lest he did not describe his sensations with the most appropriate expressions. He must always remain in doubt whether he has not been deceived, at least to some extent. These obstacles to the knowledge of the truth, which can never be thoroughly surmounted in our investigations of the artificial morbid symptoms that occur in others from the ingestion of medicines, cease entirely when we make the trials on ourselves. He who makes these trials on himself knows for certain what he has felt, and each trial is a new inducement for him to investigate the powers of other medicines. He thus becomes more and more practised in the art of observing, of such importance to the physician, by continuing to observe himself, the one on whom he can most rely and who will never deceive him; and this he will do all the more zealously as these experiments on himself promise to give him a reliable knowledge of the true value and significance of the instruments of cure that are still to a great degree unknown to our art. Let it not be imagined that such slight indispositions caused by taking medicines for the purpose of proving them can be in the main injurious to the health. Experience shows on the contrary, that the organism of the prover becomes, by these frequent attacks on his health, all the more expert in repelling all external influences inimical to his frame and all artificial and natural morbific noxious agents, and becomes more hardened to resist everything of an injurious character, by means of these moderate experiments on his own person with medicines. His health becomes more unalterable; he becomes more robust, as all experience shows.

EXPLANATION

- The best provings of the pure effects of simple medicines in altering the human health & of artificial d/s & symptoms they develop in the healthy individual, is done by a healthy, unprejudiced and sensitive physician on himself.
- The physician should note them with caution & care
- He knows the things he has experienced with greatest certainty.

So a healthy, unprejudiced & sensitive physician is the best prover.

Footnote:
- The trials made by the physician on himself have many advantages.

    1. The changes of health & morbid states he has himself experienced from them, become the most reliable & incontrovertible fact.
    2. By such observations on himself he understands his own sensations, his mode of thinking & his disposition & he will be also trained to be a good observer.
    3. All our observations on others are not nearly so interesting & reliable as those made on ourselves.

It may occur that the experimenter does not feel exactly what he is saying or may not be able to describe his sensations with most appropriate expressions.

All these obstacles are removed if the trials are made by physician himself on him.

- ✦ He knows for certain what he has felt, the powers of other medicines.
- ✦ Like this he becomes more & more practised in the art of observing.
- ✦ The organism who becomes a prover, becomes more expert in repelling all external influences & all artificial & natural morbific noxious agents, his health becomes more unalterable, he becomes more robust.

§ 142

HIGHER ART OF JUDGEMENT

But how some symptoms1 of the simple medicine employed for a curative purpose can be distinguished amongst the symptoms of the original malady, even in diseases, especially in those of a chronic character that usually remain unaltered, is a subject appertaining to the higher art of judgement, and must be left exclusively to masters in observation.

1 Symptoms which, during the whole course of the disease, might have been observed only a long time previously, or never before, consequently new ones, belonging to the medicine.

EXPLANATION

- Among the symptoms of the original malady how some symptoms, of the simple medicine [which is employed for a curative purpose], can be distinguished, it must be left to the masters in observing, to the higher art of judgement.
- Especially in those d/s of a chronic character that usually remain unaltered.

Footnote:
Symptoms during the whole course of the d/s, belonging to the medicine which have been observed a long time previously or never before [new ones].

§ 143

MATERIA MEDICA PURA

If we have thus tested on the healthy individual a considerable number of simple medicines and carefully and faithfully registered all the disease elements and symptoms they are capable of

developing as artificial disease-producers, then only have we a true materia medica – a collection of real, pure, reliable1 modes of action of simple medicinal substances, a volume of the book of nature, wherein is recorded a considerable array of the peculiar changes of the health and symptoms ascertained to belong to each of the powerful medicines, as they were revealed to the attention of the observer, in which the likeness of the (homoeopathic) disease elements of many natural diseases to be hereafter cured by them are present, which, in a word, contain artificial morbid states, that furnish for the similar natural morbid states the only true, homoeopathic, that is to say, specific, therapeutic instruments for effecting their certain and permanent cure.

1 Latterly it has been the habit to entrust the proving of medicines to unknown persons at a distance, who were paid for their work, and the formation so obtained was printed. But by so doing, the work which is of all others the most important, which is to form the basis of the only true healing art, and which demands the greatest moral certainty and trustworthiness seems to me, I regret to say, to become doubtful and uncertain in its results and to lose all value.

EXPLANATION

- For a true materia medica- - a collection of real, pure, reliable modes of action of simple medicinal substances, a volume of the book of nature, careful & faithful record of all the d/s elements & symptoms they develop as artificial d/s -producers need to be made.
- In this materia media a considerable array of the peculiar changes of the health and symptoms that belong to each of the powerful medicines, should be recorded as they were revealed to the attention of the observer.
- It contains artificial morbid states, that provide homeopathic I.e- specific therapeutic instruments for the similar natural morbid states, for effecting their certain & permanent cure.

Footnote:
Recently it has become habit to trust the proving of medicines by unknown persons who are far away. They were paid for their work & the information they gave was printed, but Hahnemann says that it is not moral & trustworthly it seems doubtful & unceratin in its results & loses all value.

- ✦ By this way the work, which is the most important to form the basis of the only true healing art becomes doubtful & uncertain.

§ 144

BUILDING OF MATERIAL MEDICA

From such a materia medica everything that is conjectural, all that is mere assertion or imaginary should be strictly excluded; everything should be the pure language of nature carefully and honestly interrogated.

EXPLANATION

- In this materia medica everything should be the pure language of nature, carefully & honestly interrogated.
- It must not contain everything that is formed on basis of, mere assertion or imaginary incomplete information.

§ 145

REMEDY

Of a truth, it is only by a very considerable store of medicines accurately known in respect of these their pure modes of action in altering the health of man, that we can be placed in a position to discover a homoeopathic remedy, a suitable artificial (curative) morbific analogue for each of the infinitely numerous morbid states in nature, for every malady in the world.1 In the meantime, even now – thanks to the truthful character of the symptoms, and to the abundance of disease elements which every one of the powerful medicinal substances has already shown in its action on the healthy body – but few disease remain, for which a tolerably suitable homoeopathic remedy may not be met with among those now proved as to their pure action,2 which, without much disturbance, restores health in a gentle, sure and permanent manner - infinitely more surely and safely than can be effected by all the general and special therapeutics of the old allopathic medical art with its unknown composite remedies, which do but alter and aggravate but cannot cure chronic diseases, and rather retard than promote recovery from acute diseases and frequently endanger life.

1 At first, about forty years ago, I was the only person who made the provings of the pure powders of medicines the most important of his occupations. Since then I have been assisted in this by some young men, who instituted experiments on themselves, and whose observations I have critically revised. Following these some genuine work of this kind was done by a few others. But what shall we not be able to effect in the way of curing in the whole extent of the infinitely large domain of disease, when numbers of accurate and trustworthy observers shall have rendered their services in enriching this, the only true materia medica, by careful experiments on themselves! The healing art will then come near the mathematical sciences in certainty.

2 See the second note to §109.

EXPLANATION

- All the general & special therapeutics of the old allopathic medical art has unknown composite remedies.
- They alter & aggravate the chronic d/s but cannot cure them.
- They retard recovery from acute d/s & frequently endanger life.

- Homeopathy, without much disturbance, restores health in a gentle, sure & permanent manner. It infinitely more surely & safely restores health better in every way than old allopathic medical art.
- Medicines accurately known of their pure modes of action help in altering the health of man for each of the infinitely numerous morbid states in nature, for every malady in the world.
- Few d/s remain, for which a suitable Homeopathic remedy may not be available with among those proved medicine.
- Thanks to the truthful character of the symptoms & abundance of d/s elements which every one of the powerful medicinal substance has shown in its action on the healthy body.

Footnote:
Hahnemann says that 40 years ago, 'I was the only person who made proving of medicines.'

Since then many young men assisted him who conducted experiments on themselves & I revised their observation.

The infinitely large domain of d/s can be cured, when numbers of accurate & trustworthy observers shall have given their services in enriching this, the only true materia medica by careful experiments on themselves

§ 146

3RD POINT INFORMATION

The third point of the business of a true physician relates to the judicious employment of the artificial morbific agents (medicines) that have been proved on healthy individuals to ascertain their pure action in order to effect the homoeopathic cure of natural diseases.

EXPLANTATION

- The third point important for a true physician to follow is to employ medicines [the artificial morbific agents] that have been proved on healthy individuals to ascertain their pure action.
- This is important in order to effect the homeopathic cure of natural d/s.

§ 147

SPECIFIC REMEDY

Whichever of these medicines that have been investigated as to their power of altering man's health we find to contain in the symptoms observed from its use the greatest similarity to the

totality of the symptoms of a given natural disease, this medicine will and must be the most suitable, the most certain homoeopathic remedy for the disease; in it is found the specific remedy of this case of disease.

EXPLANATION

- In a given case of disease, the treatment is based on the totality of the symptoms of a given natural disease.
- The medicine with greatest similarity to the totality of the symptoms of a given natural d/s is the most suitable, the most certain homoeopathic remedy for the d/s.
- In it is found the specific remedy of this case of d/s.

§ 148

NATURAL D/S CURED BY DYNAMIC AGENCY

The natural disease is never to be considered as a noxious material situated somewhere within the interior or exterior of man (§ 11-13) but as one produced by an inimical spirit-like (conceptual) agency which, like a kind of infection (note to § 11) disturbs in its instinctive existence of the spirit-like (conceptual) principle of life within the organism torturing it as an evil spirit and compelling it to produce certain ailments and disorders in the regular course of its life. These are known as symptoms (disease). If, now, the influence of this inimical agency that not only caused but strives to continue this disorder, be taken away as is done when the physician administers an artificial potency, capable of altering the life principle in the most similar manner (a homoeopathic medicine) which exceeds in energy even in the smallest dose the similar natural disease (§§ 33, 279), then the influence of the original noxious morbid agent on the life principle is lost during the action of this stronger similar artificial disease. Thence the evil no longer exists for the life principle – it is destroyed. If, as has been said, the selected homoeopathic remedy is administered properly, then the acute natural disease which is to be overruled if recently developed, will disappear imperceptibly in a few hours.

An older, more chronic disease will yield somewhat later together with all traces of discomfort, by the use of several doses of the same more highly potentized remedy or after careful selection1 of one or another more similar homoeopathic medicine. Health, recovery, follow in imperceptible, often rapid transitions. The life principle is freed again and capable of resuming the life of the organism in health as before and strength returns.

1 But this laborious, sometimes very laborious, search for and selection of the homoeopathic remedy most suitable in every respect to each morbid state, is an operation which, notwithstanding all the admirable books for facilitating it, still demands the study of the original sources themselves, and at the same time a great amount of circumspection and serious deliberation, which have their

best rewards in the consciousness of having faithfully discharged our duty. How could his laborious, care-demanding task, by which alone the best way of curing diseases is rendered possible, please the gentlemen of the new mongrel sect, who assume the honorable name of homoeopathists, and even seem to employ medicines in form and appearance homoeopathic, but determined upon by them anyhow (quidquid in buccam venit), and who, when the unsuitable remedy does not immediately give relief, in place of laying the blame on their unpardonable ignorance and laxity in performing the most and important and serious of all human affairs, ascribe it to homoeopathy, which they accuse of great imperfection (if the truth be told, its imperfection consists in this, that the most suitable homoeopathic remedy for each morbid condition does not spontaneously fly into their mouths like roasted pigeons, without any trouble on their own part). They know, however, from frequent practice, how to make up for the inefficiency of the scarcely half homoeopathic remedy by the employment of allopathic means, that come much more handy to them, among which one or more dozens of leeches applied to the affected part, or little harmless venesections to the extent of eight ounces, and so forth, play an important part; and should the patient, in spite of all this, recover, they extol their venesections, leeches, etc., alleging that, had it not been for these, the patient would not have been pulled through, and they give us to understand, in no doubtful language, that these operations, derived without much exercise of genius from the pernicious routine of the old school, in reality contributed the best share towards the cure. But if the patient die under the treatment, as not unfrequently happens, they seek to console the friends by saying that "they themselves were witnesses that everything conceivable had been done for the lamented deceased". Who would do this frivolous and pernicious tribe the honour to call them, after the name of the very laborious but salutary art, homoeopathic physicians? May the just recompense await them, that, when taken ill, they may be treated in the same manner!

EXPLANATION

- We should not consider the natural d/s a noxious material which is situated within the interior or exterior of man [aph 11-13].
- Natural d/s is produced by an inimical spirit -like agency which, like a kind of infection disturbs the spirit -like principle of life within the organism.
- This agency torture the vital principle as an evil spirit & forces it to produce certain ailments & disorders in the regular course of its life. These are known as symptoms[d/s]
- When the physician administers an artificial potency of stronger similar artificial d/s, the influence of the original noxious morbid agent on the life principle is lost.
- Now the evil is destroyed and the life principle is freed again and is capable of resuming the life of organism in health & strength returns in a few hours, in an acute natural d/s.
- In case of an older, more chronic d/s the process is time consuming together with the discomfort in between.
- In chronic d/s several doses of the same more highly potentized remedy or one or another more similar homeopathic medicine is given after careful selection.
- The life principle is freed & now capable of resuming the life of organism in health as before & the strength returns.

Footnote:
- The search & selection of the homeopathic remedy which is the most suitable to each morbid state is very laborious taste.
- It demands the study of the original sources themselves and also great amount of inquiry of the case.
- This laborious care -demanding task is the best way of curing d/s,
  But some gentlemen of the new mongrel sect, employ the homeopathic medicines determined by them anyhow, when this unsuitable remedy does not immediately give relief they blame it to homeopathy, that it is imperfect.
- They now employ allopathic means e.g- one or more dozens of leeches, applied to the affected part or venesections etc
- But if the patient die under the treatment, they console the attendant saying that, 'they did everything that could be done." How can they be called Homeopathic physician?

§ 149

LONG STANDING D/S

Diseases of long standing (and especially such as are of a complicated character) require for their cure a proportionately longer time. More especially do the chronic medicinal dyscrasia so often produced by allopathic bungling along with the natural disease left uncured by it, require a much longer time for their recovery; often, indeed, are they incurable, in consequence of the shameful robbery of the patient's strength and juices (venesections, purgatives, etc.), on account of long continued use of large doses of violently acting remedies given on the basis of empty, false theories for alleged usefulness in cases of disease appearing similar, also in prescribing unsuitable mineral baths, etc., the principal feat performed by allopathy in its so-called methods of treatment.

EXPLANATION

- Long standing d/s & especially complicated d/s require a longer time for their cure.
- Chronic medicinal dyscrasia are often produced by allopathic wrong mode of treatment.
- The natural d/s is left uncured by it, these cases require a much longer time for their recovery, often they become incurable.
- The procedures like use of venesections, purgatives etc reduce patients strength & juices by their long continued use of large doses of violent remedies.
- These remedies are given on the basis of empty, false theories. They prescribe unsuitable mineral baths etc the principal feat performed by allopathic treatment.
- These all are of no use, the d/s is not cured.

§ 150

INDISPOSITION

If a patient complain of one or more trivial symptoms, that have been only observed a short time previously, the physician should not regard this as a fully developed disease but requires serious medical aid. A slight alteration in the diet and regimen will usually suffice to dispel such an indisposition.

EXPLANATION

- In some cases where the patient complains of 1 or more trivial symptoms, short time previously, here the physician should not regard it as a fully developed d/s that requires serious medical aid, sometimes a slight alteration in the diet & regimen is enough to remove such indisposition.

E.g. A patient comes to you & says that he is having headache since today morning and on case taking it is due to watching TV late night, just give him advise to sleep & take rest. This is a case of indisposition.

§ 151

VIOLENT SYMPTOMS

But if the patient complain of a few violent sufferings, the physician will usually find, on investigation, several other symptoms besides, although of a slighter character, which furnish a complete picture of the disease.

EXPLANATION

- But if the patient complains of a few violent sufferings. In this case on investigation, physician will find several other symptoms also & a complete picture of the d/s will be formed.
- Now proper homeopathic remedy can be employed.

§ 152

ACUTE D/S

The worse of the acute disease is, of so much the more numerous and striking symptoms is it generally composed, but with so much the more certainly may a suitable remedy for it be found, if there be a sufficient number of medicines known, with respect to their positive action, to choose from. Among the lists of symptoms of many medicines it will not be difficult to find one from whose separate disease elements an antitype of curative artificial disease, very like the totality of the symptoms of the natural disease, may be constructed, and such a medicine is the desired remedy.

EXPLANATION

The acute d/s-

- In acute diseases, the worse the d/s is, the more humerous & striking symptoms it produces.
- Now to select the suitable remedy, there should be a sufficient number of medicines known, from which we have to choose the right one.
- Now among the lists of symptoms of many medicines, we have to choose the very like the totality of the symptoms of the natural d/s & such a medicine is the desired remedy.
- So we have to choose the most suitable remedy based on the totality of the symptoms.

§ 153

CHARACTERISTIC SYMPTOMS

In this search for a homoeopathic specific remedy, that is to say, in this comparison of the collective symptoms of the natural disease with the list of symptoms of known medicines, in order to find among these an artificial morbific agent corresponding by similarity to the disease to be cured, the more striking, singular, uncommon and peculiar (characteristic) signs and symptoms1 of the case of disease are chiefly and most solely to be kept in view; for it is more particularly these that very similar ones in the list of symptoms of the selected medicine must correspond to, in order to constitute it the most suitable for effecting the cure. The more general and undefined symptoms: loss of appetite, headache, debility, restless sleep, discomfort, and so forth, demand but little attention when of that vague and indefinite character, if they cannot be more accurately described, as symptoms of such a general nature are observed in almost every disease and from almost every drug.

1 Dr. von Bonninghausen, by the publication of the characteristic symptoms of homoeopathic medicines and his repertory has rendered a great service to Homoeopathy as well as Dr. J. H. G. Jahr in his handbook of principal symptoms.

EXPLANATION

- While searching for a homeopathic specific remedy some symptoms are given more attention, these are the more striking, singular, uncommon & peculiar [characteristic] signs & symptoms of the case of d/s.
  E.g. The more general & undefined symptoms like loss of appetite, headache, debility, restless, sleep.discomfort etc, require little attention when of vague & indefinite character.
- This is because they are observed in almost every d/s & from almost every drug, so we have to compare from the collective symptoms of the natural d/s with the list of symptoms of known medicines.
- This way an artificial morbific agent [medicine]corresponding by the similarity to the d/s to be cured is found out.

Footnote:
Dr. von Bonninghausen, by the publication of the characteristic symptoms of homoeopathic medicines and his repertory has rendered a great service to Homoeopathy as well as Dr. J. H. G. Jahr in his handbook of principal symptoms.

§ 154

HOMOEOPATHIC MEDICINES CURE ACUTE DISEASE WITHOUT MUCH DISTURBANCE

If the antitype constructed from the list of symptoms of the most suitable medicine contain those peculiar, uncommon, singular and distinguishing (characteristic) symptoms, which are to be met with in the disease to be cured in the greatest number and in the greatest similarity, this medicine is the most appropriate homoeopathic specific remedy for this morbid state; the disease, if it be not one of very long standing, will generally be removed and extinguished by the first dose of it, without any considerable disturbance.

EXPLANATION

- Now from the list of symptoms, the antitype of the most suitable medicine containing those peculiar uncommon, singular & characteristic symptoms in the greatest number & in the greatest similarity is selected.
- This medicine is the most appropriate homeopathic specific remedy for this morbid state.
- If the d/s is not of very long standing, it will be removed by the first dose of it, without any considerable disturbance.

§ 155

APPROPRIATE DOSE

I say without any considerable disturbance. For in the employment of this most appropriate homoeopathic remedy it is only the symptoms of the medicine that correspond to the symptoms of the disease that are called into play, the former occupying the place of the latter (weaker) in the organism, i.e., in the sensation of the life principle, and thereby annihilating them by overpowering them; but the other symptoms of the homoeopathic medicine, which are often very numerous, being in no way applicable to the case of disease in question, are not called into play at all. The patient, growing hourly better, feels almost nothing of them at all, because the excessively minute dose requisite for homoeopathic use is much too weak to produce the other symptoms of the medicine that are not homoeopathic to the case, in those parts of the body that are free from disease, and consequently can allow only the homoeopathic symptoms to act on the parts of the organism that are already most irritated and excited by the similar symptoms of the disease, in order that the sick life principle may react only to a similar but stronger medicinal disease, whereby the original malady is extinguished.

EXPLANATION

- In aphorism 154, he says without any considerable disturbances, this is explained here, while employing the most appropriate homeopathic remedy, the symptoms of the medicine that correspond to the symptoms of the d/s are called into play.
- It means the other symptoms of the homeopathic medicine which are often very numerous.
- The patient feels almost nothing of them because of the excessive minute dose of the remedy.
- This minute dose is too weak to produce the other symptoms of the medicine that are not homeopathic to the case.

- The minute dose don't produce other symptoms in those parts of the body that are free from d/s & can only allow the homoeopathic symptoms to act on the parts of the organism that are most irritated & excited by the similar symptoms of the d/s.
- Now the sick life principle may react only to a similar but stronger medicinal d/s, and the original malady is extinguished & the patient is cured.

§ 156

HOMOEOPATHIC RECOVERY

There is, however, almost no homoeopathic medicine, be it ever so suitably chosen, that, especially if it should be given in an insufficiently minute dose, will not produce, in very irritable and sensitive patients, at least one trifling, unusual disturbance, some slight new symptom while its action lasts; for it is next to impossible that medicine and disease should cover one another symptomatically as exactly as two triangles with equal sides and equal angles. But this (in ordinary circumstances) unimportant difference will be easily done away with by the potential activity (energy) of the living organism, and is not perceptible by patients not excessively delicate; the restoration goes forward, notwithstanding, to the goal of perfect recovery, if it be not prevented by the action of heterogeneous medicinal influences upon the patient, by errors of regimen or by excitement of the passions.

EXPLANATION

- Homeopathic medicine, even if suitably chosen & given in an insufficiently minute dose will always produce at least one trifling, unusual disturbance, some slight new symptom while its action lasts, in very irritable & sensitive patients.
- The medicine & the d/s would cover one another symptomatically as exactly as two triangles with equal sides & angles, it means like two triangles with equal sides & angles exactly cover each other there is no medicine & d/s that would cover each other exactly by their symptoms, but this [in ordinary circumstances], unimportant difference is easily done away by the potential energy of the living organism & is not perceptible [felt]by patients who are not excessively delicate.
- The restoration of health goes towards perfect recovery provided no medicinal influence or error of regimen or excitement of the passions, prevent recovery.
- Use of medicinal substances, taking diet that is restricted etc prevents recovery of the patient.

§ 157

HOMOEOPATHIC AGGRAVATION

But though it is certain that a homoeopathically selected remedy does, by reason of its appropriateness and the minuteness of the dose, gently remove and annihilate the acute disease analogous to it, without manifesting its other unhomoeopathic symptoms, that is to say, without the production of new, serious disturbances, yet it usually, immediately after ingestion – for the first hour, or for a few hours – causes a kind of slight aggravation when the dose has not been sufficiently small and (where the dose has been somewhat too large, however, for a considerable number of hours), which has so much resemblance to the original disease that it seems to the patient to be an aggravation of his own disease. But it is, in reality, nothing more than an extremely similar medicinal disease, somewhat exceeding in strength the original affection.

EXPLANATION

- A Homeopathically selected remedy by its appropriateness & the minuteness of the dose, gently remove & annihilate the acute d/s analogous to it.
- It means no new, serious symptoms or disturbance is produced.

But if the dose is not sufficiently small, it produces for the first hour, or a few hours a kind of slight aggravation immediately after ingestion.

- When the dose is too large it produces aggravation for a considerable number of hours.
- This aggravation is similar to the original d/s & it seems that the patient is having aggravation of his own d/s.

But in reality, it is an extremely similar medicinal d/s, which is exceeding in strength from the original affection. There is no aggravation of the original d/s.

§ 158

HOMEOPATHIC AGGRAVATION DIRECTS TO CURE

This slight homoeopathic aggravation during the first hours – a very good prognostic that the acute disease will most probably yield to the first dose – is quite as it ought to be, as the medicinal disease must naturally be somewhat stronger than the malady to be cured if it is to overpower and extinguish the latter, just as a natural disease can remove and annihilate another one similar to it only when it is stronger than the latter (§§ 43 – 48).

EXPLANATION

- This slight homeopathic aggravation during the first hours is a very good prognostic sign that the acute d/s will be cured in the first dose itself.
- This is as expected because the medicinal d/s must be somewhat stronger than the d/s to be cured, so that it can extinguish the original d/s.
- A natural d/s can remove & annihilate another one similar to it only when it is stronger than the original d/s **(§§ 43 – 48)**.
- So this slight aggravation is normal & directs us towards cure.

§ 159

SMALLER THE DOSE SLIGHT THE AGGRAVATION

The smaller the dose of the homoeopathic remedy is in the treatment of acute diseases so much the slighter and shorter is the apparent increase of the disease during the first hours.

EXPLANATION

- This Homeopathic aggravation is dependent on the dose of the Homeopathic remedy.
- The smaller the dose of medicine used in the treatment of acute d/s, the slighter & shorter the apparent increase of the d/s during the first hours.
- The slighter & shorter the duration of homeopathic aggravation.

§ 160

LARGE DOSES ARE HARMFUL

But as the dose of a homoeopathic remedy can scarcely ever be made so small that it shall not be able to relieve, overpower, indeed completely cure and annihilate the uncomplicated natural disease of not long standing that is analogous to it (§ 249, note), we can understand why a does of an appropriate homoeopathic medicine, not the very smallest possible, does always,

during the first hour after its ingestion, produce a perceptible homoeopathic aggravation of this kind.1

1 This exaltation of the medicinal symptoms over those disease symptoms analogous to them, which looks like an aggravation, has been observed by other physicians also, when by accident they employed a homoeopathic remedy. When a patient suffering from itch complains of an increase of the eruption after sulphur, his physician who knows not the cause of this, consoles him with the assurance that the itch must first come out properly before it can be cured; he knows not, however, that this is a sulphur eruption, that assumes the appearance of an increase of the itch.

"The facial eruption which the viola tricolor cured was aggravated by it at the commencement of its action," Leroy tells us (Heilk, fur Mutter, p.406), but he knew not that the apparent aggravation was owing to the somewhat too large dose of the remedy, which in this instance was to a certain extent homoeopathic. Lysons says (Med. Transact., vol ii, London, 1772), "The bark of the elm cures most certainly those skin diseases which it increases at the beginning of its action." Had he not given the bark in the monstrous doses usual in the allopathic system, but in the quite small doses requisite when the medicine shows similarity of symptoms, that is to say, when it is used homoeopathically, he would have effected a cure without, or almost without, seeing this apparent increase of the disease (homoeopathic aggravation).

EXPLANATION

- The dose of a homeopathic remedy can never be made so small otherwise it will not be able to review, overpower & completely cure & annihilate the uncomplicated natural d/s of not long standing [aph 249] nature.
- A dose of an appropriate homeopathic medicine, not the very smallest possible, always produces a perceptible homeopathic aggravation during the first hour after its ingestion.

Footnote:
These medicinal symptoms over those d/s symptoms similar to them, which look like an aggravation were observed by other physician also.

E.g. When a patient suffering from itch was given sulphur, he complained of an increase of the eruption.

- This is a sulphur eruption, that assumes the appearance of an increase of the itch.
- Leroy said that the. 'Facial eruption cured by viola tricolor was aggravated in the starting but he did not know that this was due to too large dose of the remedy [Homeopathic remedy]
- Lysan says 'The bark of elm cures those skin d/s which it increases at the beginning of its action' 'Here also he used monstrous doses.

§ 161

HOMEOPATHIC AGGRAVATION IN ACUTE AND CHRONIC DISEASES

When I here limit the so-called homoeopathic aggravation, or rather the primary action of the homoeopathic medicine that seems to increase somewhat the symptoms of the original disease, to the first or few hours, this is certainly true with respect to diseases of a more acute character and of recent origin, but where medicines of long action have to combat a malady of, considerable or of very long standing, where no such apparent increase of the original disease ought to appear during treatment and it does not so appear if the accurately chosen medicine was given in proper small, gradually higher doses, each somewhat modified with renewed dynamization (§ 247). Such increase of the original symptoms of a chronic disease can appear only at the end of treatment when the cure is almost or quite finished.

EXPLANATION

- The Homeopathic aggravation or rather the primary action of the homeopathic medicine is increase in the symptoms of the original d/s, occurs in the first hours.
  This is certainly true for d/s of a more acute character & of recent origin.
- But where medicine of long action have to treat a malady of considerable or of a very long standing. In these cases no such apparent increase of the original d/s appear during treatment, in such cases it does not appear if the accurately chosen medicine was given in proper small and then gradually higher doses, each modified with renewed dynamization[aph-247]
- Such increase of the original symptoms of a chronic d/s can appear only at the end of treatment when the cure is almost or quite finished.

So, in short in acute case this aggravation or increase in symptoms of the original d/s occurs in the first or few first hours, whereas in chronic cases it appears at the end of the treatment when cure is almost finished.

§ 162

PARTIAL SELECTION OF SIMILIMUM

Sometimes happens, owing to the moderate number of medicines yet known with respect to their true, pure action, that but a portion of the symptoms of the disease under treatment are to be met with in the list of symptoms of the most appropriate medicine, consequently this imperfect medicinal morbific agent must be employed for lack of a more perfect one.

EXPLANATION

- Sometime we have to employ the imperfect medicinal morbific agent because of lack of a more perfect one.
- It happens due to moderate number of medicine known with respect to their, true pure action.
- In these cases, a portion of the symptoms of the d/s under treatment is matched with the list of symptoms of the most appropriate medicine, that seems similar to it.
- This is because we have no other choice left but to employ the most similar among the known remedies.

§ 163

ACCESSORY SYMPTOMS

In this case we cannot indeed expect from this medicine a complete, untroubled cure; for during its use some symptoms appear which were not previously observable in the disease, accessory symptoms of the not perfectly appropriate remedy. This does by no means prevent a considerable part of the disease (the symptoms of the disease that resemble those of the medicine) from being eradicated by this medicine, thereby establishing a fair commencement of the cure, but still this does not take place without those accessory symptoms, which are, however, always moderate when the dose of the medicine is sufficiently minute.

EXPLANATION

- In above case we cannot expect a complete, undisturbed cure.
- During the use of imperfect medicine some symptoms appear which were not previously observable in the d/s [the accessory symptoms of the not perfect remedy]

- This leads to eradication of the similar symptoms of the d/s that resemble medicine and produces a fair commencement of the cure.
- The accessory symptoms are always moderate when the dose of the medicine is sufficiently minute.

§ 164

UNCOMMON, CHARACTERISTIC SYMPTOMS

The small number of homoeopathic symptoms present in the best selected medicine is no obstacle to the cure in cases where these few medicinal symptoms are chiefly of an uncommon kind and such as are peculiarly distinctive (characteristic) of the disease; the cure takes place under such circumstances without any particular disturbance.

EXPLANATION

- In cases where small number of homeopathic symptoms are present in the best selected medicines and these few medicine symptoms are of an uncommon kind & distinctive [characteristic] of the d/s.
- In these cases these small but characteristic symptoms are no obstacle to the cure.
- In these cases, the cure takes place without any particular disturbance.

§ 165

UNHOMEOPATHIC MEDICINE

If, however, among the symptoms of the remedy selected, there be none that accurately resemble the distinctive (characteristic), peculiar, uncommon symptoms of the case of disease, and if the remedy correspond to the disease only in the general, vaguely described, indefinite states (nausea, debility, headache, and so forth), and if there be among the known medicines none more homoeopathically appropriate, in that case the physician cannot promise himself any immediate favorable result from the employment of this unhomoeopathic medicine.

EXPLANATION

- If among the symptoms of the remedy which we have selected, there is no characteristic, peculiar, uncommon symptoms of the case of the d/s, and if the remedy corresponds to the d/s,

only in general, vague symptoms like nausea, debility, headache etc, and if there is none more homeopathically appropriate medicine known.
- In this case the physician cannot expect of any immediate favourable result by employment of this unhomeopathic medicine.

§ 166

RARE CASE

Such a case is, however, very rare, owing to the increased number of medicines whose pure effects are now known, and the bad effects resulting from it, when they do occur, are diminished whenever a subsequent medicine, of more accurate resemblance, can be selected.

EXPLANATION

- Such a case [aph-165] is very rare because of the increased number of medicines whose pure effects are now known.
- When the bad effects result from it they are diminished when a subsequent medicine, which resembles more accurately can be selected.
- When any bad effects occur, a more similar medicine is selected.

§ 167

IMPERFECT HOMOEPATHIC REMEDY

Thus if there occur, during the use of this imperfectly homoeopathic remedy first employed, accessory symptoms of some moment, then, in the case of acute diseases, we do not allow this first dose to exhaust its action, nor leave the patient to the full duration of the action of the remedy, but we investigate afresh the morbid state in its now altered condition, and add the remainder of the original symptoms to those newly developed in tracing a new picture of the disease.

EXPLANATION

- During the use of this imperfect homeopathic remedy given first, if accessory symptoms occur.
- Then, in the case of acute d/s, take the case as a fresh case and now from the totality of the symptoms form a new picture of disease.

- Here in the case of acute d/s, we don't wait for the action of the first dose to exhaust & we don't leave the patient for full duration of the action of the remedy.
- We investigate, the case as a fresh one and add the newly developed symptoms to the remaining original symptoms & trace a new picture of the d/s.
New totality of symptoms= Newly developed symptoms + Remaining original symptoms.

§ 168

FOLLOW-UP

We shall then be able much more readily to discover, among the known medicines, an analogue to the morbid state before us, a single dose of which, if it do not entirely destroy the disease, will advance it considerably on the way to be cured. And thus we go on, if even this medicine be not quite sufficient to effect the restoration of health, examining again and again the morbid state that still remains, and selecting a homoeopathic medicine as suitable as possible for it, until our object, namely, putting the patient in the possession of perfect health, is accomplished.

EXPLANATION

- This way we will be able to discover homoeopathic medicine for the morbid state now present..
- A single dose of the medicine will advance the d/s on the way to be cured, if not complete cure, and thus we go on this way, if even this medicine is not sufficient to restore health.
- We examine the case again & again for the symptoms that remain.
- Now we select a homeopathic medicine as suitable as possible for it, until our object of curing the patient to perfect health is accomplished.

§ 169

ANALOGOUS MEDICINES

If, on the first examination of a disease and the first selection of a medicine, we should find that the totality of the symptoms of the disease would not be effectually covered by the disease elements of a single medicine – owing to the insufficient number of known medicines, – but that two medicines contend for the preference in point of appropriateness, one of which is more homoeopathically suitable for one part, the other for another part of the symptoms of the disease,

it is not advisable, after the employment of the more suitable of the two medicines, to administer the other without fresh examination, and much less to give both together (§ 272, note) for the medicine that seemed to be the next best would not, under the change of circumstances that has in the meantime taken place, be suitable for the rest of the symptoms that then remain; in which case, consequently, a more appropriate homoeopathic remedy must be selected in place of the second medicine for the set of symptoms as they appear on a new inspection.

EXPLANATION

- If in case we examine a d/s & select a medicine & we find that the totality of the symptoms of the d/s is not covered by a single medicine, but two medicines one of which is more homeopathically suitable for one part, the other medicine for another part of the symptoms of the d/s.
- Now if out of the two medicines the more suitable is administered.
- After this never give the other medicine or never give both of medicine together [aph272note]
- We should not give the second similar medicine because after administration of the first similar medicine, now the d/s picture is changed.
  Now the remaining symptoms + New symptoms = New picture d/s
- Now a more appropriate homeopathic medicine must be selected for the set of symptoms after fresh case taking.

§ 170

FRESH CASE

Hence in this as in every case where a change of the morbid state has occurred, the remaining set of symptoms now present must be inquired into, and (without paying any attention to the medicine which at first appeared to be the next in point of suitableness) another homoeopathic medicine, as appropriate as possible to the new state now before us, must be selected. If it should so happen, as is not often the case, that the medicine which at first appeared to be the next best seems still to be well adapted for the morbid state that remains, so much the more will it merit our confidence, and deserve to be employed in preference to another.

EXPLANATION

- Hence in this case or every case where a change of the morbid state has occurred, take a fresh case.
- The remaining symptoms must be inquired and another homeopathic medicine, as similar as possible to the new state, must be selected.
- If in case [not often it occurs], the second medicine which we chose in the starting [aph-169], which at first appeared to be the next best remedy is similar to the morbid state at present.
- In this case we can employ this second remedy in preference to another.

§ 171

ANTIPSORIC MEDICINES

In non-venereal chronic disease, those, therefore, that arise from psora, we often require, **in order to effect a cure, to give several antipsoric remedies in succession, every successive one being homoeopathically chosen in consonance with the group of symptoms remaining after completion of the action of the previous remedy.**

EXPLANATION

- In non-venereal chronic diseases, which most commonly arise from psora, we have to give antipsoric remedies.
- Here several anti-psoric remedies are given one-after another in succession.
- Each successive remedy is chosen homoeopathically based on group of symptoms remaining after the completion of the action of the previous remedy.

§ 172

TOO FEW SYMPTOMS

A similar difficulty in the way of the cure occurs from the symptoms of the disease being too few – a circumstances that deserves our careful attention, for by its removal almost all the difficulties that can lie in the way of this most perfect of all possible modes of treatment (except that its apparatus of known homoeopathic medicines is still incomplete) are removed.

EXPLANATION

- In a case of d/s where too few symptoms of the d/s are present it becomes difficult to cure.
- It deserves our careful attention.
- By careful attention the most perfect of all possible modes of treatment is successful.
- We should also know that the apparatus[remedy]of known Homeopathic medicines is still incomplete, even then it is the most perfect of all modes of the treatment known.

§ 173

ONE SIDED DISEASES

The only diseases that seem to have but few symptoms, and on that account to be less amenable to cure, are those which may be termed one-sided, because they display only one or two principal symptoms which obscure almost all the others. They belong chiefly to the class of chronic diseases.

EXPLANATION

- Diseases which have few symptoms are termed one-side d/s
- They are less amenable to cure, as they display only one or two principal symptoms which make [obscure] almost all the other symptoms, difficult to see.
- They chiefly belong to the class of chronic d/s.

§ 174

TYPES OF ONE-SIDED DISEASES

Their principal symptom may be either an internal complaint (e.g. a headache of many years' duration, a diarrhoea of long standing, an ancient cardialgia, etc.), or it may be an affection more of an external kind. Diseases of the latter character are generally distinguished by the name of local maladies.

EXPLANATION

- The one-sided d/s either have an internal complaint or external affection.
- The principal symptom may be an internal complaint.

E.g- A headache of many years duration.
A diarrhoea of long standing
An ancient cardalgia etc.

- Or the principal symptom maybe an affection of an external kind called local maladies.

§ 175

ONE-SIDED DISEASE WITH INTERNAL COMPLAIN

In one-sided diseases of the first kind it is often to be attributed to the medical observer's want of discernment that he does not fully discover the symptoms actually present which would enable him to complete the sketch of the portrait of the disease.

EXPLANATION

- In one-sided d/s of the first kind it is medical observer's ability to judge & discover the symptoms actually present.
- This will enable him to complete the sketch of the portrait of the d/s.

§ 176

CAREFUL INITIAL EXAMINATION OF ONE SIDED D/S

There are, however, still a few diseases, which, after the most careful initial examination (§§ 84-98), present but one or two severe, violent symptoms, while all the others are but indistinctly perceptible.

EXPLANATION

- There are a few diseases which after the most careful initial examination [aph-84-98], only present one or two severe, violent symptoms.
- While all the other symptoms are not clearly noticed, it requires an investigation of the case.

§ 177

SELECTION OF MEDICINE

In order to meet most successfully such a case as this, which is of very rare occurrence, we are in the first place to select, guided by these few symptoms, the medicine which in our judgment is the most homoeopathically indicated.

EXPLANATION

- In one-sided d/s of the first kind, which is of very rare occurrence, we need to follow this way.
- In the first place select a medicine, based on these few symptoms, which appears the most homeopathically indicated.
- It means select a homeopathic remedy which seems the most similar to these few symptoms.

§ 178

EFFECT OF MEDICINE ON ONE-SIDED DISEASE

It will, no doubt, sometimes happen that this medicine, selected in strict observance of the homoeopathic law, furnishes the similar artificial disease suited for the annihilation of the malady present; and this is much more likely to happen when these few morbid symptoms are very striking, decided, uncommon and peculiarly distinctive (characteristic).

EXPLANATION

- After employing the medicine, based on homeopathic law, we have selected sometimes annihilation of the malady occurs.
- This is likely to happen when these few morbid symptoms are very striking, uncommon & characteristic symptoms.

§ 179

PARTIALLY SUITABLE MEDICINES

More frequently, however, the medicine first chosen in such a case will be only partially, that is to say, not exactly suitable, as there was no considerable number of symptoms to guide to an accurate selection.

EXPLANATION

- More frequently, the medicine first chosen in such a case will be partially suitable, as there was no considerable number of symptoms to guide to an accurate selection therefore the medicine chosen will be only partially suitable.

§ 180

APPEARANCE OF ACCESSORY SYMPTOMS

In this case the medicine, which has been chosen as well as was possible, but which, for the reason above stated, is only imperfectly homoeopathic, will, in its action upon the disease that is only partially analogous to it – just as in the case mentioned above (§ 162, et seq.) where the limited number of homoeopathic remedies renders the selection imperfect – produce accessory symptoms, and several phenomena from its own array of symptoms are mixed up with the patient's state of health, which are, however, at the same time, symptoms of the disease itself, although they may have been hitherto never or very rarely perceived; some symptoms which the patient had never previously experienced appear, or others he had only felt indistinctly become more pronounced.

EXPLANATION

- In these cases as the medicine chosen is imperfectly homeopathic so it produces accessory symptoms and several phenomena, from its own array of symptoms are mixed up with the patient's state of health.
- These symptoms are symptoms of the disease itself although they were never or very rarely perceived till employment of the remedy.
- Some symptoms appear which the patient had never experienced previously or others he had not felt clearly they become more pronounced.

§ 181

ACCESSORY SYMPTOMS DUE TO MEDICINE

Let is not be objected that the accessory phenomena and new symptoms of this disease that now appear should be laid to the account of the medicament just employed. They owe their origin to it1 certainly, but they are always only symptoms of such a nature as this disease was itself capable of producing in this organism, and which were summoned forth and induced to make their appearance by the medicine given, owing to its power to cause similar symptoms. In a word, we have to regard the whole collection of symptoms now perceptible as belonging to the disease itself, as the actual existing condition, and to direct our further treatment accordingly.

1 When they were not caused by an important error in regimen, a violent emotion, or a tumultuous revolution in the organism, such as the occurrence or cessation of the menses, conception, childbirth, and so forth.

EXPLANATION

- The accessory phenomena & new symptoms of the d/s that appear now are due to the medicine just employed.
- The medicine, due to its power to cause similar symptoms, induced the symptoms this disease was itself capable of producing in this organism.
- So in short these symptoms are the symptoms of the d/s itself which are induced by the given partially homeopathic medicine.
- Now we should observe the whole collection of symptoms and direct our further treatment accordingly.

Footnote:-
- These symptoms are due to the medicine employed which brings out that symptoms of the d/s, but condition is that they should not be caused by an error in regimen, a violent emotion or a tumultuous revolution in the organism like occurrence or cessation of menses, conception, childbirth etc.

§ 182

DISCOVERY OF REMEDY

Thus the imperfect selection of the medicament, which was in this case almost inevitable owing to the too limited number of the symptoms present, serves to complete the display of the symptoms of the disease, and in this way facilitates the discovery of a second, more accurately suitable, homoeopathic medicine.

EXPLANATION

- Thus this imperfectly selected homeopathic remedy which was given due to too limited number of the symptoms present, brings out the symptoms of the d/s.
- In this way this medicine facilitates the discovery of a second, more accurately suitable, homeopathic medicine by bringing larger symptoms of the disease to the surface.

§ 183

SEARCH SUITABLE REMEDY

Whenever, therefore, the dose of the first medicine ceases to have a beneficial effect (if the newly developed symptoms do not, by reason of their gravity, demand more speedy aid – which, however, from the minuteness of the dose of homoeopathic medicine, and in very chronic diseases, is excessively rare), a new examination of the disease must be instituted, the status morbi as it now is must be noted down, and a second homoeopathic remedy selected in accordance with it, which shall exactly suit the present state, and one which shall be all the more appropriate can then be found, as the group of symptoms has become larger and more complete.1

1 In cases where the patient (which, however, happens excessively seldom in chronic, but not infrequently in acute, diseases) feels very ill, although his symptoms are very indistinct, so that this state may be attributed more to the benumbed state of the nerves, which does not permit the patient's pains and sufferings to be distinctly perceived, this torpor of the internal sensibility is removed by opium, and in its secondary action the symptoms of the disease become distinctly apparent.

EXPLANATION

- When the dose of the first medicine stops to have a beneficial effect [if the newly developed symptoms don't demand aid due to the minuteness of the dose of the Homoepathic medicine & in very chronic d/s is excessively rare], a new examination of the d/s must be started.
- The new morbid state must be noted down & a second homeopathic remedy is selected according to it.
- The second homeopathic remedy which exactly suits the present state and which is more appropriate can be found, as now the group of symptoms has become larger & more complete. Now the more suitable homeopathic remedy can be found & employed.

Footnote:
In cases where the patient feels very ill which happens very seldom [rare], in chronic d/s but frequently occurs in acute d/s.

Here he feels very ill though his symptoms are very indistinct due to benumbed state of nerves, which do not permit patient's pains & sufferings to be clearly perceived. This is removed by opium & it in its secondary action the d/s symptoms become distinctly apparent.

§ 184

CONTINUE AS PREVIOUS TILL COMPLETE CURE

In like manner, after each new dose of medicine has exhausted its action, when it is no longer suitable and helpful, the state of the disease that still remains is to be noted anew with respect to its remaining symptoms, and another homoeopathic remedy sought for, as suitable as possible for the group of symptoms now observed, and so on until the recovery is complete.

EXPLANATION

- In the similar manner, after each new dose of medicine has completed its action & it is no longer suitable & helpful.
- Now the symptoms that remain are noted as a new case & another homeopathic remedy is found out.
- This homeopathic remedy should be as suitable as possible for the group of symptoms now observed & so on this is repeated until the recovery is complete.

§ 185

LOCAL MALADIES

Among the one-sided disease an important place is occupied by the so-called local maladies, by which term is signified those changes and ailments that appear on the external parts of the body. Till now the idea prevalent in the schools was that these parts were alone morbidly affected, and that the rest of the body did not participate in the disease – a theoretical, absurd doctrine, which has led to the most disastrous medical treatment.

EXPLANATION

- Now let us take the one-sided d/s of the second kind called local maladies.
- Local maladies means those changes & ailments that appear on the external parts of the body.
- Till now the theoretical, absurd doctrine had the idea that these parts are alone affected & the rest of the body has nothing to do with it [it dose not participate in the d/s]& this has led to the most disastrous medical treatments.

§ 186

ACUTE LOCAL MALADIES

Those so-called local maladies which have been produced a short time previously, solely by an external lesion, still appear at first sight to deserve the name of local disease. But then the lesion must be very trivial, and in that case it would be of no great moment. For in the case of injuries accruing to the body from without, if they be at all severe, the whole living organism sympathizes; there occur fever, etc. The treatment of such diseases is relegated to surgery; but this is right only in so far as the affected parts require mechanical aid, whereby the external obstacles to the cure, which can only be expected to take place by the agency of the vital force, may be removed by mechanical means, e.g., by the reduction of dislocations, by needles and bandages to bring together the lips of wounds, by mechanical pressure to still the flow of blood from open arteries, by the extraction of foreign bodies that have penetrated into the living parts, by making an opening into a cavity of the body in order to remove an irritating substance or to procure the evacuation of effusions or collections of fluids, by bringing into apposition the broken extremities of a fractured bone and retaining them in exact contact by an appropriate bandage, etc. But when in such injuries the whole living organism requires, as it always does, active dynamic aid to put it in a position to accomplish the work of healing, e.g. when the violent fever resulting from extensive contusions, lacerated muscles, tendons and blood-vessels requires to be removed by medicine given internally, or when the external pain of scalded or burnt parts needs to be homoeopathically subdued, then the services of the dynamic physician and his helpful homoeopathy come into requisition.

EXPLANATION

- These local maladies, produced a short time previously, solely by an external lesion still appear at first sight as local d/s, but if it is a local d/s it must be very trivial [it must be of little important or not worth considering]
  But as we will see below that whole living organism is affected, so the term local d/s does not seem suitable for it.

Example:- In case of injuries occuring to the body, the whole living organism sympathizes & there occurs fever etc.

Usually the treatment of such d/s is submitted to surgery but this is right if the affected parts require mechanical aid where external obstacles to cure may be removed by mechanical means.

E, g- By reduction of dislocation, by needles & bandages to bring lips of wounds together, by mechanical pressure to stop the flow of blood from open arteries, by extraction of foreign bodies which has penetrated into the living parts, making opening into cavity to remove an irritating substances or evacuate effusions or collections of fluids, by bringing broken fractured bone together etc.

But in such injuries the whole living organism requires active dynamic aid to put the body in a position to accomplish the work of healing & this needs homeopathic treatment by the dynamic physician.

E.g- When the violent fever results from extensive contusions, lacerated muscles, tendons & blood-vessels & it needs to removed by medicines given internally.

E.g-When the external pain of scalded or burnt parts needs homoeopathic treatment.

§ 187

LOCAL MALADIES CONTINUED

But those affections, alterations and ailments appearing on the external parts, that do not arise from any external injury or that have only some slight external wound for their immediate exciting cause, are produced in quite another manner; their source lies in some internal malady. To consider them as mere local affections, and at the same time to treat them only, or almost only, as it were surgically, with topical applications – as the old school have done from the remotest ages – is as absurd as it is pernicious in its results.

EXPLANATION

Those affections and ailments which don't arise from any external injury or slight external wound act as an immediate exciting cause, their source lies in some internal malady.

So we should not consider them as more local affections.

They should not be treated surgically, with topical application or other similar remedies as the old school have done but this has resulted in harmful results.

§ 188

LOCAL MALADIES CONTINUED

These affections were considered to be merely topical, and were therefore called local diseases, as if they were maladies exclusively limited to those parts wherein the organism took little or no part, or affections of these particular visible parts of which the rest of the living organism, so to speak, knew nothing.1

1 One of the many great and pernicious blunders of the old school.

EXPLANATION

- These affections were considered only topical & therefore called local diseases.
- According to them those maladies were exclusively limited to those parts and rest of the organism took no part or little part in it, as if it was not affected.

Footnote:
This theory was one of the many great & harmful blunders[mistake]of the old school.

§ 189

CLARIFICATION OF MISCONCEPTION

And yet very little reflection will suffice to convince us that no external malady (not occasioned by some important injury from without) can arise, persist or even grow worse without some internal cause, without the co-operation of the whole organism, which must consequently be in a diseased state. It could not make its appearance at all without the consent of the whole of the rest of the health, and without the participation of the rest of the living whole (of the

vital force that pervades all the other sensitive and irritable parts of the organism); indeed, it is impossible to conceive its production without the instrumentality of the whole (deranged) life; so intimately are all parts of the organism connected together to form an indivisible whole in sensation and functions. No eruption on the lips, no whitlow can occur without previous and simultaneous internal ill-health.

EXPLANATION

- All the parts of the organism are connected together to form an indivisible whole in sensations & functions.
- No external malady [expect important injury] can arise or grow worse without internal cause.
- The whole of the rest of the health & rest of the living whole, participates in its appearance.
- Unless the whole life is deranged it is impossible for it to appear.
- Thus even an eruption on the lips, whitlow occurs due to previous & simultaneous internal ill-health.

§ 190

MANAGEMENT BY INTERNAL REMEDY

All true medical treatment of a disease on the external parts of the body that has occurred from little or no injury from without must, therefore, be directed against the whole, must effect the annihilation and cure of the general malady by means of internal remedies, if it is wished that the treatment should be judicious, sure, efficacious and radical.

EXPLANATION

In these cases if we want that the treatment should be judicious, sure efficacious & radical then it requires internal remedies [homeopathically similar].

A d/s on the external parts of the body that has occured from little or no injury requires treatment against the whole organism.

For annihilation & cure of the general malady, internal remedy is the only cure, that is sure, efficacious, judicious & radical.

§ 191

NO EXTERNAL REMEDY REQUIRED

This is confirmed in the most unambiguous manner by experience, which shows in all cases that every powerful internal medicine immediately after its ingestion causes important changes in the general health of such a patient, and particularly in the affected external parts (which the ordinary medical school regards as quite isolated), even in a so-called local disease of the most external parts of the body, and the change it produces is most salutary, being the restoration to health of the entire body, along with the disappearance of the external affection (without the aid of any external remedy), provided the internal remedy directed towards the whole state was suitable chosen in a homoeopathic sense.

EXPLANATION

- In these cases the internal remedy should be directed towards the whole state & suitably chosen in a homoeopathic sense.
- When powerful internal medicine is given to the patient, after its ingestions, important changes in the general health of patient occurs with disappearance of the external affection.
- Here no aid of any external remedy was given due to deranged vital energy.
- The patient's health is restored along with disappearance of external affection if the internal remedy is suitably chosen.

§ 192

TREATMENT OF LOCAL DISEASES

This is best effected when, in the investigation of the case of disease, along with the exact character of the local affection, all the changes, sufferings and symptoms observable in the patient's health, and which may have been previously noticed when no medicines had been used, are taken in conjunction to form a complete picture of the disease before searching among the medicines, whose peculiar pathogenetic effects are known, for a remedy corresponding to the totality of the symptoms, so that the selection may be truly homoeopathic.

EXPLANATION

- In these cases the investigation of the case of d/s should include all the changes, sufferings & symptoms observable in the patient's health, along with exact character of the local affection.
- It should also include previously noticed symptoms when no medicine had been used, thus a complete picture of the d/s should be made & based on the totality of the symptoms proper homeopathic remedy should be selected.

§ 193

LOCAL AFFECTION IS A STRIKING SYMPTOM

By means of this medicine, employed only internally (and, if the disease be but of recent origin, often by the very first dose of it), the general morbid state of the body is removed along with the local affection, and the latter is cured at the same time as the former, proving that the local affection depended solely on a disease of the rest of the body, and should only be regarded as an inseparable part of the whole, as one of the most considerable and striking symptoms of the whole disease.

EXPLANATION

- These medicines, employed internally remove the general morbid state of the body along with the local affection.
- The local affection is cured at the same time as the general morbid state.
- This proves that local affection depended solely on the d/s of the rest of the body & it should be regarded as an inseparable part of the whole.
- Local affection should be regarded as one of the most considerable & striking symptoms of the whole d/s.

§ 194

EXTERNAL AFFECTION AND PSORA

It is not useful, either in acute local diseases of recent origin or in local affections that have already existed a long time, to rub in or apply externally to the spot an external remedy, even though it be the specific and, when used internally, salutary by reason of its homoeopathicity, even although it should be at the same time administered internally; for the acute topical affections (e.g., inflammations of the individual parts, erysipelas, etc.), which have not been caused by external injury of proportionate violence, but by dynamic or internal causes, yield most surely to internal remedies homoeopathically adapted to the perceptible state of the health present in the exterior and interior, selected from the general store of proved medicines,1 and generally without any other aid; but if these diseases do not yield to them completely, and if there still remain in the affected spot and in the whole state, notwithstanding good regimen, a relic of disease which the vital force is not competent to restore to the normal state, then the acute disease was (as not infrequently happens) a product of psora which had hitherto remained latent in the interior, but has now burst forth and is on the point of developing into a palpable chronic disease.

As, for instance, aconite, rhus, belladonna, mercury, etc.

EXPLANATION

- Here Hahnemann says that it is not useful to rub or apply external remedy to the spot externally either in acute local d/s of recent origin or in local affections of long time.
- For the acute topical affections e.g- Inflammations of individual parts, erysipelas etc, which are not caused by external injury of proportionate violence but are due to dynamic or internal causes.
- They yield to internal remedies homeopathically selected from proved medicines & without any other aid.
- If these d/s still remain in the affected spot and in the whole state, a relic of d/s which vital force is not able to restore to the normal state it means that the acute d/s was a product of psora.
- This psora remained latent in the interior till now, but it has now burst & is on the point of developing into a palpable chronic d/s.

§ 195

ANTI-PSORIC TREATMENT

In order to effect a radical cure in such cases, which are by no means rare, after the acute state has pretty well subsided, an appropriate antipsoric treatment (as is taught in my work on Chronic Diseases) must then be directed against the symptoms that still remain and the morbid state of health to which the patient was previously subject. In chronic local maladies that are not obviously venereal, the antipsoric internal treatment is, moreover, alone requisite.

EXPLANATION

- In above cases, after the acute state has subsided, an appropriate antipsoric treatment is given.
- It must be directed against the symptoms that still remain & the morbid state of health to which the patient was previously subject.
- In chronic local maladies that are not veneral the antipsoric internal treatment is alone that is required.

§ 196

SELECTION OF MEDICINE

It might, indeed, seen as though the cure of such diseases would be hastened by employing the medicinal substance which is known to be truly homoeopathic to the totality of the symptoms, not only internally, but also externally, because the action of a medicine applied to the seat of the local affection might effect a more rapid change in it.

EXPLANATION

- We might think that the cure of such disease would be faster if the truely homeopathic medicine, based on the totality of symptoms, is applied internally as well as externally.
- We would think this because the action of a medicine applied to the local affection might effect a more rapid change in it.
  But this is not correct, why so this we will see in next aphorism.

§ 197

LOCAL DISEASE NO EXTERNAL APPLICATION

This treatment, however, is quite inadmissible, not only for the local symptoms arising from the miasm of psora, but also and especially for those originating in the miasm of syphilis or sycosis, for the simultaneous local application, along with the internal employment, of the remedy in diseases whose chief symptom is a constant local affection, has this great disadvantage, that, by such a topical application, this chief symptom (local affection)1 will usually be annihilated sooner than the internal disease, and we shall now be deceived by the semblance of a perfect cure; or at least it will be difficult, and in some cases impossible, to determine, from the premature

disappearance of the local symptom, if the general disease is destroyed by the simultaneous employment of the internal medicine.

1 Recent itch eruption, chancre, condylomata, as I have indicated in my book of Chronic Diseases.

EXPLANATION

- This treatment as discussed in [aph-196], that the homeopathic medicine is given both externally & internally is not admissible [not correct]
- The simultaneous local application, along with internal employment of the remedy has a great disadvantage.
- By such a topical application, this chief symptom i.e- local affection will be annihilated [removed], sooner than internal d/s is cured.
- Due to premature disappearance of the local symptom, it would be difficult or in some cases impossible to determine that if the general d/s is destroyed by the simultaneous employment of the internal medicine.
- In short we can say that by external application of homeopathic remedy the local affection will disappear sooner than the internal d/s. we would not be able to know the effect of internal malady as the chief symptom [local affection] is removed by external application of the remedy.
- Therefore this treatment is not admissible for the local symptoms arising from the miasm of psora & also for those originating from miasm of syphilis or sycosis.

§ 198

TOPICAL EMPLOYMENT OF MEDICINE

The mere topical employment of medicines, that are powerful for cure when given internally, to the local symptoms of chronic miasmatic diseases is for the same reason quite inadmissible; for if the local affection of the chronic disease be only removed locally and in a one-sided manner, the internal treatment indispensable for the complete restoration of the health remains in dubious obscurity; the chief symptom (the local affection) is gone, and there remain only the other, less distinguishable symptoms, which are less constant and less persistent than the local affection, and frequently not sufficiently peculiar and too slightly characteristic to display after that, a picture of the disease in clear and peculiar outlines.

EXPLANATION

- Here Hahnemann says that only topical employment of medicines for the local symptoms of chronic miasmatic d/s is also not admissible for the same reason as above.

- If the local affection of a chronic d/s is removed locally & in a one-sided manner, the internal treatment for complete restoration of the health remains uncertain.

Because now the chief symptom [local affection] is gone & now only less constant, less distinguishable symptoms remain that are not characteristic to display a correct & clear picture of the d/s.

§ 199

PARTIAL SELECTION OF SIMILIMUM

If the remedy perfectly homoeopathic to the disease had not yet been discovered1 at the time when the local symptoms were destroyed by a corrosive or desiccative external remedy or by the knife, then the case becomes much more difficult on account of the too indefinite (uncharacteristic) and inconstant appearance of the remaining symptoms; for what might have contributed most to determine the selection of the most suitable remedy, and its internal employment until the disease should have been completely annihilated, namely, the external principal symptom, has been removed from our observation.

1 As was the case before my time with the remedies for the condylomatous disease (and the antipsoric medicines).

EXPLANATION

When local symptoms are destroyed by a corrosive or desiccative external remedy or by the knife, before Homoepathic remedy haa been discovered.

Then the case becomes much more difficult to cure.

Because now uncharacteristic & inconstant symptoms remains as the external principal symptom has been removed from our observation.

§ 200

INTERNAL DYNAMIC REMEDY

Had it still been present to guide the internal treatment, the homoeopathic remedy for the whole disease might have been discovered, and had that been found, the persistence of the local affection during its internal employment would have shown that the cure was not yet completed; but were it cured on its seat, this would be a convincing proof that the disease was

completely eradicated, and the desired recovery from the entire disease was fully accomplished – an inestimable, indispensable advantage to reach a perfect cure.

EXPLANATION

- If the local affection would be present, it would guide the homeoapthic remedy for the whole d/s and guide the internal treatment.
- If the local affection was present during internal employment of the remedy this would guide us if the cure is fully accomplished or not.
- It would guide us & be a convincing proof that the d/s was completely eradicated & desired recovery from the entire d/s was fully accomplished.

And disappearance of local affection during treatment would give us information that the cure was perfect to restore the vital energy to health.

§ 201

DAMAGE OF [VITAL-FORCE]

It is evident that man's vital force, when encumbered with a chronic disease which it is unable to overcome by its own powers instinctively, adopts the plan of developing a local malady on some external part, solely for this object, that by making and keeping in a diseased state this part which is not indispensable to human life, it may thereby silence the internal disease, which otherwise threatens to destroy the vital organs (and to deprive the patient of life), and that it may thereby, so to speak, transfer the internal disease to the vicarious local affection and, as it were, draw it thither. The presence of the local affection thus silences, for a time, the internal disease, though without being able either to cure it or to diminish it materially.1 The local affection, however, is never anything else than a part of the general disease, but a part of it increased all in one direction by the organic vital force, and transferred to a less dangerous (external) part of the body, in order to allay the internal ailment. But (as has been said) by this local symptom that silences the internal disease, so far from anything being gained by the vital force towards diminishing or curing the whole malady, the internal disease, on the contrary, continues, in spite of it, gradually to increase and Nature is constrained to enlarge and aggravate the local symptom always more and more, in order that it may still suffice as a substitute for the increased internal disease and may still keep it under. Old ulcers on the legs get worse as long as the internal psora is uncured, the chancre enlarges as long as the internal syphilis remains uncured, the fig warts increased and grow while the sycosis is not cured whereby the latter is rendered more and more difficult to cure, just as the general internal disease continues to increase as time goes on.

1 The issues of the old-school do something similar; as artificial ulcers on external parts, they silence some internal chronic diseases, but only for a short time, as long as they cause a painful irritation to which the sick organism is not used, without being able to cure them; but, on the other hand, they weaken and destroy the general health much more than is done by most of the metastases effected by the instinctive vital force.

EXPLANATION

- When man's vital force is blocked with a chronic d/s, it is unable to overcome the d/s by its own powers.
- So the body adopts the plan of developing a local malady on some external part.
- The body does so that it may silence the internal d/s which would destroy the vital organs & deprive the patient of life.
- It transfers the internal d/s to local affection of external part which is not vital or absolutely necessary for the human life.
- Thus the presence of the local affection thus silences the internal d/s for a time, though it is not able to cure it or to diminish it materially [116footnote].
- This local affection is a part of the general d/s which by the organic vital force is increased all in one direction & transferred to a less dangerous [external]part of the body, in order to diminish the internal ailments.
- Though local symptoms silence the internal d/s but the internal d/s continues to increase & it's nature keeps to enlarge & aggravate the local symptoms more & more as the internal d/s is increased.
- As the internal d/s is increased the local symptom is aggravated in order that it may still be enough as a substitute for the increased internal d/s & still keep it under.
  E.g- Old ulcers on the legs get worse as long as the internal psora is uncured.
- The chancre enlarges as long as the internal syphilis remains uncured.
- The wart increase & grow while the sycosis is not cured.
- As the time goes on and no homeopathic aid is given the case becomes more & more difficult to cure as the general internal d/s continues to increase with time.

Footnote:
The old-school practitioners do the similar.
They silence some internal chronic d/s as artificial ulcers on external parts but for a very short-time, till they cause a painful irritation to the sick organism.

- ✦ This does not cure them but they weaken & destroy the general health much more.

§ 202

LOCAL MALADIES & ALLOPATHIC TREATMENT

If the old-school physician should now destroy the local symptom by the topical application of external remedies, under the belief that he thereby cures the whole disease, Nature makes up for its loss by rousing the internal malady and the other symptoms that previously existed in a latent state side by side with the local affection; that is to say, she increases the internal disease. When this occurs it is usual to say, though incorrectly that the local affection has been driven back into the system or upon the nerves by the external remedies.

EXPLANATION

- The old-school physician destroy the local symptom by the topical application of external remedies & believes that whole disease is cured.
- In reality nature makes up for its loss & rouses the internal malady & now other symptoms appears.
- These symptoms existed in latent state side by side with local affection.
- This process increases the internal d/s.

§ 203

LOCAL MALADIES & EXTERNAL TREATMENT

Every external treatment of such local symptoms, the object of which is to remove them from the surface of the body, while the internal miasmatic disease is left uncured, as, for instance, driving off the skin the psoric eruption by all sorts of ointments, burning away the chancre by caustics and destroying the condylomata on their seat by the knife, the ligature or the actual cautery; this pernicious external mode of treatment, hitherto so universally practised, has been the most prolific source of all the innumerable named or unnamed chronic maladies under which mankind groans; it is one of the most criminal procedures the medical world can be guilty of, and yet it has hitherto been the one generally adopted, and taught from the professional chairs as the only one.1

1 For any medicines that might at the same time be given internally served but to aggravate the malady, as these remedies possessed no specific power of curing the whole disease, but assailed the organism, weakened it and inflicted on it, in addition, other chronic medicinal diseases.

EXPLANATION

- External treatment of local symptoms with objective to remove them from the surface of the body while the internal miasmatic d/s is left uncured is a harmful mode of treatment.
  e.g- Removing psoric eruption by all sorts of ointments, burning away the chancre by caustics, destroying condylomata on their seat by the knife, the ligature or the actual cautery are all harmful external mode of treatment, but universally practised till now.
- It is one of the most criminal procedures & source of all innumerable named or unnamed chronic maladies.
  Yet it has been adopted & taught by the professionals.

Footnote:
These external remedies don't possess specific power of curing the whole d/s but weaken the organism & in addition inflicts other chronic medicinal d/s

§ 204

CHRONIC D/S

If we deduct all chronic affections, ailments and diseases that depend on a persistent unhealthy mode of living, (§ 77) as also those innumerable medicinal maladies (v. § 74) caused by the irrational, persistent, harassing and pernicious treatment of diseases often only of trivial character by physicians of the old school, most the remainder of chronic diseases result from the development of these three chronic miasms, internal syphilis, internal sycosis, but chiefly and in infinitely greater proportion, internal psora, each of which was already in possession of the whole organism, and had penetrated it in all directions before the appearance of the primary, vicarious local symptom of each of them (in the case of psora the scabious eruption, in syphilis the chancre or the bubo, and in sycosis the condylomata) that prevented their outburst; and these chronic miasmatic diseases, if deprived of their local symptom, are inevitably destined by mighty Nature sooner or later to become developed and to burst forth, and thereby propagate all the nameless misery, the incredible number of chronic diseases which have plagued mankind for hundreds and thousands of years, none of which would so frequently have come into existence had physicians striven in a rational manner to cure radically and to extinguish in the organism these three miasms by the internal homoeopathic medicines suited for each of them, without employing topical remedies for their external symptoms. (See note to § 282).

EXPLANATION

The chronic affections, ailments & d/s depend on:-

1. A persistent unhealthy mode of living [aph-77]
2. Medicinal maladies [aph-74], caused by the irrational persistent, harassing & harmful treatment of d/s by physicians of the old school.
3. Rest most of the chronic d/s result from the development of three chronic miasms.
   A] Internal syphilis
   B] Internal sycosis
   C] Mostly by internal psora.

- Each of these infections, psora, syphilis, sycosis is already in possession of the whole organism & penetrates it in all directions before appearance of the primary/local symptom of each of them that prevented their outburst.
- In case of psora the scabious eruption
- In syphilis the chancre or the bubo & in sycosis the condylomata.
- In these chronic miasmatic d/s, if local symptoms are removed, they develop & burst & propagate all the nameless misery, a number of chronic d/s.
- If the physician would rely solely on giving proper internal homeoapthic remedies for each [see note to aph- 282], they would be able to remove these three miasms in the organism, but they relyed on employing local remedies for the external symptoms.

§ 205

CHRONIC DISEASE MANIFESTATION

The homoeopathic physician never treats one of these primary symptoms of chronic miasms, nor yet one of their secondary affections that result from their further development, by local remedies (neither by those external agents that act dynamically,1 nor yet by those that act mechanically), but he cures, in cases where the one or the other appears, only the great miasm on which they depend, whereupon its primary, as also its secondary symptoms disappear spontaneously; but as this was not the mode pursued by the old-school practitioners who preceded him in the treatment of the case, the homoeopathic physician generally, alas!, finds that the primary symptoms2 have already been destroyed by them by means of external remedies, and that he has now to do more with the secondary ones, i.e., the affections resulting from the breaking forth and development of these inherent miasms, but especially with the chronic disease evolved from internal psora, the internal treatment of which, as far as a single physician can elucidate it by many years of reflection, observation and experience, I have endeavored to point out in my work on Chronic Diseases, to which I must refer the reader.

1 I cannot therefore advise, for instance, the local extirpation of the so-called cancer of the lips and face (the product of highly developed psora, not infrequently in conjunction with syphilis) by means of the arsenical remedy of Frere Cosme, not only because it is excessively painful and often fails, but more for this reason, because, if this dynamic remedy should indeed succeed in freeing the affected part of the body from the malignant ulcer locally, the basic malady is thereby not diminished in the slightest, the preserving vital force is therefore necessitated to transfer the field of operation of the great internal malady to some more important part (as it does in every case of metastasis), and the consequence is blindness, deafness, insanity, suffocative asthma, dropsy, apoplexy, etc. But this ambiguous local liberation of the part from the malignant ulcer by the topical arsenical remedy only succeeds, after all, in those cases where the ulcer has not yet attained any great size, and when the vital force is still very energetic; but it is just in such a state of things that the complete internal cure of the whole original disease is also still practicable.

The result is the same without previous cure of the inner miasm when cancer of the face or breast is removed by the knife alone and when encysted tumors are enucleated; something worse ensues, or at any rate death is hastened. This has been the case times without number, but the old school still goes blindly on in the same way in every new case, with the same disastrous results.

2 Itch eruption, chancre (bubo), condylomata.

EXPLANATION

- The Homeopathic physician never treats one of these primary symptoms of the chronic miasms.
- It also never treats one of their secondary affections due to result of local remedies use.
- He cures only the great miasm on which they depend, by which its primary, as also its secondary symptoms disappear spontaneously.
- But the old-school practitioners, destroy characteristic primary symptoms by means of external remedies, now the homeopathic physician is left with the secondary symptoms, those affections which result from the break forth & development of these miasms and especially the chronic d/s evolved from internal psora.
- Hahnemann refer's the reader to read his work on 'chronic d/s'.

Footnote:
So Hahenamnn says that we cannot advise, local extirpation by arsenic remedy of so called cancer of the lips & face which is the product of highly developed psora.

- ✦ The arsenic remedy is excessively painful & often fails and it frees local affected part from malignant ulcer locally only but the basic malady is not removed.
- ✦ The result is that the vital force now transfers the internal malady to some more important part as it does in every case of metastasis.
- ✦ The consequence is blindness, deafness, insanity, suffocative asthma, dropsy, apoplexy etc.
- ✦ This topical arsenical remedy is only successful in those cases where ulcer is not of great size & the vital force is still very energetic & internal cure is practicable.
- ✦ The result is same without previous cure of inner miasm, by removal of cancer of the face or breast by knife alone & the patient health worses & death is hastened.

- But the old school follows their procedure in the same way in every new case & same disastrous results occur.
- Primary symptoms are the eruption chancre [bubo], condylomata.

§ 206

DETERMINE THE MIASM & TREAT ACCORDINGLY

Before commencing the treatment of a chronic disease, it is necessary to make the most careful investigation1 as to whether the patient has had a venereal infection (or an infection with condylomatous gonorrhoea); for then the treatment must be directed towards this alone, when only the signs of syphilis (or of the rarer condylomatous disease) are present, but this disease is very seldom met with alone nowadays. If such infection have previously occurred, this must also be borne in mind in the treatment of those cases in which psora is present, because in them the latter is complicated with the former, as is always the case when the symptoms are not those of pure syphilis; for when the physician thinks he has a case of old venereal disease before him, he has always, or almost always, to treat a syphilitic affection accompanied mostly by (complicated with) psora, for the internal itch dyscrasia (the psora) is far the most frequent fundamental cause of chronic diseases. At times, both miasms may be complicated also with sycosis in chronically diseased organisms, or, as is much more frequently the case, psora is the sole fundamental cause of all other chronic maladies, whatever names they may bear, which are, moreover, so often bungled, increased and disfigured to a monstrous extent by allopathic unskillfulness.

1 In investigations of this nature we must not allow ourselves to be deceived by the assertions of the patients of their friends, who frequently assign as the cause of chronic, even of the severest and most inveterate diseases, either a cold caught (a thorough wetting, drinking cold water after being heated) many years ago, or a former fright, a sprain, a vexation (sometimes even a bewitchment), etc. These causes are much too insignificant to develop a chronic disease in a healthy body, to keep it up for years, and to aggravate it year by year, as is the case with all chronic diseases from developed psora. Causes of a much more important character than those remembered noxious influences must lie at the root of the initiation and progress of a serious, obstinate disease of long standing; the assigned causes could only rouse into activity the latent chronic miasm.

EXPLANATION

Therefore before commencing the treatment of a chronic d/s, careful investigation of the case should be done.

See weather the patient had a venereal infection [or an infection with condylomatous gonorrhoea], the treatment will be directed towards this alone when only signs of syphilis or of the rarer condylomatous d/s are present, the treatment will be towards it.

- If such infection has occurred in the past & now the case has psora, here the psora is complicated with syphilis or sycosis.
- Now the treatment is anti-syphilitic followed by treatment of psora.
- In chronically d/s organisms sometimes boths miasms may be complicated with sycosis.
- Psora is the sole fundamental cause of all other chronic d/s which are often increased by allopathic diastrous treatment.

Footnote 1:
While investigating the case of this nature we must not be believe in something that is false by the assertions of the patients or their friends, who frequently assign either a cold caught (a thorough wetting, drinking cold water after being heated) many years ago, or a former fright, a sprain, a vexation (sometimes even a bewitchment), etc, as the cause of chronic, even of the severest and most inveterate diseases.

These causes are much too insignificant to develop a chronic disease in a healthy body, to keep it up for years and to aggravate it year by year, as is the case with all chronic diseases from developed psora.

Causes of a much more important character than those remembered noxious influences must lie at the root of the initiation and progress of a serious, obstinate disease of long standing;

The assigned causes told by patient or their friends could only activate the latent chronic miasm but the real cause must be found out.

§ 207

EFFECT OF ALLOPATHIC TREATMENT

When the above information has been gained, it still remains for the homoeopathic physician to ascertain what kinds of allopathic treatment had up to that date been adopted for the chronic disease, what perturbing medicines had been chiefly and most frequently employed, also what mineral baths had been used and what effects these had produced, in order to understand in some measure the degeneration of the disease from its original state, and, where possible, to correct in part these pernicious artificial operations, or to enable him to avoid the employment of medicines that have already been improperly used.

EXPLANATION

- Now after the proper investigation when all the above information has been obtained, now the physician enquires about the type of allopathic treatment taken for the chronic d/s.
- The medicine which were used, ask about the mineral baths used & the effects they produced.
- It will help to understand the degeneration of the d/s from its original state and if possible to correct these harmful artificial operation and help him avoid the employment of improper medicines.

§ 208

OBSTACLES TO CURE

The age of the patient, his mode of living and diet, his occupation, his domestic position, his social relation and so forth, must next be taken into consideration, in order to ascertain whether these things have tended to increase his malady, or in how far they may favor or hinder the treatment. In like manner the state of his disposition and mind must be attended to, to learn whether that presents any obstacles to the treatment, or requires to be directed encouraged or modified.

EXPLANATION

- Enquire the age of the patient, his mode of living and diet, his occupation, his domestic position, his social relation etc to know weather these things have increased his malady or how they may favour or hinder the treatment of the case.
- Also the state of his disposition and mind must be noted to learn if there is any obstacle to the treatment or he requires to be directed, encouraged or modified.

§ 209

FORMATION OF THE PORTRAIT OF THE D/S

After this is done, the physician should endeavor in repeated conversations with the patient to trace the picture of his disease as completely as possible, according to the directions given above, in order to be able to elucidate the most striking and peculiar (characteristic) symptoms, in accordance with which he selects the first antipsoric or other remedy having the greatest symptomatic resemblance, for the commencement of the treatment, and so forth.

EXPLANATION

- After this, the physician should have conversations with the patient to get the complete picture of his disease.
- Like this we will be able to make clear, the most striking & characteristic symptoms.
- On the basis of the totality of symptoms we now select the first antipsoric or other remedy which is the most similar to the case.

§ 210

ONE SIDED D/S DIFFICULT TO TREAT

Of psoric origin are almost all those diseases that I have above termed one-sided, which appear to be more difficult to cure in consequence of this one-sidedness, all their other morbid symptoms disappearing, as it were, before the single, great, prominent symptom. Of this character are what are termed mental diseases. They do not, however, constitute a class of disease the condition of the disposition and mind is always altered;1 and in all cases of disease we are called on to cure the state of the patient's disposition is to be particularly noted, along with the totality of the symptoms, if we would trace an accurate picture of the disease, in order to be able therefrom to treat it homoeopathically with success.

1 How often, for instance, do we not meet with a mild, soft disposition in patients who have for years been afflicted with the most painful diseases, so that the physician feels constrained to esteem and compassionate the sufferer! But if he subdue the disease and restore the patient to health – as is frequently done in homoeopathic practice – he is often astonished and horrified at the frightful alteration in his disposition. He often witnesses the occurrence of ingratitude, cruelty, refined malice and propensities most disgraceful and degrading to humanity, which were precisely the qualities possessed by the patient before he grew ill.

Those who were patient when well often become obstinate, violent, hasty, or even intolerant and capricious, or impatient or disponding when ill; those formerly chaste and modest often frequently become lascivious and shameless. A clear-headed person not infrequently becomes obtuse of intellect, while one ordinarily weak-minded becomes more prudent and thoughtful; and a man slow to make up his mind sometimes acquires great presence of mind and quickness of resolve, etc.

EXPLANATION

Almost all diseases that he has termed one sided are of psoric origin, they are more difficult to cure because of this one sidedness.(See §173).

- Similar are the mental diseases.
- Mental diseases do not constitute a class of diseases separately because all corporeal diseases have altered condition of the disposition & mind.
- In all cases of diseases we have to cure the state of the patient's disposition along with the totality of the symptoms.
- This way an accurate picture of the disease will be formed in order to treat it homoeopathically with success.

Footnote:
- The patient who have been suffering from the most painful diseases for years we find a mild, soft disposition in them.
- After the patient is restored to health the physician is often surprised & horrified by the frightful alteration in his disposition.

For eg. When the patient was healthy he was normal & when he becomes ill there occurs ingratitude, cruelty, he harms others & actions became disgraceful to humanity.

Eg:- These people who were patient when well often become obstinate (stubborn), violent, hasty or impatient when ill.

Eg:- A man slow to make up his mind acquires great presence of mind & quickness to resolve etc.

§ 211

GOOD OBSERVATION FOR SELECTION OF REMEDY

This holds good to such an extent, that the state of the disposition of the patient often chiefly determines the selection of the homoeopathic remedy, as being a decidedly characteristic symptom which can least of all remain concealed from the accurately observing physician.

EXPLANATION

- The accurately observing physician observes the state of the disposition of the patient & it often chiefly decides the homeopathic remedy.
- It forms a characteristic symptom of the d/s on the basis of which a homoeopathic remedy can be selected.

§ 212

POWERFUL MEDICINAL SUBSTANCES

The Creator of therapeutic agents has also had particular regard to this main feature of all diseases, the altered state of the disposition and mind, for there is no powerful medicinal substance in the world which does not very notably alter the state of the disposition and mind in the healthy individual who tests it, and every medicine does so in a different manner.

EXPLANATION

- While drug proving, the creator of therapeutic agents, gives particular importance to the altered state of the disposition & mind.
- Every powerful medicinal substance in the world alters the state of the disposition & mind in the healthy individual who tests it.
- Every medicine alters disposition & mind in a different manner.

§ 213

SELECTION OF HOMEOPATHY IN SUCH D/S

We shall, therefore, never be able to cure conformably to nature – that is to say, homoeopathically – if we do not, in every case of disease, even in such as are acute, observe, along with the other symptoms, those relating to the changes in the state of the mind and disposition, and if we do not select, for the patient's relief, from among the medicines a disease-force which, in addition to the similarity of its other symptoms to those of the disease, is also capable of producing a similar state of the disposition and mind.1

1 Thus aconite will seldom or never effect a rapid or permanent cure in a patient of a quiet, calm, equable disposition; and just as little will nux vomica be serviceable where the disposition is mild and phlegmatic, pulsatilla where it is happy, gay and obstinate, or ignatia where it is imperturbable and disposed neither to be frightened nor vexed.

EXPLANATION

- If we want to cure conformably to nature that is, homeopathically, we need to observe the changes in the state of the mind & disposition along with the other symptoms, even in acute cases.
- So we need to select a medicine which in addition to the similarity of its other symptoms of the d/s is also capable of producing a similar state of the disposition & mind.

Footnote:

- For this reason aconite will seldom or never effect a rapid or permanent cure in a patient who is of quiet, calm & equable disposition.
- Similarly nux-vomica never effect cure in a patient where disposition is mild & phlegmatic.
- Similarly pulsatilla never effect cure in one who is happy, gay & obstinate.

§ 214

TREATMENT OF MENTAL D/S

The instructions I have to give relative to the cure of mental diseases may be confined to a very few remarks, as they are to be cured in the same way as all other diseases, namely, by a remedy which shows, by the symptoms it causes in the body and mind of a healthy individual, a power of producing a morbid state as similar as possible to the case of disease before us, and in no other way can they be cured.

EXPLANATION

- Here Hahnemann says that mental d/s are to be cured in the same way as all other d/s.
- Here also remedy is chosen which shows, a power of producing a morbid state as similar as possible to the case of d/s.

§ 215

MENTAL & CORPOREAL D/S

Almost all the so-called mental and emotional diseases are nothing more than corporeal diseases in which the symptom of derangement of the mind and disposition peculiar to each of them is increased, while the corporeal symptoms decline (more or less rapidly), till it a length attains the most striking one-sidedness, almost as though it were a local disease in the invisible subtle organ of the mind or disposition.

EXPLANATION

- Almost all the so-called mental & emotional d/s are corporeal d/s in which the symptom of derangement of the mind & disposition is increased while the corporeal symptoms decline.
- Later it attains the one-sidedness nature, as it were a local d/s in the invisible subtle organ of the mind or disposition I.e- Mainly the affection of mind & disposition observable.

§ 216

MENTAL DISEASES

The cases are not rare in which a so-called corporeal disease that threatens to be fatal – a suppuration of the lungs, or the deterioration of some other important viscus, or some other disease of acute character, e.g., in childbed, etc. – becomes transformed into insanity, into a kind of melancholia or into mania by a rapid increase of the psychical symptoms that were previously present, whereupon the corporeal symptoms lose all their danger; these latter improve almost to perfect health, or rather they decrease to such a degree that their obscured presence can only be detected by the observation of a physician gifted with perseverance and penetration. In this manner they become transformed into a one-sided and, as it were, a local disease, in which the symptom of the mental disturbance, which was at first but slight, increases so as to be the chief symptom, and in a great measure occupies the place of the other (corporeal) symptoms, whose intensity it subdues in a palliative manner, so that, in short, the affections of the grosser corporeal organs become, as it were, transferred and conducted to the almost spiritual, mental and emotional organs, which the anatomist has never yet and never will reach with his scalpel.

EXPLANATION

- Now let the discuss the mental symptoms in details.
- The cases of corporeal d/s that are fatal [e.g- a suppuration of lungs or other important viscus or some other d/s of acute character etc], becomes transformed into insanity, into a kind of melancholia or into mania. Here a rapid increase of psychial symptoms present previously, occurs & the corporeal symptoms lose all their danger.
- These corporeal symptoms improve almost to perfect health or they decrease to such a degree that only a attentive physician can observe them.
- This way they transform into a one-sided local d/s, in which the symptom of the mental disturbances[which at first were slight]increase so much that they become the chief symptom & occupies the place of other [corporeal] symptoms and palliates their intensity.
- In short we can say that the affection of the grosser corporeal organs become transferred to the spiritual mental & emotional organs & these mental & emotional organs can never be reach by anatomist with his scalpel.

§ 217

DISEASE PORTRAIT= MENTAL+ PHYSICAL SYMPTOMS

In these diseases we must be very careful to make ourselves acquainted with the whole of the phenomena, both those belonging to the corporeal symptoms, and also, and indeed particularly, those appertaining to the accurate apprehension of the precise character of the chief symptom, of the peculiar and always predominating state of the mind and disposition, in order to discover, for the purpose of extinguishing the entire disease, among the remedies whose pure effects are known, a homoeopathic medicinal pathogenetic force – that is to say, a remedy which in its list of symptoms displays, with the greatest possible similarity, not only the corporeal morbid symptoms present in the case of disease before us, but also especially this mental and emotional state.

EXPLANATION

In these diseases wre must observe & become known with the whole of the phenomena belonging to corporeal symptoms and particularly to chief symptom of the peculiar & predominating state of the mind & disposition.

So that a homoeopathic medicinal pathogenetic force can be selected.

A remedy which has the greatest possible similarity to corporeal morbid symptoms & especially the mental & emotional state is selected for cure.

§ 218

HISTORY OF THE PATIENT

To this collection of symptoms belongs in the first place to accurate description of all the phenomena of the previous so-called corporeal disease, before it degenerated into a one-sided increase of the physical symptom, and became a disease of the mind and disposition. This may be learned from the report of the patient's friends.

EXPLANATION

In this case, we should ask the patient's friends about the symptoms that were present in the starting, I.e- description of all the phenomena of previous corporeal d/s, before it degenerated into a one-sided increase of the psychial symptom & became a d/s of the mind & disposition.

Enquire about the corporeal symptoms previously present.

§ 219

PAST & PRESENT SYMPTOMS

A comparison of these previous symptoms of the corporeal disease with the traces of them that still remain, though they have become less perceptible (but which even now sometimes become prominent, when a lucid interval and a transient alleviation of the psychical disease occurs), will serve to prove them to be still present, though obscured.

EXPLANATION

- When we compare these previous symptoms of the corporeal d/s with the traces of them that are still present though less perceptible.
- We find that they prove to be still present though concealed.

§ 220

SELECTION OF MEDICINE IN CHRONIC D/S

By adding to this the state of the mind and disposition accurately observed by the patient's friends and by the physician himself, we have thus constructed the complete picture of the disease, for which in order to effect the homoeopathic cure of the disease, a medicine capable of producing strikingly similar symptoms, and especially an analogous disorder of the mind, must be sought for among the antipsoric remedies, if the physical disease have already lasted some time.

EXPALNATION

To the above corporeal symptoms, the state of the mind & disposition is accurately observed by the physician & patient's friends are also enquired by the physician.

Like this we construct the complete picture of the d/s, so that a medicine capable of producing similar symptoms & especially symptoms of mind must be chosen among the antipsoric remedies.

§ 221

MANAGEMENT OF ACUTE MENTAL D/S

If, however, insanity or mania (caused by fright, vexation, the abuse of spirituous liquors, etc.) have suddenly broken out as an acute disease in the patient's ordinary calm state, although it almost always arises from internal psora, like a flame bursting forth from it, yet when it occurs in this acute manner it should not be immediately treated with antipsoric, but in the first place with remedies indicated for it out of the order class of proved medicaments (e.g., aconite, belladonna, stramonium, hyoscyamus, mercury, etc.) in highly potentized, minute, homoeopathic doses, in order to subdue it so far that the psora shall for the time revert to its former latent state, wherein the patient appears as if quite well.

EXPLANATION

- However, if the insanity or mania which is caused by fright, vexation, abuse of spirituous liquors etc, has suddenly broken out as an acute d/s in the patient who was in a calm state.
- In these cases when it occurs in this acute manner it should not be immediately treated with antipsoric.
  But in the first place it must be treated with remedies indicated for it.
  e.g- Aconite, belladona, stramonium, hysoscyamus, mercury etc.
- These are given in highly potentized, minute homeopathic doses, so that the psora revert to its former latent state, the patient appears as if quite well.

§ 222

RADICAL TREATMENT

But such a patient, who has recovered from an acute mental or emotional disease by the use of these non-antipsoric medicines, should never be regarded as cured; on the contrary, no time should be lost in attempting to free him completely,1 by means of a prolonged antipsoric treatment, from the chronic miasm of the psora, which, it is true, has now become once more latent but is quite ready to break out anew; if this be done, there is no fear of another similar attack, if he attend faithfully to the diet and regimen prescribed for him.

1 It very rarely happens that a mental or emotional disease of long standing ceases spontaneously (for the internal dyscrasia transfers itself again to the grosser corporeal organs); such are the few

cases met with now and then, where a former inmate of a madhouse has been dismissed apparently recovered. Hitherto, moreover, all madhouses have continued to be chokefull, so that the multitude of other insane persons who seek for admission into such institutions could scarcely find room in them unless some of the insane in the house died. Not one is ever really and permanently cured in them! A convincing proof, among many others, of the complete nullity of the non-healing art hitherto practised, which has been ridiculously honored by allopathic ostentation with the title of rational medicine. How often, on the other hand, has not the true healing art, genuine pure homoeopathy, been able to restore such unfortunate beings to the possession of their mental and corporeal health, and so give them back again to their delighted friends and to the world!

EXPLANATION

- Now we should not waste time and give him the antipsoric remedy for complete cure,
  Because if we leave the patient at this stage he is not cured completely.
  Though psora has been latent but it may break anytime.
  After proper treatment, there is no fear of another similar attack, if he follows faithfully to the diet & regimen prescribed for him.

Footnote:
- It is very rare, that a mental or emotional d/s of long standing ceases on its own because the internal dyscrasia transfers itself again to the grosser corporeal organs.
- No patient in a psychiatry hospital ever is seen really & permanently cured.
- The allopathic treatment is a non-healing art though practised till now.
- Homeopathy has been able to restore such patients to their mental & corporeal health & given them back to the world, cured.

§ 223

ANTIPSORIC TREATMENT IS A MUST

But if the antipsoric treatment be omitted, then we may almost assuredly expect, from a much slighter cause than brought on the first attack of the insanity, the speedy occurrence of a new and more lasting the severe fit, during which the psora usually develops itself completely, and passes into either a periodic or continued mental derangement, which is then more difficult to be cured by antipsorics.

EXPLANATION

Now let us see what happens if the antipsoric treatment is omitted[not given]
   The first attack of the insanity which was brought by much slighter cause.

Now the new & more lasting & severe fit occur speedly from the same cause.

During this the psora usually develops completely & now passes into periodic or continued mental derangement, now this is more difficult to be cured by antipsoric.

So it is neccessary to employ antipsoric treatment there in, so that this does not happen & the case is cured gently.

§ 224

MENTAL D/S OF DOUBTFUL ORIGIN

If the mental disease be not quite developed, and if it be still somewhat doubtful whether it really arose from a corporeal affection, or did not rather result from faults of education, bad practices, corrupt morals, neglect of the mind, superstition or ignorance; the mode of deciding this point will be, that if it proceed from one or other of the latter causes it will diminish and be improved by sensible friendly exhortations, consolatory arguments, serious representations and sensible advice, whereas a real moral or mental malady, depending on bodily disease, would be speedily aggravated by such a course, the melancholic would become still more dejected, querulous, inconsolable and reserved, the spiteful maniac would thereby become still more exasperated, and the chattering fool would become manifestly more foolish.1

1 It would seem as though the mind, in these cases, felt with uneasiness and grief the truth of these rational representations and acted upon the body as it wished to restore the lost harmony, but that the body, by means of its disease, reacted upon the organs of the mind and disposition and put them in still greater disorder by a fresh transference of its sufferings on to them.

EXPLANATION

Now whether the mental d/s is due to some other cause or it really arose from a corporeal affection, we can find it out from some points.

- The other causes are faults of education, bad practices, corrupt morals, neglect of mind, superstition or ignorance.
- If the cause of mental malady is from above ones so it is improved by friendly exhortations, consolatory arguments, serious representations & sensible advice.
- Whereas a real moral or mental malady which depends on bodily d/s will be speedily aggravated by such a process.
- The melancholic becomes still more querulous, sad[dejected], inconsolable & reserved.
- The [spitedul]malicious becomes still more annoyed [exasperated].
- The chattering fool would become more foolish.

Footnote:
The body by means of its d/s reacts upon the organs of the mind & disposition & puts them in greater disorder by a fresh transference of its sufferings on to them.

- ✦ Don't think that these uneasiness & grief of mind is body reaction to restore the lost harmony.

§ 225

EMOTIONAL DISEASES

There are, however, as has just been stated, certainly a few emotional diseases which have not merely been developed into that form out of corporeal diseases, but which, in an inverse manner, the body being but slightly indisposed, originate and are kept up by emotional causes, such as continued anxiety, worry, vexation, wrongs and the frequent occurrence of great fear and fright. This kind of emotional diseases in time destroys the corporeal health, often to a great degree.

EXPLANATION

- There are a few emotional d/s which have not been developed into that form out of corporeal d/s.
- Here the cause is emotional e.g- continued anxiety, worry, vexation, wrongs & great fear & fright.
- In these, the body which is slightly indisposed, these emotional d/s originate & are kept up by these emotional causes.
- This kind of emotional d/s in time destroys the corporeal health, to a great degree.

§ 226

TREATMENT OF EMOTIONAL D/S

It is only such emotional diseases as these, which were first engendered and subsequently kept up by the mind itself, that, while they are yet recent and before they have made very great inroads on the corporeal state, may, by means of psychical remedies, such as a display of confidence, friendly exhortations, sensible advice, and often by a well-disguised deception, be rapidly changed into a healthy state of the mind (and with appropriate diet and regimen, seemingly into a healthy state of the body also.)

EXPLANATION

- In above such emotional diseases which are first arisen & subsequently kept up by the mind itself.
- When these emotional d/s are recent & before they are have made very great inroads on the corporeal state, they can be rapidly changed into a healthy state of the mind by means of psychial remedies.
- The psychial remedies include a display of confidence, friendly [exhoratations] urging someone to do something, advice & often by a well-disguised deception [making someone believe]
- And with appropriate diet & regimen, it also changes the body to healthy state.

§ 227

RADICAL ANTIPSORIC TREATMENT

But the fundamental cause in these cases also is a psoric miasm, which was only not yet quite near its full development, and for security's sake, the seemingly cured patient should be subjected to a radical, antipsoric treatment, in order that he may not again, as might easily occur, fall into a similar state of mental disease.

EXPLANATION

- But in these cases also, the fundamental cause is a psoric miasm which was not quite near its full development.
- Therefore for safety, the seemingly cured patient should be given a radical antipsoric treatment, so that he may not again fall into a similar state of mental d/s.

§ 228

COMPLETE CURE OF MENTAL AND EMOTIONAL D/S

In mental and emotional diseases resulting from corporeal maladies, which can only be cured by homoeopathic antipsoric medicine conjoined with carefully regulated mode of life, an appropriate psychical behavior towards the patient on the part of those about him and of the physician must be scrupulously observed, by way of an auxiliary mental regimen. To furious mania we must oppose clam intrepidity and cool, firm resolution – to doleful, querulous lamentation, a mute display of commiseration in looks and gestures – to senseless chattering, a silence not wholly inattentive – to disgusting and abominable conduct and to conversation of a similar character, total inattention. We must merely endeavor to prevent the destruction and injury of surrounding objects, without reproaching the patient for his acts, and everything must be arranged in such a way that the necessity for any corporeal punishments and tortures1 whatever may be avoided. This is so much the more easily effected, because in the administration of the medicine – the only circumstance in which the employment of coercion could be justified – in the homoeopathic system the small doses of the appropriate medicine never offend the taste, and may consequently be given to the patient without his knowledge in his drink, so that all compulsion is unnecessary.

1 It is impossible to marvel at the hard-heartedness and indiscretion of the medical men in many establishments for patients of this kind, who, without attempting to discover the true and only efficacious mode of curing such disease, which is by homoeopathic medicinal (antipsoric) means, content themselves with torturing these most pitiable of all human beings with the most violent blows and other painful torments. By this unconscientious and revolting procedure they debase themselves beneath the level of the turnkeys in a house of correction, for the latter inflict such chastisement as the duty devolving on their office, and on criminals only, whilst the former appear, from a humiliating consciousness of their uselessness as physicians, only to vent their spite at the supposed incurability of mental diseases in harshness towards the pitiable, innocent sufferers, for they are too ignorant to be of any use and too indolent to adopt a judicious mode of treatment.

EXPLANATION

- In mental & emotional d/s which result from corporeal maladies, can be cured by homeopathic antipsoric medicine along with proper mode of life, and [psychial]behaviour towards the patient of those about him & of the physician must be observed.
- Liked for furious mania we must oppose calm fearlessness[intrepidity]& cool
- Firm resolution to doleful [sorrowful person], querulous lamentation, a mute display of commiseration in looks & gestures -to senseless chattering.
- A silence not wholly inattentive to disgusting & abominable[very bad & shocking] conduct etc.
- We must try hard [endeavor]to prevent the destruction & injury of surrounding objects but not reproach the patient for his acts.
  And should avoid any corporeal punishments & tortures.
- In the homeopathic system the small doses of the appropriate medicine never offend the taste & so they can be given to the patient in his drive without his knowledge, this way employment of practice of persuading someone forcefully [coercion], is avoided to force him take medicine.

Footnote:
We often see the irrational behaviour of the medical men in many establishments for patients of this kind.

- ✦ They don't discover the true & only efficacious mode of curing such d/s, which is by homeopathic medicines[antipsoric].
- ✦ They instead of this, torture these human beings with painful & violent blows.
- ✦ This is never a mode of treatment of mental d/s of pitiable, innocent sufferers as they are too lazy to adopt a judicious mode of treatment.

§ 229

BEHAVIOR OF PHYSICIAN WITH THE PATIENT

On the other hand, contradiction, eager explanations, rude corrections and invectives, as also weak, timorous yielding, are quite out of place with such patients; they are equally pernicious modes of treating mental and emotional maladies. But such patients are most of all exasperated and their complaint aggravated by contumely, fraud, and deceptions that they can detect. The physician and keeper must always pretend to believe them to be possessed of reason.

All kinds of external disturbing influences on their senses and disposition should be if possible removed; there are no amusements for their clouded spirit, no salutary distractions, no means of instruction, no soothing effects from conversation, books or other things for the soul that pines or frets in the chains of the diseased body, no invigoration for it, but the care; it is only when the bodily health is changed for the better that tranquillity and comfort again beam upon their mind.1

1 Foot-note in Sixth Edition only.
The treatment of the violent insane manic and melancholic can take place only in an institution specially arranged for their treatment but not within the family circle of the patient.

EXPLANATION

- On the other hand, contradiction, rude correctious etc, are equally harmful modes of treating mental and emotional maladies.
- Such patients are most annoyed and their complaints aggravated if they detect any fraud or insulting language etc.
- The physician & keeper must always pretend to believe them to be of reason.
- All kinds of external disturbing influences on their senses & disposition should be removed.
- There is no means of instruction, no soothing effects from conversation, books or other things for the soul, no way to make one feel healthy, but only way is care.
- By proper homoeopathic cure the bodily health is changed, for the better comfort upon their mind.

Footnote:
The treatment of the violent insane maniac & melancholic patient can take place only in an institution arranged for their treatment & not within the family circle of the patient.

§ 230

RADICAL TREATMENT OF MENTAL D/S

If the antipsoric remedies selected for each particular case of mental or emotional disease (there are incredibly numerous varieties of them) be quite homoeopathically suited for the faithfully traced picture of the morbid state, which, if there be a sufficient number of this kind of medicines known in respect of their pure effects, is ascertained by an indefatigable search for the most appropriate homoeopathic remedy all the more easily, as the emotional and mental state, constituting the principal symptom of such a patient, is so unmistakably perceptible, – then the most striking improvement in no very long time, which could not be brought about by physicking the patient to death with the largest oft – repeated doses of all other unsuitable (allopathic) medicines. Indeed, I can confidently assert, from great experience, that the vast superiority of the homoeopathic system over all other conceivable methods of the treatment is nowhere displayed in a more triumphant light than in mental and emotional diseases of long standing, which originally sprang from corporeal maladies or were developed simultaneously with them.

EXPLANATION

- Here Hahnemann says that he can confidently declare from his experience, that the homoeopathic system is very superior than other methods of treatment, mainly in mental & emotional d/s of long standing cases. These mental & emotional d/s originally sprang from corporeal maladies or developed simultaneously with corporeal maladies.
- The appropriate homoeopathic remedy produces the most striking improvement which cannot be brought by using the largest repeated doses of all other unsuitable [allopathic] medicine.
- The search for homeopathic remedy is more easily as in the emotional & mental state, the principal symptom of such a patient is unmistakably perceptible.
- So that the correct picture of the morbid state can be obtained & the antipsoric remedies can be selected appropriately.

§ 231

INTERMITTENT DISEASE

The intermittent disease deserve a special consideration, as well those that recur at certain periods – like the great number of intermittent fevers, and the apparently non-febrile affections that recur at intervals like intermittent fevers – as also those in which certain morbid states alternate at uncertain intervals with morbid states of a different kind.

EXPLANATION

- Now intermittent d/s & those that recur at certain periods deserve a special attention.
- Those d/s which recur at certain periods like great number of intermittent fever & apparently non-febrile affections that recur at intervals like intermittent fevers.
- And also those in which certain morbid states alternate with morbid states of a different kind at uncertain intervals called alternating d/s. All the above d/s deserve a special consideration.

§ 232

ALTERNATING DISEASE

These latter, alternating diseases, are also very numerous,1 but all belong to the class of chronic diseases; they are generally a manifestation of developed psora alone, sometimes, but seldom, complicated with a syphilitic miasm, and therefore in the former case may be cured by antipsoric medicines; in the latter, however, in alternation with antisyphilitics as taught in my work on the Chronic Diseases.

1 Two or three states may alternate with one another. Thus, for instance, in the case of double alternating diseases, certain pains may occur persistently in the legs, etc., immediately on the disappearance of a kind of ophthalmia, which latter again appears as soon as the pain in the limbs has gone off for the time – convulsions and spasms may alternate immediately with any other affection of the body or some part of it – in a case of threefold alternating states in a common indisposition, periods of apparent increase of health and unusual exaltation of the corporeal and mental powers (extravagant gaiety, extraordinary activity of the body, excess of comfortable feeling, inordinate appetite, etc.) may occur, after which, and quite unexpectedly, gloomy, melancholy humor, intolerable hypochondriacal derangement of the disposition, with disorder of several of the vital operations, the digestion, sleep, etc., appear, which again, and just as suddenly, give place to the habitual moderate ill-health; and so also several and very various alternating states. When the new state makes its appearance, there is often no perceptible trace of the former one. In other cases only slight traces of the former alternating state remain when the new one occurs; few of the symptoms of the first state remain on the appearance and during the continuance of the second. Sometimes the morbid alternating states are quite of opposite natures, as for instance, melancholy periodically alternating with gay insanity or frenzy.

EXPLANATION

- The last one I.e-alternating d/s are also very large in number but all belong to the class of chronic d/s.
- They are generally a manifestation of developed psora alone but maybe complicated with a syphilitic miasm.
- If they are manifestation of developed psora alone they are cured by antipsoric medicines.
- If they are complicated with a syphilitic miasm, antipsoric remedy in alteration with antisyphiltics brings cure [as taught in Hahnemann's work on the 'chronic d/s'.

Footnote:-
In alternating d/s two or three states may alternate with one another.

Eg- In case of double alternating d/s.

A patient has a kind of ophthalmia when it disappears, certain pains appear immediately in legs, when this pain in limbs is gone the opthalmia reappear again.

Eg - In a case of threefold alternating states, periods of apparent increase of health & unusual state of extreme happiness [exaltation]of the corporeal & mental powers may occur, after this gloomy. melancholy humor, intolerable hypochondriacal derangement of the disposition with disorder of digestion, sleep etc, appear & which suddenly give place to the habitual moderate ill-health & very several alternating state.

- when the new state makes its appearance, there is often no trace of the former one present.
- In some cases only slight traces of former alternating state remain when the new one occurs.
- Sometimes the morbid alternating sates are quite of opposite natures e.g- Melancholy alternating with gay insanity or frenzy [a state of great emotion that is not under control]

§ 233

TYPICAL INTERMITTENT D/S

The typical intermittent disease are those where a morbid state of unvarying character returns at a tolerably fixed period, while the patient is apparently in good health, and takes its departure at an equally fixed period; this is observed in those apparently non-febrile morbid states that come and go in a periodical manner (at certain times), as well as in those of a febrile character, to wit, the numerous varieties of intermittent fevers.

EXPLANATION

- In the typical intermittent d/s a morbid state of unvarying [unchanging]character returns at a fixed period, while the patient is apparently in good health & goes away at an equally fixed period.

- This is observed in those apparently non-febrile morbid sates that come & go in a periodical manner [at certain times]and also in febrile morbid states, the numerous varieties of intermittent fevers.
- The details we will study in following aphorisms.

§ 234

NON FEBRILE TYPICAL INTERMITTENT DISEASES

Those apparently non-febrile, typical, periodically recurring morbid states just alluded to observed in one single patient at a time (they do not usually appear sporadically or epidemically) always belong to the chronic diseases, mostly to those that are purely psoric, are but seldom complicated with syphilis, and are successfully treated by the same means; yet it is sometimes necessary to employ as an intermediate remedy a small dose of a potentized solution of cinchona bark, in order to extinguish completely their intermittent type.

EXPLANATION

These apparently non-febrile, typical, periodically recurring morbid states are observed in one single patient at a time.

- They don't usually appear sporadically or epidemically.
- These belong to chronic d/s, most of which are purely psoric but seldom complicated with syphilis.
- Sometimes it becomes necessary to employ a small dose of a potentized solution of cinchona bark, as an intermittent type can be extinguished completely.

§ 235

INTERMITTENT FEVER

With regard to the intermittent fevers,1 that prevail sporadically or epidemically (not those endemically located in marshy districts), we often find every paroxysm likewise composed of two opposite alternating states (cold, heat – heat, cold), more frequently still of three (cold, heat, sweat). Therefore the remedy selected for them from the general class of proved (common, not antipsoric) medicines must either (and remedies of this sort are the surest) be able likewise to produce in the healthy body two (or all three) similar alternating states, or else must correspond

by similarity of symptoms, in the most homoeopathic manner possible, to the strongest, best marked, and most peculiar alternating state (either to the cold stage, or to the hot stage, or to the sweating state, each with its accessory symptoms, according as the one or other alternating state is the strongest and most peculiar); but the symptoms of the patient's health during the intervals when he is free from fever must be the chief guide to the most appropriate homoeopathic remedy.2

1 The pathology hitherto in vogue, which is still in the stage of irrational infancy, recognizes but one single intermittent fever, which it likewise termed ague, and admits of no varieties but such as are constituted by the different intervals at which the paroxysms recur, quotidian, tertian, quartan etc. But there are much more important differences among them than what are marked by the periods of their recurrence; there are innumerable varieties of these fevers, some of which cannot even be denominated ague, as their fits consist solely of heat; others, again, are characterised by cold alone, with or without subsequent perspiration; yet others which exhibit general coldness of the surface, with a sensation on the patient's part, or whilst the body feels externally hot, the patient feels cold; others, again, in which one paroxysm consists entirely of a rigor or simple chilliness followed by an interval of health, while the next consists of heat alone, followed or not by perspiration; others, again, in which the heat comes first and the cold stage not till that is gone; others, again, wherein after a cold or hot stage apyrexia ensues, and then perspiration comes on like a second fit, often many hours subsequently; others, again, in which no perspiration at all comes on, and yet others in which the whole attack consists of perspiration alone, without any cold or hot stage, or in which the perspiration is only present during the heat; and there are innumerable other differences, especially in regard to the accessory symptoms, such as headache of a peculiar kind, bad taste of the mouth, nausea, vomiting, diarrhoea, want of or excessive thirst, peculiar pains in the body or limbs, disturbed sleep, deliria, alterations of temper, spasms, etc., before, during or after the sweating stage, and countless other varieties. All these are manifestly intermittent fevers of very different kinds, each of which, as might naturally be supposed, requires a special (homoeopathic) treatment. It must be confessed that they can almost all be suppressed (as is often done) by enormous doses of bark and of its pharmaceutical preparation, the sulphate of quinine; that is to say, their periodical recurrence (their typus) may be extinguished by it, but the patients who suffered from intermittent fevers for which cinchona bark is not suitable, as is the case with all those epidemic intermittent fevers that traverse whole countries and even mountainous districts, are not restored to health by the extinction of the typus; on the contrary, they now remain ill in another manner, and worse, often much worse, than before; they are affected by peculiar, chronic bark dyscrasias, and can scarcely be restored to health even by a prolonged treatment by the true system of medicine – and yet that is what is called curing, forsooth!

2 Dr. von Bonninghausen, who has rendered more services to our beneficent system of medicine than any other of my disciples, has best elucidated this subject, which demands so much care, and has facilitated the choice of the efficient remedy for the various epidemics of fever, in his work entitled Versuch einer homoopathischen Therapie der Wechselfieber, 1833, Muster bi Regensberg.

EXPLANATION

- In intermittent fevers, present sporadically or epidemically (not those endemically located in marshy districts)we often find that every paroxysm is composed of two opposite alternating sates [cold, heat-heat, cold], more frequently of three states[cold, heat, sweat]

- Therefore the remedy selected for them from proved medicines [not antipsoric] must either be able to produce two or all three similar alternating states in the healthy body, or either must correspond by similarity of symptoms to the strongest, best marked & most peculiar alternating state & either to the cold stage or to the hot stage or to the sweating state, each with its accessory symptoms whichever alternating state is the strongest & most peculiar.
- In these intermittent fevers, the symptoms of the patients's health during the intervals when he is free from fever must be the chief guide to the most appropriate homeopathic remedy.

Footnote 1:

The pathology till now recognizes it as one single intermittent fever, which it termed ague and admits of no varieties but constituted by the different intervals at which paroxysm recur, quotidian, tertian, quartan etc.

- There are much more important differences among the intermittent fever, there are innumerable varieties of these fever.
- Some consist solely of heat as their fits others characterised by cold alone, with or without subsequent perspiration, others exhibit general coldness of surface, with a sensation of heat on parts of body or in some cases the body feels externally hot, the patient feels cold.
- in others, one paroxysm consists entirely of a rigor or simple chilliness, followed by an interval of health while next consist of heat alone, followed or not by perspiration.
- In some others heat comes first & the cold stage not till that is gone.
- In others, after a cold or hot state apyrexia ensues & then perspiration comes like a second fit often many hours subsequently.
- In others no perspiration comes on & in others whole attack consist of perspiration without any cold or hot stage & there are many other differences, especially in regard to the accessory symptoms, like headache, bad taste of mouth, nausea, vomiting, diarrhoea, want of or excessive thirst, peculiar pains in the body or limbs, disturbed sleep etc before, during or after the cold stage, before, during or after the hot stage, before, during or after the sweating stages etc.
- All the above are intermittent fevers of very different kinds & each of which requires a special [homeopathic treatment].
- They can almost all be suppressed [as is often done], by enormous doses of bark & sulphate of quinine [its pharmaceutical preparation], it means their periodical recurrence [their typhus], may be extinguished by it, but the patients who suffered from intermittent fevers for which cinchona bark is not suitable,[epidemic intermittent fevers], are not restored to health by the extinction of the typus but they now remain ill in another manner & worse than before. They are affected by peculiar, chronic bark dyscrasias & the restoration of health even by a prolonged treatment by true system of medicine is not successful & yet that is what is called curing, indeed[forsooth].

Footnote 2:

Dr. Von Bonninghausen has given more service to the homeopathic system of medicine than any other of Hahnemann's disciples. He has best elucidated this subject & has helped in the choice of the efficient remedy for the various epidemics of fever, in his work 'Versuch einer homeopathischen therapic der wechselfieber' 1833, Munster bei Regensberg.

§ 236

APPROPRIATE TIME FOR ADMINISTRATION OF MEDICINE

The most appropriate and efficacious time for administering the medicine in these cases is immediately or very soon after the termination of the paroxysm, as soon as the patient has in some degree recovered from its effects; it has then time to effect all the changes in the organism requisite for the restoration of health, without any great disturbance or violent commotion; whereas the action of a medicine, be it ever so specifically appropriate, if given immediately before the paroxysm, coincides with the natural recurrence of the disease and causes such a reaction in the organism, such a violent contention, that an attack of that nature produces at the very least a great loss of strength, if it do not endanger life.1 But if the medicine be given immediately after the termination of the fit, that is to say, at the period when the apyretic interval has commenced and a long time before there are any preparations for the next paroxysm, then the vital force of the organism is in the best possible condition to allow itself to be quietly altered by the remedy, and thus restored to the healthy state.

   1 This is observed in the fatal cases, by no means rare, in which a moderate dose of opium given during the cold stage quickly deprived the patients of life.

EXPLANATION

- In these cases, most appropriate & efficacious time for administering the medicine is immediately or very soon after the paroxysm has terminated.
- As soon as the patient has recovered in some degree from its effects, it has time to effect all the change in the organism requisite for restoration of health, this can occur without any great disturbance or violent state of confusion, this is so because during this period the apyretic interval has commenced & a long time before there are any preparations for the next paroxysm, then the vital force of the organism is in the best possible condition to allow itself to be quietly altered by the remedy & thus restored to the healthy state.
- Whereas even if appropriate specific remedy is given immediately before the paroxysm it coincides with the natural recurrence of the d/s & causes such a reaction in the organism.
- Such a violent reaction[contention] produces a great loss of strength, if it does not endanger life.

Footnote:
This is observed in the fatal cases in which a moderate dose of opium given during the cold stage quickly caused patient to die.

§ 237

TIME FOR PRESCRIBING MEDICINE WHEN THERE IS SHORT INTERVAL BETWEEN PAROXYSMS

But if the stage of apyrexia be very short, as happens in some very bad fevers, or if it be disturbed by some of the after sufferings of the previous paroxysm, the dose of the homoeopathic medicine should be administered when the perspiration begins to abate, or the other subsequent phenomena of the expiring paroxysm begin to diminish.

EXPLANATION

But if this stage of apyrexia [when there is no fever] is very short as it happens in some very bad fevers or if it is disturbed by some after sufferings of the previous paroxysm.

- ✦ In these cases the dose of the homeopathic medicine should be administered when the perspiration begins to become less intense [abate] or the other subsequent phenomena of expiring paroxysm begin to diminish.

§ 238

REPETITION OF MEDICINE

Not infrequently, the suitable medicine has with a single dose destroyed several attacks and brought about the return of health, but in the majority of cases, another dose must be administered after such attack. Better still, however, when the character of the symptoms has not changed, doses of the same medicine given according to the newer discovery of repetition of doses (see note to § 270), may be given without difficulty in dynamizing each successive dose with 10-12 successions of the vial containing the medicinal substance. Nevertheless, there are at times cases, though seldom, where the intermittent fever returns after several days' well being. This return of the same fever after a healthy interval is only possible when the noxious principle that first caused the fever, is still acting upon the convalescent, as is the case in marshy regions. Here a permanent restoration can often take place only by getting away from this causative factor, as is possible by seeking a mountainous retreat, if the cause was a marshy fever.

EXPLANATION

- The suitable medicine destroys several attacks & brings the return of health in first dose.
- But in majority of cases, an other dose must be administered after each attack.
- When the character of the symptoms has not changed, doses of the same medicine is given by dynamizing each successive dose with 10-12 successions of the vial according to the newer discovery of repetition of doses.
- At times there are cases, where the intermittent fever returns after several days of well being
- This is possible only when the noxious principle that first caused the fever, is still acting upon the convalescent [patient who is recovering] as is the case in marshy regions.
- Here permanent restoration of health can occur only by getting away from the causative factor, if the cause was a marshy fever going to mountains can restore health of the patient.

§ 239

EVERY MEDICINE CAUSES DIFFERENT PECULIAR FEVER

As almost every medicine causes in its pure action a special, peculiar fever and even a kind of intermittent fever with its alternating states, differing from all other fevers that are caused by other medicines, homoeopathic remedies may be found in the extensive domain of medicines for all the numerous varieties of natural intermittent fevers and, for a great many of such fevers, even in the moderate collection of medicines already proved on the healthy individual.

EXPLANATION

Every medicine causes a special peculiar fever in its pure action & even a kind of intermittent fever with its alternating states.

Each medicine differs from all other fevers that are caused by other medicines.

Therefore homeopathic remedies may be found for all the numerous varieties of natural intermittent fevers and for a great many of such fevers.

§ 240

INTERMITTENT FEVER & ANTIPSORIC MEDICINE

But if the remedy found to be the homoeopathic specific for a prevalent epidemic of intermittent fever do not effect a perfect cure in some one or other patient, if it be not the influence of a marshy district that prevents the cure, it must always be the psoric miasm in the background, in which case antipsoric medicines must be employed until complete relief is obtained.

EXPLANATION

- Now if the following condition arises.
- The remedy of which was found to be homoeopathically specific for a epidemic of intermittent fever, don't cure in some one or other patient & if it be not due to noxious principle I.e- influence of a marshy district that prevents the cure, so it means that it must always be the psoric miasm in the background.
- In these cases antipsoric medicines must be employed until complete relief is obtained.

§ 241

INTERMITTENT GENUS EPIDEMICUS

Epidemics of intermittent fever, in situations where none are endemic, are of the nature of chronic diseases, composed of single acute paroxysms; each single epidemic is of a peculiar, uniform character common to all the individuals attacked, and when this character is found in the totality of the symptoms common to all, it guides us to the discovery of the homoeopathic (specific) remedy suitable for all the cases, which is almost universally serviceable in those patients who enjoyed tolerable health before the occurrence of the epidemic, that is to say, who were not chronic sufferers from developed psora.

EXPLANATION

The epidemics of intermittent fever [where none are endemic], are of the nature of chronic d/s.

They are composed of single acute paroxysms each single epidemy is of a peculiar, uniform character which is common to all the individuals attacked.

§ 242

PSORIC INTERMITTENT FEVER

If, however, in such an epidemic intermittent fever the first paroxysms have been left uncured, or if the patients have been weakened by improper allopathic treatment; then the inherent psora that exists, alas! in so many persons, although in a latent state, becomes developed, takes on the type of the intermittent fever, and to all appearance continues to play the part of the epidemic intermittent fever, so that the medicine, which would have been useful in the first paroxysms (rarely an antipsoric), is now no longer suitable and cannot be of any service. We have now to do with a psoric intermittent fever only, and this will generally be subdued by minute and rarely repeated doses of sulphur or hepar sulphuris in a high potency.

EXPLANATION

- If in such epidemic intermittent fever, the first paroxysm are left uncured or if the patient have been weakened by improper allopathic treatment then the psora which was in a latent state becomes developed.
- This developed psora in all appearances continues to play the part of the epidemic intermittent fever.
- Now the medicine, which was useful in the first paroxysm is now, no longer suitable & cannot be of any benefit.
- Now for this psoric intermittent fever, minute & rarely repeated doses of sulphur or hepar sulpharis in a high potency subdue it.

§ 243

TREATMENT OF PERNICIOUS INTERMITTENT FEVER

In those often very pernicious intermittent fevers which attack a single person, not residing in a marshy district, we must also at first, as in the case of acute diseases generally, which they resemble in respect to their psoric origin, employ for some days, to render what service it may, a homoeopathic remedy selected for the special case from the other class of proved (not antipsoric) medicines; but if, notwithstanding this procedure, the recovery is deferred, we know that we have psora on the point of its development, and that in this case antipsoric medicines alone can effect a radical cure.

EXPLANATION

- In very harmful intermittent fevers which attack a single person, who is not residing in a marshy district, we should employ a homeopathic remedy selected for the special case from the other class of proved medicines[not antipsoric], for some days[as we do in the case of acute d/s]
  But if the recovery dose not occur this means, we have to treat psora on the point of its development & antipsoric medicines alone can affect a radical cure.we have to employ antipsoric medicines.

§ 244

ENDEMIC INTERMITTENT FEVER

The intermittent fevers endemic in marshy districts and tracts of country frequently exposed to inundations, give a great deal of work to physicians of the old school, and yet a healthy man may in his youth become habituated even to marshy districts and remain in good health, provided he preserves a faultless regimen and his system is not lowered by want, fatigue or pernicious passions. The intermittent fevers endemic there would at the most only attack him on his first arrival; but one or two very small doses of a highly potentized solution of cinchona bark would, conjointly with the well-regulated mode of living just alluded to, speedily free him from the disease. But persons who, while taking sufficient corporeal exercise and pursuing a healthy system of intellectual occupations and bodily regimen, cannot be cured of marsh intermittent fever by one or a few of such small doses of cinchona – in such persons psora, striving to develop itself, always lies at the root of their malady, and their intermittent fever cannot be cured in the marshy district without antipsoric treatment.1 It sometimes happens that when these patients exchange, without delay, the marshy district for one that is dry and mountainous, recovery apparently ensues (the fever leaves them) if they be not yet deeply sunk in disease, that is to say, if the psora was not completely developed in them and can consequently return to its latent state; but they will never regain perfect health without antipsoric treatment.

1 Large, oft-repeated doses of cinchona bark, as also concentrated cinchona remedies, such as the sulphate of quinine, have certainly the power of freeing such patients from the periodical fits of the marsh ague; but those thus deceived into the belief that they are cured remain diseased in another way, frequently with an incurable Quinin intoxication (see §276 note.)

EXPLANATION

- The intermittent fevers endemic in marshy districts & country exposed to inundations. A healthy man in his youth may become habituated even to marshy districts & remain in good health, if he follows good regimen & his system is not lowered by fatigue or harmful passions.
- The intermittent fevers endemic there, could attack him only once on his first arrival & one or two very small doses of highly potentized solution of cinchona and well-regulated mode of living, help speedily free him from d/s but even by above measures, in such persons psora always lies at the root of their malady & needs antipsoric treatment for cure.
- It sometimes happens that when these patients without delay, move to a place that is dry & mountainous, the recovery ensues and the fever leaves them.
- This recovery occurs in those in which the psora was not completely developed & psora returns to its latent state but for perfect health they always require antipsoric treatment.

Footnote:
Large, oft-repeated doses of cinchona bark, & its remedies, such as sulphate of quinine have power of freeing periodical fits of marsh argue of such patients but those who believed that they are cured remaied diseased in another way, frequently with an incurable quinin intoxixation

§ 245

DIET, REGIMEN & MODE OF EMPLOYING MEDICINE

Having thus seen what attention should, in the homoeopathic treatment, be paid to the chief varieties of diseases and to the peculiar circumstances connected with them, we now pass on to what we have to say respecting the remedies and the mode of employing them, together with the diet and regimen to be observed during their use.

Every perceptibly progressive and strikingly increasing amelioration in a transient (acute) or persistent (chronic) disease, is a condition which, as long as it lasts, completely precludes every repetition of the administration of any medicine whatsoever, because all the good the medicine taken continues to effect is new hastening towards its completion. Every new dose of any medicine whatsoever, even of the one last administered, that has hitherto shown itself to be salutary, would in this case disturb the work of amelioration.

EXPLANTATION

- As we have seen what attention should be paid to the chief varieties of d/s & to the peculiar circumstances connected with them.
- Now we will study about remedies & the mode of employing them.
- We will also see the regimen to be observed during their use.

§ 246

MODE OF EMPLOYING REMEDIES IN CHRONIC D/S

Every perceptibly progressive and strikingly increasing amelioration during treatment is a condition which, as long as it lasts, completely precludes every repetition of the administration of any medicine whatsoever, because all the good the medicine taken continues to effect is now hastening towards its completion. This is not infrequently the cause in acute diseases, but in more chronic diseases, on the other hand, a single dose of an appropriately selected homoeopathic remedy will at times complete even with but slowly progressive improvement and give the help which such a remedy in such a case can accomplish naturally within 40, 50, 60, 100 days. This is, however, but rarely the case; and besides, it must be a matter of great importance to the physician as well as to the patient that were it possible, this period should be diminished to one-half, one-quarter, and even still less, so that a much more rapid cure might be obtained. And this may be very happily affected, as recent and oft-repeated observations have taught me under the following conditions: firstly, if the medicine selected with the utmost care was perfectly homoeopathic; secondly, if it is highly potentized, dissolved in water and given in proper small dose that experience has taught as the most suitable in definite intervals for the quickest accomplishment of the cure but with the precaution, that the degree of every dose deviate somewhat from the preceding and following in order that the vital principle which is to be altered to a similar medicinal disease be not aroused to untoward reactions and revolt as is always the case1 with unmodified and especially rapidly repeated doses.

1 What I said in the fifth edition of the organon, in a long note to this paragraph in order to prevent these undesirable reactions of the vital energy, was all the experience I then had justified. But during the last four or five years, however, all these difficulties are wholly solved by my new altered but perfected method. The same carefully selected medicine may now be given daily and for months, if necessary in this way, namely, after the lower degree of potency has been used for one or two weeks in the treatment of chronic disease, advance is made in the same way to higher degrees, (beginning according to the new dynamization method, taught herewith with the use of the lowest degrees).

EXPLANATION

- During treatment progressive & strikingly increasing amelioration, completely precludes the repetition of any medicine because all the good the medicine continues to effect is now hastening towards its completion.
- This is frequently the case in acute d/s, but in chronic d/s, a single dose of an appropriately selected homeopathic remedy produce slowly progressive improvement & take within 40,50,60,100 days.
- The physician as well as patient want a much more rapid cure & this period should be diminished to one-half, one-quarter & even still less.
- This can be accomplished under following conditions.
  A] Firstly, the selected medicine was perfectly homeopathic.
  B] Secondly, if it is highly potentized, dissolved in water & given in proper small dose at definite intervals, the degree of every dose deviates some what from preceding & following doses so that the vital principle is not aroused to untoward reactions & revolt, which occurs when unmodified & rapidly repeated doses are given.

Footnote:
Hahnemann said in the fifth edition of the organon that he has written a long note to this paragraph, how to prevent these undesirable reactions of the vital energy, was according to the experience he had justified.

- ✦ But during the last 4 or 5 years all these difficulties are wholly solved by his new altered but perfect method.
- ✦ The same carefully selected medicine can now be given daily & for months, in this way like for 1 or 2 weeks, lower degree of potency is used & later the potency is increased in the treatment of chronic d/s.

§ 247

REPETITION OF THE DOSE

It is impractical to repeat the same unchanged dose of a remedy once, not to mention its frequent repetition (and at short intervals in order not to delay the cure). The vital principle does not accept such unchanged doses without resistance, that is, without other symptoms of the medicine to manifest themselves than those similar to the disease to be cured, because the former dose has already accomplished the expected change in the vital principle and a second dynamically wholly similar, unchanged dose of the same medicine no longer finds, therefore, the same conditions of the vital force. The patient may indeed be made sick in another way by receiving other such unchanged doses, even sicker than he was, for now only those symptoms of the given remedy remain active which were not homoeopathic to the original disease, hence no step towards cure can follow, only a true aggravation of the condition of the patient. But if the succeeding dose is changed slightly every time, namely potentized somewhat higher (§§ 269-270) then the vital principle may be altered without difficulty by the same medicine (the sensation of natural disease diminishing) and thus the cure brought nearer.1

1 We ought not even with the best chosen homoeopathic medicine, for instance one pellet of the same potency that was beneficial at first, to let the patient have a second or third dose, taken dry. In the same way, if the medicine was dissolved in water and the first dose proved beneficial, a second or third and even smaller dose from the bottle standing undisturbed, even in intervals of a few days, would prove no longer beneficial, even though the original preparation had been potentized with ten succussions or as I suggested later with but two succussions in order to obviate this disadvantage and this according to above reasons. But through modification of every dose in its dynamiztion degree, as I herewith teach, there exists no offence, even if the doses be repeated more frequently, even if the medicine be ever so highly potentized with ever so many succussions. It almost seems as if the best selected homoeopathic remedy could best extract the morbid disorder from the vital force and in chronic disease to extinguish the same only if applied in several different forms.

EXPLANATION

- It is impractical to repeat the same unchanged dose of a remedy once.
- The vital principle does not accept such unchanged doses without resistance I.e- it mainfests the other symptoms of the medicine other than those similar to the d/s to be cured.

- This is because the former dose has already produced the expected change in the vital principle.
- A second dynamically wholly similar, unchanged dose of the same medicine, now does not finds the same conditions of the vital force.
- The patient may be made sick, even sicker than he was because now only those symptoms of the medicine remain active which were not Homeopathic to the original d/s
- Hence no cure can follow & only a true aggravation of the patients occur.
- But if the succeeding dose is changed slightly every time it is potentized somewhat higher [aph=269-270], then the vital principle maybe altered without difficulty by the same medicine & thus cure is brought nearer.

Footnote:
Even with the best chosen Homeopathic remedy if one pellet of the same potency that was beneficial at first, we cannot let the patient have a second or third dose, taken dry.

- But by the, modification of every dose in its dynamization degree, even if the doses are repeated more frequently, it can be repeated.
- The best selected homeopathic remedy could best extract the morbid disorder from the vital force & in chronic d/s to extinguish the morbid disorder only if it is applied in several different forms.

§ 248

HOW IS REPITITION OF MEDICINE DONE

For this purpose, we potentize anew the medicinal solution1 (with perhaps 8, 10, 12 successions) from which we give the patient one or (increasingly) several teaspoonful doses, in long lasting diseases daily or every second day, in acute diseases every two to six hours and in very urgent cases every hour or oftener. Thus in chronic diseases, every correctly chosen homoeopathic medicine, even those whose action is of long duration, may be repeated daily for months with ever increasing success. If the solution is used up (in seven to fifteen days) it is necessary to add to the next solution of the same medicine if still indicated one or (though rarely) several pellets of a higher potency with which we continue so long as the patient experiences continued improvement without encountering one or another complaint that he never had before in his life. For if this happens, if the balance of the disease appears in a group of altered symptoms then another, one more homoeopathically related medicine must be chosen in place of the last and administered in the same repeated doses, mindful, however, of modifying the solution of every dose with thorough vigorous successions, thus changing its degree of potency and increasing it somewhat. On the other hand, should there appear during almost daily repetition of the well indicated homoeopathic remedy, towards the end of the treatment of a chronic disease, so-called (§ 161) homoeopathic aggravations by which the balance of the morbid symptoms seem to again increase somewhat (the medicinal disease, similar to the original, now alone persistently manifests itself). The doses in that case must then be reduced still further and repeated in longer intervals and possibly stopped several days, in order to see if the convalescence need no further medicinal aid. The apparent symptoms (Schein – Symptome) caused by the excess of the homoeopathic medicine will soon disappear and leave undisturbed health in its wake. If only a small vial say a dram of dilute alcohol is used in the treatment, in which is contained and dissolved through succussion one globule of the medicine which is to be used by olfaction every two, three or four days, this also must be thoroughly succussed eight to ten times before each olfaction.

1 Made in 40, 30, 20, 15 or 8 tablespoons of water with the addition of some alcohol or a piece of charcoal in order to preserve it. If charcoal is used, it is suspended by means of a thread in the vial and is taken out when the vial is succussed. The solution of the medicinal globule (and it is rarely necessary to use more than one globule) of a thoroughly potentized medicine in a large quantity of water can be obviated by making a solution in only 7-8 tablespoons of water and after thorough succussion of the vial take from it one tablespoon and put it in a glass of water (containing about 7 to 8 spoonfuls), this stirred thoroughly and then given a dose to the patient. If he is unusually excited and sensitive, a teaspoon of this solution may be put in a second glass of water, thoroughly stirred and teaspoonful doses or more be given. There are patients of so great sensitiveness that a third or fourth glass, similarly prepared, may be necessary. Each such prepared glass must be made fresh daily. the globule of the high potency is best crushed in a few grains of sugar of milk which the patient can put in the vial and be dissolved in the requisite quantity of water.

EXPLANTATION

We potentize the medicinal solution with perhaps 8,10,12 successions & from which we give the patient one or increasingly several teaspoonful doses.

- In long lasting d/s repetition can be daily or every second day
- In acute d/s every 2-6 hours & in very urgent cases every hour or more oftener.
- Thus in chronic d/s, even those homeopathic medicine whose action is of long duration may be repeated daily for months with ever increasing success.
- If the solution is used up in 7 to 15 days, now it is necessary to add to the next solution of the same medicine one or [though rarely] several pellets of a higher potency. we continue it as long as the patient experiences continued improvement & we don't get one or another complaint that he never had before in his life.
- If this happens, one more homeopathically related medicine is chosen & administered in the same repeated doses by modifying the solution of every dose with vigorous successions, which changes its degree of potency.
- If in the treatment of chronic d/s during daily repetition of well indicated homeopathic remedy. homeopathic aggravations occur, here the dose must be reduced still further & repeated in longer intervals & stopped for several days, in order to see if the period of recovery need no further medicinal aid.

- The apparent symptoms [schein-symptome] caused by the excess of the homepathic medicine will soon disappear and leaves health undisturbed.
- Even if the medicine is given through olfaction every 2,3, or 4 days, it also must be thoroughly succussed 8-10 times before each olfaction.

Footnote:
Medicinal solution is made in 40,30,20,15 or 8 tablespoonfuls of water with some alcohol or a piece of charcoal in order to preserve it.

- If charcoal is used, it is suspended by means of a thread in the vial & is taken out when the vial is succussed.
- The solution of the medicinal globule is made in 7-8 tablespoonfuls of water.
- Thorough succussion of the vial is done, now take 1 tablespoonful & put it in a glass of water containing about 7-8 spoonfuls of water.
- Then stir it thoroughly & give a dose to the patient.
- If the patient is unusually excited & sensitive a teaspoonful of above solution is put in second glass of water, stirred & teaspoonful doses or more can be given.
- If patients are of great sensitivity then a third or fourth glass can be prepared similarly.
- Each such prepared glass must be made fresh daily.
- The globule of the high potency is best crushed in a few grains of sugar of milk which patient can put in the vial & dissolve it in the required quantity of water.

§ 249

ANTIDOTE

Every medicine prescribed for a case of disease which, in the course of its action, produces new and troublesome symptoms not appertaining to the disease to be cured, is not capable of effecting real improvement,1 and cannot be considered as homoeopathically selected; it must, therefore, either, if the aggravation be considerable, be first partially neutralized as soon as possible by an antidote before giving the next remedy chosen more accurately according to similarity of action; or if the troublesome symptoms be not very violent, the next remedy must be given immediately, in order to take the place of the improperly selected one.2

1 As all experience shows that the dose of the specially suited homoeopathic medicine can scarcely be prepared too small to effect perceptible amelioration in the disease for which it is appropriate (§§ 275-278), we should act injudiciously and hurtfully were we when no improvement, or some, though it be even slight, aggravation ensues, to repeat or even increase the dose of the same medicine, as is done in the old system, under the delusion that it was not efficacious on account of its small quantity (its too small dose). Every aggravation by the production of new symptoms – when nothing untoward has occurred in the mental or physical regimen – invariably proves unsuitableness on the part of the

medicine formerly given in the case of disease before us, but never indicates that the dose has been too weak.

2 The well informed and conscientiously careful physician will never be in a position to require an antidote in his practice if he will begin, as he should, to give the selected medicine in the smallest possible dose. Like minute doses of a better chosen remedy will re-establish order throughout.

EXPLANATION

- If a medicine prescribed for a case of d/s produces new & troublesome symptoms, not related to the d/s to be cured, it means it is not homeopathically selected & is not capable of effecting real improvement.
- Now if the aggravation is considerable, proper antidote is given to neutralize it. Now next remedy is chosen more accurately according to the similarity of action.
  But if the troublesome symptoms are not very violent, the next remedy must be given immediately, in order to take the place of the improperly selected one.

Footnote:
Dose of the suited homeoapathic medicine can scarcely be prepared to small to effect perceptible amelioration in the d/s.[aph -275-276]

- When there is no improvement or some aggravation occurs, we should not repeat or increase the dose of the same medicine, as is done in the old system. They believe that the medicine was not efficacious due to its small quantity or its too small dose.
- If the mental or physical regimen is proper & aggravation occurs & new symptoms appear it means the medicine was unsuitable but it never indicates that the dose has been too weak.
- A careful physician, if he will begin to give the selected medicine in the smallest possible dose, he will never require an antidote in his practice.
- A similar minute dose of a better chosen remedy will re-establish order throughout.

§ 250

ACUTE DISEASE & WRONG SELECTION

When, to the observant practitioner who accurately investigates the state of the disease, it is evident, in urgent cases after the lapse of only six, eight or twelve hours, that he has made a bad selection in the medicine last given, in that the patient's state is growing perceptibly, however slightly, worse from hour to hour, by the occurrence of new symptoms and sufferings, it is not only allowable for him, but it is his duty to remedy his mistake, by the selection and administration of a homoeopathic medicine not merely tolerably suitable, but the most appropriate possible for the existing state of the disease (§ 167).

EXPLANATION

- When after giving the medicine he notices that after 6,8 or 12 hours, new symptoms & sufferings are present & patients state is growing slightly worse from hour to hour.
- His duty is to remedy his mistake of bad selection in the medicine last given.
- He must now select the most appropriate homeoapthic medicine & administer it according to the existing state of the d/s[167].

§ 251

ALTERNATING ACTION

There are some medicines (e.g., ignatia, also bryonia and rhus, and sometimes belladonna) whose power of altering man's health consists chiefly in alternating actions – a kind of primary-action symptoms that are in part opposed to each other. Should the practitioner find, on prescribing one of these, selected on strict homoeopathic principles, that no improvement follows, he will in most cases soon effect his object by giving (in acute diseases, even within a few hours) a fresh and equally small dose of the same medicine.1

1 As I have more particularly described in the introduction to "Ignatia" (in the first volume of the Materia Medica Pura).

EXPLANATION

- There are some medicine e.g- Ignatia, bryonia, rhus & sometimes belladonna, whose power of altering man's health is chiefly in alternating action.
- Alternating actions are a kind of primary -action symptoms that are in part opposed to each other.
- If the homeopathic practitioner finds that no improvement follows on prescribing a remedy selected on strict homeopathic principles.
- He will give a fresh & equally small dose of the same medicine.

§ 252

REMOVAL OF OBSTACLE IN THE WAY OF CURE

But should we find, during the employment of the other medicines in chronic (psoric) diseases, that the best selected homoeopathic (antipsoric) medicine in the suitable (minutest) dose does not effect an improvement, this is a sure sign that the cause that keeps up the disease still persists, and that there is some circumstances in the mode of life of the patient or in the situation in which he is placed, that must be removed in order that a permanent cure may ensue.

EXPLANATION

- But if during employment of the other medicines best selected antipsoric medicine in the suitable minutest dose does not effect an improvement in chronic [psoric]d/s.
- This is a sure sign that there is some cause like mode of life of the patient or in the situation he is placed that keeps up the d/s still persistent, they must be removed in order that a permanent cure may ensure.

§ 253

SIGNS OF AGGRAVATION & AMELIORATION

Among the signs that, in all diseases, especially in such as are of an acute nature, inform us of a slight commencement of amelioration or aggravation that is not perceptible to every one, the state of mind and the whole demeanor of the patient are the most certain and instructive. In the case of ever so slight an improvement we observe a greater degree of comfort, increased calmness and freedom of the mind, higher spirits – a kind of return of the natural state. In the case of ever so small a commencement of aggravation we have, on the contrary, the exact opposite of this: a constrained helpless, pitiable state of the disposition, of the mind, of the whole demeanor, and of all gestures, postures and actions, which may be easily perceived on close observation, but cannot be described in words.1

1 The signs of improvement in the disposition and mind, however, may be expected only soon after the medicine has been taken when the dose has been sufficiently minute (i.e., as small as possible), an unnecessary large dose of even the most suitable homoeopathic medicine acts too violently, and at first produces too great and too lasting a disturbance of the mind and disposition to allow us soon to perceive the improvement in them. I must here observe that this so essential rule is chiefly transgressed by presumptuous tryos in homoeopathy, and by physicians who are converted to homoeopathy from the ranks of the old school. From old prejudices these persons abhor the smallest doses of the lowest dilutions of medicine in such cases, and hence they fail to experience the great advantages and blessings of that mode of proceeding which a thousandfold experience has shown to be the most salutary; they cannot effect all that homoeopathy is capable of doing, and hence they have no claim to be considered its adherents.

EXPLANATION

- The best signs, especially in d/s of acute nature, which tell us of a slight commencement of amelioration or aggravation is the state of mind & the whole outward behaviour of the patient.
- In the case of even slight an improvement we will observe a greater degree of comfort, increased calmness & freedom of the mind, higher spirits -a kind of return of the natural state.
- In the case of ever so small aggravation we observe the contrary, the exact opposite of above.

Footnote:

When the dose is sufficiently minute I.e- as small as possible, the signs of improvement in the disposition & mind, may be expected only soon after the medicine has been taken.

- An unnecessarily larger dose of even the most suitable homeopathic medicine acts too violently.
- This larger dose produces too great & too lasting disturbance of the mind & disposition at first & then improvement is perceived in them.
- Hahnemann says here that this so essential rule is chiefly not followed by a beginner in Homeopathy and by physician who are converted to homeopathy from the ranks of the old school, they fail to experience the great advantages & blessings of that mode of proceeding which by experience is the most beneficial to the patient. Hence they cannot be considered as followers of homeopathy.

§ 254

HOW TO IDENTIFY WHETHER AGGRAVATION /AMELIORATION

The other new or increased symptoms or, on the contrary, the diminution of the original ones without any addition of new ones, will soon dispel all doubts from the mind of the attentively observing and investigating practitioner with regard to the aggravation or amelioration; though there are among patients persons who are either incapable of giving an account of this amelioration or aggravation, or are unwilling to confess it.

EXPLANATION

An attentively observing & investigating practitioner will be able to perceive whether aggravation or amelioration proceeds after giving the medicine.

- He observes whether the other new symptoms or increased symptoms or the diminution of the original symptoms without any addition of new ones appear & accordingly makes clear in his mind in regard to the aggravation or amelioration.
- But there are some, patients who are either not able to give the details of this amelioration or aggravation or they are unwilling to confess it.

§ 255

FOLLOW UP-RECORDINGS

But even with such individuals we may convince ourselves on this point by going with them through all the symptoms enumerated in our notes of the disease one by one, and finding that they complain of no new unusual symptoms in addition to these, and that none of the old symptoms are worse. If this be the case, and if an improvement in the disposition and mind have already been observed, the medicine must have effected positive diminution of the disease, or, if sufficient time have not yet elapsed for this, it will soon effect it. Now, supposing the remedy is perfectly appropriate, if the improvement delay too long in making its appearance, this depends either on some error of conduct on the part of the patient, or on other interfering circumstances.

EXPLANATION

- But even with such patients we can find out whether improvement has occured or not.
- We ask about the symptoms of patient one by one & find that no new unusual symptoms are added to these & none of the old symptoms are worse.
- If none of these has occured it means their is improvement in the disposition & mind & the medicine has affected positive diminution of the d/s or if sufficient time has not passed, it will soon effect it.
- Now if the improvement delays too long, this depends either on error of conduct by the patient or on other circumstances that interface cure.

§ 256

SIGN OF WRONG SIMILIMUM

On the other hand, if the patient mention the occurrence of some fresh accidents and symptoms of importance – signs that the medicine chosen has not been strictly homoeopathic – even though he should good-naturedly assure us that he feels better, as is not infrequently the case in phthisical patients with lung abscess, we must not believe this assurance, but regard his state as aggravated as it will soon be perfectly apparent it is.

EXPLANATION

- If the patient mentions the occurence of some fresh accidents & symptoms which are important means that the medicine chosen has not been strictly homeopathic.
- In some cases like the case in phthisical patients with lung abscess if above occurs but the patient assures us that he is feeling better. We must not believe this assurances, but regards his state as aggravation which will soon be observable.

§ 257

FAVORITE REMEDY

The true physician will take care to avoid making favorite remedies of medicines, the employment of which he has, by chance, perhaps found often useful, and which he has had opportunities of using with good effect. If he do so, some remedies or rarer use, which would have been more homoeopathically suitable, consequently more serviceable, will often be neglected.

EXPLANTATION

- The true physician should take care to avoid making favourite remedies of medicines.
- This may be found often useful but by chance only.
- If we do so, some remedies which are of rarer use & which maybe more Homeopathically suitable in a given case will often be neglected.

§ 258

NEVER BE PREJUDISED

The true practitioner, moreover, will not in his practice with mistrustful weakness neglect the employment of those remedies that he may now and then have employed with bad effects, owing to an erroneous selection (from his own fault, therefore), or avoid them for other (false) reasons, as that they were unhomoeopathic for the case of disease before him; he must bear in mind the truth, that of medicinal agents that one alone invariably deserves the preference in every case of disease which correspond most accurately by similarity to the totality of the characteristic symptoms, and that no paltry prejudices should interfere with this serious choice.

EXPLANATION

- The true practitioner will not neglect to employ those remedies which he used in past but it produced bad effects. The cause can be from his own fault or avoid them for other false reasons, as they were unhomeopathic for the case of d/s before him.
- He will not hasitate to use them, because of above reason, if it is the most similar based on totality of symptoms in the given case, he will employ it.
- No prejudices should interfere with this serious choice.

§ 259

DIET & REGIMEN DURING IN CURE

Considering the minuteness of the doses necessary and proper in homoeopathic treatment, we can easily understand that during the treatment everything must be removed from the diet and regimen which can have any medicinal action, in order that the small dose may not be overwhelmed and extinguished or disturbed by any foreign medicinal irritant.1

1 The softest tones of a distant flute that in the still midnight hours would inspire a tender heart with exalted feelings and dissolve it in religious ecstasy, are inaudible and powerless amid discordant cries and the noise of day.

EXPLANTATION

- As the doses used are minute, so during the treatment everything must be removed from the diet & regimen which can have any medicinal action.
- So that the small dose may not be over whelmed and extinguished or disturbed by any foreign medicinal irritant..

Footnote:
Here he has given an example to explain above aphorism.

- ✦ The softest tones of a distant flute can inspire a tender heart with feelings during the midnight hours but the same tone becomes powerless & inaudible amongst cries & the noise of daytime.

§ 260

DIET AND REGIMEN

Hence the careful investigation into such obstacles to cure is so much the more necessary in the case of patients affected by chronic diseases, as their diseases are usually aggravated by such noxious influences and other disease-causing errors in the diet and regimen, which often pass unnoticed.1

1 Coffee; fine Chinese and other herb teas; beer prepared with medicinal vegetable substances unsuitable for the patient's state; so-called fine liquors made with medicinal spices; all kinds of punch; spiced chocolate; odorous waters and perfumes of many kinds; strong-scented flowers in the apartment; tooth powders and essences and perfumed sachets compounded of drugs; highly spiced dishes and sauces; spiced cakes and ices; crude medicinal vegetables for soups; dishes of herbs, roots and stalks of plants possessing medicinal qualities; asparagus with long green tips, hops, and all vegetables possessing medicinal properties, celery, onions; old cheese, and meats that are in a state of decomposition, or that passes medicinal properties (as the flesh and fat of pork, ducks and geese, or veal that is too young and sour viands), ought just as certainly to be kept from patients as they should avoid all excesses in food, and in the use of sugar and salt, as also spirituous drinks, undiluted with water, heated rooms, woollen clothing next the skin, a sedentary life in close apartments, or the frequent indulgence in mere passive exercise (such as riding, driving or swinging), prolonged suckling, taking a long siesta in a recumbent posture in bed, sitting up long at night, uncleanliness, unnatural debauchery, enervation by reading obscene books, reading while lying down, Onanism or imperfect or suppressed intercourse in order to prevent conception, subjects of anger, grief or vexation, a passion for play, over-exertion of the mind or body, especially after meals, dwelling in marshy districts, damp rooms, penurious living, etc. All these things must be as far as possible avoided or removed, in order that the cure may not be obstructed or rendered impossible. Some of my disciples seem needlessly to increase the difficulties of the patient's dietary by forbidding the use of many more, tolerably indifferent things, which is not to be commended.

EXPLANATION

- A careful investigation of such obstacles to cure is therefore more necessary in cases of chronic d/s.
- The chronic d/s are usually aggravated by such noxious influences & other d/s causing errors in the diet & regimen. These errors often pass unnoticed.

Footnote:
Coffee; fine Chinese and other herb teas; beer prepared with medicinal vegetable substances unsuitable for the patient's state; so-called fine liquors made with medicinal spices; all kinds of punch; spiced chocolate; odorous waters and perfumes of many kinds; strong-scented flowers in the apartment; tooth powders and essences and perfumed sachets compounded of drugs; highly spiced dishes and sauces;

spiced cakes and ices; crude medicinal vegetables for soups; dishes of herbs, roots and stalks of plants possessing medicinal qualities; asparagus with long green tips, hops, and all vegetables possessing medicinal properties, celery, onions; old cheese, and meats that are in a state of decomposition, or that passes medicinal properties (as the flesh and fat of pork, ducks and geese, or veal that is too young and sour viands), ought just as certainly to be kept from patients as they should avoid all excesses in food, and in the use of sugar and salt, as also spirituous drinks, undiluted with water, heated rooms, woollen clothing next the skin, a sedentary life in close apartments, or the frequent indulgence in mere passive exercise (such as riding, driving or swinging), prolonged suckling, taking a long siesta in a recumbent posture in bed, sitting up long at night, uncleanliness, unnatural debauchery, enervation by reading obscene books, reading while lying down, Onanism or imperfect or suppressed intercourse in order to prevent conception, subjects of anger, grief or vexation, a passion for play, over-exertion of the mind or body, especially after meals, dwelling in marshy districts, damp rooms, penurious living, etc. All these things must be as far as possible avoided or removed, in order that the cure may not be obstructed or rendered impossibl. Some, of the disciples of Hahnemann forbid the use of many more things which is not required.

§ 261

REGIMEN IN CHRONIC TREATMENT

The most appropriate regimen during the employment of medicine in chronic diseases consists in the removal of such obstacles to recovery, and in supplying where necessary the reverse: innocent moral and intellectual recreation, active exercise in the open air in almost all kinds of weather (daily walks, slight manual labor), suitable, nutritious, unmedicinal food and drink, etc.

EXPLANATION

- During the employment of medicine in chronic d/s following regimen should be employed.
  1. Removal of such obstacles to recovery.
  2. Supplying the reverse like innocent moral and intellectual recreation, active exercise in the open air in almost all kinds of weather (daily walks, slight manual labor), suitable, nutritious, unmedicinal food and drink, etc.

§ 262

DIET IN ACUTE DISEASE

In acute diseases, on the other hand – except in cases of mental alienation – the subtle, unerring internal sense of the awakened life-preserving faculty determines so clearly and precisely, that the physician only requires to counsel the friends and attendants to put no obstacles in the way of this voice of nature by refusing anything the patient urgently desires in the way of food, or by trying to persuade him to partake of anything injurious.

EXPLANATION

- On the other hand in acute d/s except in cases of mental isolation, the delicate, always accurate internal sense of the awakened life-preserving faculty determines so clearly that the physician only needs to counsel the friends & attendants to put no obstacles, if the patient urgently desires anything in the way of food or by trying to make him to eat or drink anything injurious.

§ 263

ALLOW DESIRED DIET TO THE PATIENT

The desire of the patient affected by an acute disease with regard to food and drink is certainly chiefly for things that give palliative relief: they are, however, not strictly speaking of a medicinal character, and merely supply a sort of want. The slight hindrances that the gratification of this desire, within moderate bounds, could oppose to the radical removal of the disease1 will be amply counteracted and overcome by the power of the homoeopathically suited medicine and the vital force set free by it, as also by the refreshment that follows from taking what has been so ardently longed for. In like manner, in acute diseases the temperature of the room and the heat or coolness of the bed-coverings must also be arranged entirely in conformity with the patients' wish. He must be kept free from all over-exertion of mind and exciting emotions.

1 This is, however, rare. Thus, for instance, in pure inflammatory diseases, where aconite is so indispensable, whose action would be destroyed by partaking of vegetable acids, the desire of the patient is almost always for pure cold water only.

EXPLANATION

- The patient's desire of food & drink affected by an acute d/s is mainly for things that give palliative relief.
- The slight obstacles that the satisfaction of this desire, within moderate limits, can oppose to the radical removal of the of the d/s, will be counteracted & overcome by the power of the homeopathically suited medicine & by the power of vital force set free by it.
- Desire also occur by the refreshments that follows from taking, what the body longed for zealously from a long time.
- In the same manner, in acute d/s the temperature of the room & the heat or coolness of the bed-coverings must be kept free from all over-excertion of mind & exciting emotions.

Footnote:

- This is however rare, for example- In pure inflammatory d/s where aconite is so important. The action of aconite would be destroyed by eating or drinking of vegetable acids, but the desire of the patient is almost always for pure cold water only.

§ 264

GENUINENESS OF THE MEDICINE

The true physician must be provided with genuine medicines of unimpaired strength, so that he may be able to rely upon their therapeutic powers; he must be able, himself, to judge of their genuineness.

EXPLANATION

- The true physician should be provided with genuine medicines of unimpaired strength, so that he may be able to rely upon their therapeutic powers.
- He must be able to judge the genuineness of the medicine, himself.

§ 265

EMPLOYMENT OF RIGHT MEDICINE

It should be a matter of conscience with him to be thoroughly convinced in every case that the patient always takes the right medicine and therefore he must give the patient the correctly chosen medicine prepared, moreover, by himself.

EXPLANATION

The physician should be convinced in every case that the patient always takes the right medicine, therefore he must give the patient the correctly chosen medicine prepared by himself.

§ 266

MEDICINES-VEGETABLE MEDICINE & ANIMAL KINGDOM

Substances belonging to the animal and vegetable kingdoms possess their medicinal qualities most perfectly in their raw state.1

1 All crude animal and vegetable substances have a greater or less amount of medicinal power, and are capable of altering man's health, each in its own peculiar way. Those plants and animals used by the most enlightened nations as food have this advantage over all others, that they contain a larger amount of nutritious constituents; and they differ from the others in this that their medicinal powers in their raw state are either not very great in themselves, or are diminished by the culinary processes they are subjected to in cooking for domestic use, by the expression of the pernicious juice (like the cassava root of South America), by fermentation (of the rye-flour in the dough for making bread, sour-crout prepared without vinegar and pickled gherkins), by smoking and by the action of heat (in boiling, stewing, toasting, roasting, baking), whereby the medicinal parts of many of these substances are in part destroyed and dissipated. By the addition of salt (pickling) and vinegar (sauces, salads) animal and vegetable substances certainly lose much of their injurious medicinal qualities, but other disadvantages result from these additions.

But even those plants that possess most medicinal power lose that in part or completely by such processes. By perfect desiccation all the roots of the various kinds of iris, of the horseradish, of the different species or arum and the peonies lose almost all their medicinal virtue. The juice of the most virulent plants often becomes inert, pitch-like mass, from the heat employed in preparing the ordinary extracts. By merely standing a long time, the expressed juice of the most deadly plants becomes quite powerless; even at moderate atmospheric temperature it rapidly takes on the vinous fermentation (and thereby loses much of its medicinal power), and immediately thereafter the acetous and putrid fermentation, whereby it is deprived of all peculiar medicinal properties; the fecula that is then deposited, if well washed, is quite innocuous, like ordinary starch. By the transudation that takes place when a number of green plants are laid one above the other, the greatest part of their medicinal properties is lost.

EXPLANATION

- Substances that belong to the animal & vegetable kingdom possess their medicinal qualities in their raw state, most perfectly.

Footnote:
All crude animal & vegetable substances have a medicinal power & they are capable of altering man's health, in it's own peculiar way.

- Those plants & animals used as food, contain a larger amount of nutritious constituents.
- They differ from the others in this that their medicinal power in raw state are either not very great in themselves, or are diminished by the expression of the harmful juice [like the cassava root of south america], by fermentation [making bread], by smoking & by the action of heat [in boiling, stewing, toasting, roasting, baking].
- By these processes the medicinal parts of many of these substances are destroyed & dissipated.
- By addition of salt [pickling] & vinegar [sauces, salads]animal & vegetable substances lose much of their injurious medicinal qualities but by these additions other disadvantages result.
- By standing a long time, the expressed juice of the most deadly plants becomes quite powerless[due to fermentation].
- By the transudation that occurs when a number of green plants are laid one above the other, the greatest part of their medicinal properties is lost.

§ 267

MEDICINES-INDIGENOUS PLANTS

We gain possession of the powers of indigenous plants and of such as may be had in a fresh state in the most complete and certain manner by mixing their freshly expressed juice immediately with equal parts of spirits of wine of a strength sufficient to burn in a lamp. After this has stood a day and a night in a close stoppered bottle and deposited the fibrinous and albuminous matters, the clear superincumbent fluid is then to be decanted off for medicinal use.1 All fermentation of the vegetable juice will be at once checked by the spirits of wine mixed with it and rendered impossible for the future, and the entire medicinal power of the vegetable juice is thus retained (perfect and uninjured) for ever by keeping the preparation in well-corked bottles and excluded from the sun's light.2

1 Buchholz (Taschenb. f. Scheidek. u. Apoth. a. d. J., 1815, Weimar, Abth. I, vi) assures his readers (and his reviewer in the Leipziger Literaturzeitung, 1816, No. 82, does not contradict him) that for this excellent mode of operating medicines we have to thank the campaign in Russia, whence it was (in 1812) imported into Germany. According to the noble practice of many Germans to be unjust towards their own countrymen, he conceals the fact that this discovery and those directions, which he quotes in my very words from the first edition of the Organon of Rational Medicine, § 230 and note, proceed from me, and that I first published them to the world two years before the Russian campaign (the Organon appeared in 1810). Some folks would rather assign the origin of a discovery to the deserts of Asia than to a German to whom the honor belongs. O tempora! O mores!

Alcohol has certainly been sometimes before this used for mixing with vegetable juices, e.g., to preserve them some time before making extracts of them, but never with the view of administering them in this form.

2 Although equal parts of alcohol and freshly expressed juice are usually the most suitable proportion for affecting the deposition of the fibrinous and albuminous matters, yet for plants that contain much thick mucus (e.g. Symphytum officinale, Viola tricolor, etc.), or an excess of albumen (e.g., Aethusa cynapium, Solanum nigrum, etc.), a double proportion of alcohol is generally required for this object. Plants that are very deficient in juice, as Oleander, Buxus, Taxus, Ledum, Sabina, etc., must first be pounded up alone into a moist, fine mass and the stirred up with a double quantity of alcohol, in order that the juice may combine with it, and being thus extracted by the alcohol, may be pressed out; these latter may also when dried be brought with milk-sugar to the millionfold trituration, and then be further diluted and potentized (v. § 271)

EXPLANATION

- The powers of indigenous plants in a fresh state in the most complete & certain manner can be possessed by mixing their freshly expressed juice immediately with equal parts of spirits of wine.
- The strength of spirits of wine should be of a strength sufficient to burn in a lamp
- This fresh juice mixed with equal parts of spirits of wine is kept in a close stoppered bottle for a day & a night.
- This leads to deposition of the fibrinous & albuminous matter, now the clear superincumbent fluid is then decanted into other vessel for medicinal use.
- Due to addition of the spirits of wine the fermentation of the vegetable juice is checked.
- Like this the entire medicinal power of the vegetable juice is retained [perfect uninjured]for ever by keeping the preparation in well-corked bottles.
- They are protected with wax to prevent evaporation & excluded from the sun's light.

Footnote 1:
Hahnemann says that buchholz assures his readers that for this excellent mode of preparing medicines we have to thank the campaign in russia in 1812, when it was imported into germany.

He says that 'He concealed the fact that this discovery & those directions were from my first edition of the 'Organon of rational medicine, aph-230 & note, which I first published two years back in 1810 before the ' Russian campaign'

- ✦ Alcohol was used sometimes before for mixing with vegetable juice e.g- to preserve them, some time before making extracts of them, but they were never used with the view of administering them in this form.

Footnote 2:
- Equal parts of alcohol & fresh juice are usually the most suitable proportion for affecting, deposition of the fibrinous & albuminous matter.
- Yet for plants that contain much thick mucus e.g- Symphytum officinal, viola tricolor etc or which contain an excess of albumen.

E.g- Aethsa cynapium, solanum nignum etc, we require a double proportion of alcohol.

Plants that are very deficient in juice like oleander, buxus, taxus, ledum, sabina etc. They are pounded up alone into a moist, fine mass & then stirred up with a double quantity of alcohol, so that the juice may combine with it & may be pressed out. These may later also when dried be brought with milk-sugar to the millionfold, trituration & then be further diluted & potentized.

§ 268

MEDICINES-EXOTIC SUBSTANCES

The other exotic plants, barks, seeds and roots that cannot be obtained in the fresh state the sensible practitioner will never take in the pulverized form on trust, but will first convince himself of their genuineness in their crude, entire state before making any employment of them.1

1 In order to preserve them in the form of powder, a precaution is requisite that has hitherto been usually neglected by druggists, and hence powders, even of well-dried animal and vegetable substances could not be preserved uninjured even in well-corked bottles. The entire crude vegetable substances, though perfectly dry, yet contain, as an indispensable condition of the cohesion of their texture, a certain quantity of moisture, which dose not indeed prevent the unpulverized drug from remaining in as dry a state as is requisite to preserve it from corruption, but which is quite too much for the finely pulverized state. The animal or vegetable substance which in its entire state was perfectly dry, furnishes, therefore, when finely pulverized, a somewhat moist powder, which without rapidly becoming spoilt and mouldy, can yet not be preserved in corked bottles if not previously freed from this superfluous moisture. This is the best effected by spreading out the powder in a flat tin saucer with a raised edge, which floats in a vessel full of boiling water (i.e. a water-bath), and, by means of stirring it about, drying it to such a degree that all the small atoms of it (no longer stick together in lumps, but) like dry, fine sand, are easily separated from each other, and are readily converted into dust. In this dry state the fine powders may be kept forever uninjured in well-corked and sealed bottles, in all their original complete medicinal power, without ever being injured by mites or mould; and they are best preserved when the bottles are kept protected from the daylight (in covered boxes, chests, cases). If not shut up in air-tight vessels, and not preserved from the access of the light of the sun and day, all animal and vegetable substances in time gradually lose their medicinal power more and more, even in the entire state, but still more in the form of powder.

EXPLANATION

- The other exotic plants, barks, seeds & roots that cannot be obtained in the fresh state.
- A sensible practitioner will never take their fine powdered form on trust but he will first convince himself that it is genuine in, its crude entire state, before making any medicinal use of them.

Footnote:
The entire crude vegetable substances, though are perfectly dry, yet they contain a certain quantity of moisture.

- The animal or vegetable substance though dry but when it is finely pulverized, a moist powder is obtained.
- It cannot be preserved in corked bottles.
- They need to be freed from this moisture by drying it to such a degree that all the small atoms of it are like dry, fine sand & are easily separated from each other & are easily converted into dust.
- The power is spread out in a flat tin saucer with a raised edge, which floats in a vessel full of boiling water & it is dried by stirring.
- In this dry state the fine powders may be kept forever uninjured in well-corked & sealed airtight bottles. Their original complete medicinal power is retained, they cannot be injured by mites or mould.
- These bottles are kept protected from daylight.

§ 269

DYNAMIZATION OF DRUGS

The homoeopathic system of medicine develops for its special use, to a hitherto unheard-of degree, the inner medicinal powers of the crude substances by means of a process peculiar to it and which has hitherto never been tried, whereby only they all become immeasurably and penetratingly efficacious1 and remedial, even those that in the crude state give no evidence of the slightest medicinal power on the human body.

This remarkable change in the qualities of natural bodies develops the latent, hitherto unperceived, as if slumbering2 hidden, dynamic (§ 11) powers which influence the life principle, change the well-being of animal life.3 This is effected by mechanical action upon their smallest particles by means of rubbing and shaking and through the addition of an indifferent substance, dry of fluid, are separated from each other. This process is called dynamizing, potentizing (development of medicinal power) and the products are dynamizations4 or potencies in different degrees.

1 Long before this discovery of mine, experience had taught several changes which could be brought about in different natural substances by means of friction, for instance, warmth, heat, fire, development of odor in odorless bodies, magnetization of steel, and so forth. But all these properties produced by friction were related only to physical and inanimate things, whereas it is a law of nature according to which physiological and pathogenic changes take place in the body's condition by means of forces capable of changing the crude material of drugs, even in such as had never shown any

medicinal properties. This is brought about by trituration and succussion, but under the condition of employing an indifferent vehicle in certain proportions. this wonderful physical and especially physiological and pathogenic law of nature had not been discovered before my time. No wonder then, that the present students of nature and physicians (so for unknowing) cannot have faith in the magical curative powers of the minute doses of medicines prepared according to homoeopathic rules (dynamized).

2 The same thing is seen in a bar of iron and steel where a slumbering trace of latent magnetic force cannot but be recognized in their interior. Both, after their completion by means of the forge stand upright, repulse the north pole of a magnetic needle with the lower end and attract the south pole, while the upper end shows itself as the south pole of the magnetic needle. But this is only a latent force; not even the finest iron particles can be drawn magnetically or held on either end of such a bar.

Only after this bar of steel is dynamized, rubbing it with a dull file in one direction, will it become a true active powerful magnet, one able to attract iron and steel to itself and impart to another bar of steel by mere contact and even some distance away, magnetic power and this in a higher degree the more it has been rubbed. In the same way will triturating a medicinal substance and shaking of its solution (dynamization, potentation) develop the medicinal powers hidden within and manifest them more and more or if one may say so, spiritualizes the material substance itself.

3 On this account it refers to the increase and stronger development of their power to cause changes in the health of animals and men if these natural substances in this improved state, are brought very near to the living sensitive fibre or come in contact with it (by means of intake or olfaction). Just as a magnetic bar especially if its magnetic force is increased (dynamized) can show magnetic power only in a needle of steel whose pole is near or touches it. The steel itself remains unchanged in the remaining chemical and physical properties and can bring about no changes in other metals (for instance, in brass), just as little as dynamized medicines can have any action upon lifeless things.

4 We hear daily how homoeopathic medicinal potencies are called mere dilutions, when they are the very opposite, i.e., a true opening up of the natural substances bringing to light and revealing the hidden specific medicinal powers contained within and brought forth by rubbing and shaking. The aid of a chosen, unmedicinal medium of attenuation is but a secondary condition.

Simple dilution, for instance, the solution of a grain of salt will become water, the grain of salt will disappear in the dilution with much water and will never develop into medicinal salt which by means of our well prepared dynamization, is raised to most marvellous power.

EXPLANATION

The homoeopathic system of medicine develops the inner medicinal powers of the crude substances by means of a process known as dynamization.

Even those substances that in the crude state give no evidence of the slightest medicinal power on the human body become efficacious and remedial.

This remarkable change in the qualities of natural bodies develops the hidden, as if sleeping dynamic (aphorism 11) powers which influence the life principle and change the well-being of animal life.

This process includes mechanical action upon their smallest particles by rubbing and shaking and through the addition of an indifferent substance, dry or liquid, are separated from each other. This process is called Dynamizing, potentizing (development of medicinal power) and the products are dynamizations or potencies of different degrees.

Footnote 1:-
Long before this discovery of Hahnemann, experience had taught several changes which could be brought about in different natural substances by mean of friction, for example, warmth, heat, fire, development of odour in odourless bodies, magnetization of steel etc. But all these properties produced by friction were related only to physical and inanimate things.

Whereas it is a law of nature that physiological and pathogenic changes take place in the body's condition by forces capable of changing the crude material of drugs, by the process of trituration and succussion but under the condition of employing an indifferent vehicle on certain proportions. This wonderful physical and especially physiological and pathological law of nature had not been discovered before his time.

Footnote 2:-
The same thing is seen in a bar of iron and steel. Here hidden trace of latent magnetic force cannot be recognized in their interior. Both repulse the north pole of a magnetic needle with the lower end and attract the South Pole. But this is only a latent force, it cannot draw iron magnetically.

When this bar of steel is dynamized, by rubbing it with a full file in one direction, it will become a true active powerful magnet. It will now be able to attract iron and steel to itself and impart magnetic power to another bar of steel by mere contact and even some distance away. The more it has been rubbed the higher will be the magnetic power. In the same way triturating a medicinal substance and shaking of its solution develop the medicinal powers hidden within the substance.

Footnote 3:-
It refers only to the increase and stronger development of their power to cause changes in the health of animals and men, when these natural substances in this improved State, are brought very near to the living sensitive fibre or come in contact with it by means of intake or olfaction. Just as a magnetic bar especially if it's magnetic force is increased can show magnetic power only in a needle of steel whose Pole is near or touches it. The steel itself remains unchanged in the remaining chemical and physical properties and can bring about no changes in other metals, just as dynamized medicines cannot have any action upon lifeless things.

Footnote 4:-
We daily hear people use word dilutions, we see how homoeopathic medicinal potencies are called mere dilutions but in actual it is not dilution. In dilution e.g. the solution of a grain of salt, here a grain of salt will disappear in the dilution with much water and will never develop into medicinal salt.

But homoeopathic dynamizations are the very opposite, i.e., a true opening up of the natural substances occurs which brings to light and reveals the hidden specific medicinal powers contained within and brought forth by rubbing and shaking.

§ 270

METHODS OF DYNAMIZATION

In order to best obtain this development of power, a small part of the substance to be dynamized, say one grain, is triturated for three hours with three times one hundred grains sugar of milk according to the method described below1 up to the one-millionth part in powder form. For reasons given below (b) one grain of this powder is dissolved in 500 drops of a mixture of one part of alcohol and four parts of distilled water, of which one drop is put in a vial. To this are added 100 drops of pure alcohol2 and given one hundred strong succussions with the hand against a hard but elastic body.3 This is the medicine in the first degree of dynamization with which small sugar globules4 may then be moistened5 and quickly spread on blotting paper to dry and kept in a well-corked vial with the sign of (I) degree of potency. Only one6 globule of this is taken for further dynamization, put in a second new vial (with a drop a water in order to dissolve it) and then with 100 powerful succussions.

With this alcoholic medicinal fluid globules are again moistened, spread upon blotting paper and dried quickly, put into a well-stoppered vial and protected from heat and sun light and given the sign (II) of the second potency. And in this way the process is continued until the twenty-ninth is reached. Then with 100 drops of alcohol by means of 100 succussions, an alcoholic medicinal fluid is formed with which the thirtieth dynamization degree is given to properly moistened and dried sugar globules.

By means of this manipulation of crude drugs are produced preparations which only in this way reach the full capacity to forcibly influence the suffering parts of the sick organism. In this way, by means of similar artificial morbid affection, the influence of the natural disease on the life principle present within is neutralized. By means of this mechanical procedure, provided it is carried out regularly according to the above teaching, a change is effected in the given drug, which in its crude state shows itself only as material, at times as unmedicinal material but by means of such higher and higher dynamization, it is changed and subtlized at last into spirit-like7 medicinal power, which, indeed, in itself does not fall within our senses but for which the medicinally prepared globule, dry, but more so when dissolved in water, becomes the carrier, and in this condition, manifests the healing power of this invisible force in the sick body.

1 One-third of one hundred grains sugar of milk is put in a glazed porcelain mortar, the bottom dulled previously by rubbing it with fine, moist sand. Upon this powder is put one grain of the powdered drug to be triturated (one drop of quicksilver, petroleum, etc.). The sugar of milk used for dynamization must be of that special pure quality that is crystallized on strings and comes to us in

the shape of long bars. For a moment the medicines and powder are mixed with a porcelain spatula and triturated rather strongly, six to seven minutes, with the pestle rubbed dull, then the mass is scraped from the bottom of the mortar and from the pestle for three to four minutes, in order to make it homogeneous. This is followed by triturating it in the same way 6 – 7 minutes without adding anything more and again scraping 3 – 4 minutes from what adhered to the mortar and pestle. The second third of the sugar of milk is now added, mixed with the spatula and again triturated 6 – 7 minutes, followed by the scraping for 3 – 4 minutes and trituration without further addition for 6 – 7 minutes. The last third of sugar of milk is then added, mixed with the spatula and triturated as before 6 -7 minutes with most careful scraping together. The powder thus prepared is put in a vial, well corked, protected from direct sunlight to which the name of the substance and the designation of the first product marked /100 is given. In order to raise this product to /10000, one grain of the powdered /100 is mixed with the third part of 100 grains of powdered sugar of milk and then proceed as before, but every third must be carefully triturated twice thoroughly each time for 6 -7 minutes and scraped together 3 -4 minutes before the second and last third of sugar of milk is added. After each third, the same procedure is taken. When all is finished, the powder is put in a well corked vial and labelled /10000, i.e., (I), each grain containing 1/1,000,000 the original substance. Accordingly, such a trituration of the three degrees requires six times six to seven minutes for triturating and six times 3 -4 minutes for scraping, thus one hour for every degree. After one hour such trituration of the first degree, each grain will contain 1/000; of the second 1/10,000; and in the third 1/1,000,000 of the drug used.* Mortar and spatula must be cleaned well before they are used for another medicine. Washed first with warm water and dried, both mortar and pestle, as well as spatula are then put in a kettle of boiling water for half an hour. precaution might be used to such an extent as to put these utensils on a coal fire exposed to a glowing heat.

* These are the three degrees of the dry powder trituration, which if carried out correctly, will effect a good beginning for the dynamization of the medicinal substance.

2 The vial used for potentizing is filled two-thirds full.

3 Perhaps on a leather bound book.

4 They are prepared under supervision by the confectioner from starch and sugar and the small globules freed from fine dusty parts by passing them through a sieve. Then they are put through a strainer that will permit only 100 to pass through weighing one grain, the most serviceable size for the needs of a homoeopathic physician.

5 A small cylindrical vessel shaped like a thimble, made of glass, porcelain or silver, with a small opening at the bottom in which the globules are put to be medicated. They are moistened with some of the dynamized medicinal alcohol, stirred and poured out on blotting paper, in order to dry them quickly.

6 According to first directions, one drop of the liquid of a lower potency was to be taken to 100 drops of alcohol for higher potentiation. This proportion of the medicine of attenuation to the medicine that is to be dynamized (100:1) was found altogether too limited to develop thoroughly and to a high degree the power of the medicine by means of a number of such successions without specially using great force of which wearisome experiments have convinced me.

But if only one such globule be taken, of which 100 weigh one grain, and dynamize it with 100 drops of alcohol, the proportion of 1 to 50,000 and even greater will be had, for 500 such globules can hardly absorb one drop, for their saturation. With this disproportionate higher ratio between medicine and diluting medium many successive strokes of the vial filled two-thirds with alcohol can produce a much greater development of power. But with so small a diluting medium as 100 to 1 of the medicine, if many succussions by means of a powerful machine are forced into it, medicines are then developed which, especially in the higher degrees of dynamization, act almost immediately, but with furious, even dangerous violence, especially in weakly patients, without having a lasting, mild reaction of the vital principle. But the method described by me, on the contrary, produces medicines of highest development of power and mildest action, which, however, if well chosen, touches all suffering parts curatively.* In acute fevers, the small doses of the lowest dynamization degrees of these thus perfected medicinal preparations, even of medicines of long continued action (for instance, belladonna) may be repeated in short intervals. In the treatment of chronic diseases, it is best to begin with the lowest degrees of dynamization and when necessary advance to higher, even more powerful but mildly acting degrees.

* In very rare cases, notwithstanding almost full recovery of health and with good vital strength, an old annoying local trouble continuing undisturbed it is wholly permitted and even indispensably necessary, to administer in increasing doses the homoeopathic remedy that has proved itself efficacious but potenized to a very high degree by means of many succussions by hand. Such a local disease will often then disappear in a wonderful way.

7 This assertion will not appear improbable, if one considers that by means of this method of dynamization (the preparations thus produced, I have found after many laborious experiments and counter-experiments, to be the most powerful and at the same time mildest in action, i.e., as the most perfected) the material part of the medicine is lessened with each degree of dynamization 50,000 times yet incredibly increased in power, so that the further dynamization of 125 and 18 ciphers reaches only the third degree of dynamization. The thirtieth thus progressively prepared would give a fraction almost impossible to be expressed in numbers. It becomes uncommonly evident that the material part by means of such dynamization (development of its true, inner medicinal essence) will ultimately dissolve into its individual spirit-like, (conceptual) essence. In its crude state therefore, it may be considered to consist really only of this underdeveloped conceptual essence.

EXPLANATION

In order to obtain this development of power, a small part of the substance to be dynamized, say one grain, is triturated for three hours with three times one hundred grains sugar of milk according to the method described below up to one-millionth part in powder form. For reasons given below (b) one grain of this powder is dissolved in 500 drops of a mixture of one part of alcohol and four parts of distilled water. Of this one drop is put in a vial. To this 100 drops of pure alcohol is added and given one hundred strong succussions with the hand against a hard but elastic body.

This is the medicine in the first degree of dynamization with which small sugar globules are moistened and quickly spread on blotting paper to dry and kept in a well-corked vial with the sign of (I) degree of potency.

Only one globule of this is taken for further dynamization and put in a second new vial (with a drop of water in order to dissolve it) and then with 100 drops of good alcohol and dynamized in the same way with 100 powerful succussions.

Globules are again moistened with this alcoholic medicinal fluid and spread upon blotting paper and dried quickly and put into a well-stoppered vial and protected from heat and sunlight and given the sign (II) of the second potency.

And in this way the process is continued until the twenty-ninth is reached. Then with 100 drops of alcohol by means of 100 successions, an alcoholic medicinal fluid is formed with which the thirtieth dynamization degree is given to properly moistened and dried sugar globules.

By means of this medicinal procedure, if it is carried out regularly according to the above teaching.

By means of such higher and higher dynamization, the crude substance is changed and subtilized at last into spirit-like medicinal power, which manifest the healing power of this invisible force in the sick body.

Footnote 1:
One-third of one hundred grains sugar of milk is put in a glazed porcelain mortar, the bottom dulled previously by rubbing it with fine, moist sand. Upon this powder is put one grain of the powdered drug to be triturated (one drop of quicksilver, petroleum, etc.). The sugar of milk used for dynamization must be of that special pure quality that is crystallized on strings and comes to us in the shape of long bars. For a moment the medicines and powder are mixed with a porcelain spatula and triturated rather strongly, six to seven minutes, with the pestle rubbed dull, then the mass is scraped from the bottom of the mortar and from the pestle for three to four minutes, in order to make it homogeneous. This is followed by triturating it in the same way 6 – 7 minutes without adding anything more and again scraping 3 – 4 minutes from what adhered to the mortar and pestle.

The second third of the sugar of milk is now added, mixed with the spatula and again triturated 6 – 7 minutes, followed by the scraping for 3 – 4 minutes and trituration without further addition for 6 – 7 minutes.

The last third of sugar of milk is then added, mixed with the spatula and triturated as before 6 -7 minutes with most careful scraping together. The powder thus prepared is put in a vial, well corked, protected from direct sunlight to which the name of the substance and the designation of the first product marked /100 is given. In order to raise this product to /10000, one grain of the powdered /100 is mixed with the third part of 100 grains of powdered sugar of milk and then proceed as before, but every third must be carefully triturated twice thoroughly each time for 6 -7 minutes and scraped together 3 -4 minutes before the second and last third of sugar of milk is added.

After each third, the same procedure is taken. When all is finished, the powder is put in a well corked vial and labelled /10000, i.e., (I), each grain containing 1/1,000,000 the original substance.

Accordingly, such a trituration of the three degrees requires six times six to seven minutes for triturating and six times 3 -4 minutes for scraping, thus one hour for every degree. After one hour such trituration of the first degree, each grain will contain 1/000; of the second 1/10,000; and in the third 1/1,000,000 of the drug used.* Mortar and spatula must be cleaned well before they are used for another medicine. Washed first with warm water and dried, both mortar and pestle, as well as spatula are then put in a kettle of boiling water for half an hour. precaution might be used to such an extent as to put these utensils on a coal fire exposed to a glowing heat.

These are the three degrees of the dry powder trituration, which if carried out correctly, will effect a good beginning for the dynamization of the medicinal substance.

- The vial used for potentizing is filled two-thirds full.
- Perhaps on a leather bound book.
- They are prepared under supervision by the confectioner from starch and sugar and the small globules freed from fine dusty parts by passing them through a sieve. Then they are put through a strainer that will permit only 100 to pass through weighing one grain, the most serviceable size for the needs of a homoeopathic physician.

A small cylindrical vessel shaped like a thimble, made of glass, porcelain or silver, with a small opening at the bottom in which the globules are put to be medicated. They are moistened with some of the dynamized medicinal alcohol, stirred and poured out on blotting paper, in order to dry them quickly.

According to first directions, one drop of the liquid of a lower potency was to be taken to 100 drops of alcohol for higher potentiation. This proportion of the medicine of attenuation to the medicine that is to be dynamized (100:1) was found altogether too limited to develop thoroughly and to a high degree the power of the medicine by means of a number of such successions without specially using great force of which wearisome experiments have convinced me.

But if only one such globule be taken, of which 100 weigh one grain, and dynamize it with 100 drops of alcohol, the proportion of 1 to 50,000 and even greater will be had, for 500 such globules can hardly absorb one drop, for their saturation. With this disproportionate higher ratio between medicine and diluting medium many successive strokes of the vial filled two-thirds with alcohol can produce a much greater development of power. But with so small a diluting medium as 100 to 1 of the medicine, if many successions by means of a powerful machine are forced into it, medicines are then developed which, especially in the higher degrees of dynamization, act almost immediately, but with furious, even dangerous violence, especially in weakly patients, without having a lasting, mild reaction of the vital principle. But the method described by me, on the contrary, produces medicines of highest development of power and mildest action, which, however, if well chosen, touches all suffering parts curatively.* In acute fevers, the small doses of the lowest dynamization degrees of these thus perfected medicinal preparations, even of medicines of long continued action (for instance, belladonna) may be repeated in short intervals. In the treatment of chronic diseases, it is best to begin with the lowest degrees of dynamization and when necessary advance to higher, even more powerful but mildly acting degrees.

In very rare cases, notwithstanding almost full recovery of health and with good vital strength, an old annoying local trouble continuing undisturbed it is wholly permitted and even indispensably necessary, to administer in increasing doses the homoeopathic remedy that has proved itself efficacious but potenized to a very high degree by means of many successions by hand. Such a local disease will often then disappear in a wonderful way.

This assertion will not appear improbable, if one considers that by means of this method of dynamization, the material part of the medicine is lessened with each degree of dynamization 50,000 times yet incredibly increased in power, so that the further dynamization of 125 and 18 ciphers reaches only the third degree of dynamization. The thirtieth thus progressively prepared would give a fraction almost impossible to be expressed in numbers. It becomes uncommonly evident that the material part by means of such dynamization (development of its true, inner medicinal essence) will ultimately dissolve into its individual spirit-like, (conceptual) essence. In its crude state therefore, it may be considered to consist really only of this underdeveloped conceptual essence.

§ 271

PHYSICIAN-KNOWLEDGE OF PHARMACY

If the physician prepares his homoeopathic medicines himself, as he should reasonably do in order to save men from sickness,1 he may use the fresh plant itself, as but little of the crude article is required, if he does not need the expressed juice perhaps for purposes of healing. He takes a few grains in a mortar and with 100 grains sugar of milk three distinct times brings them to the one-millionth trituration (§ 270) before further potentizing of a small portion of this by means of shaking is undertaken, a procedure to be observed also with the rest of crude drugs of either dry or oily nature.

1 Until the State, in the future, after having attained insight into the indispensability of perfectly prepared homoeopathic medicines, will have them manufactured by a competent impartial person, in order to give them free of charge to homoeopathic physicians trained in homoeopathic hospitals, who have been examined theoretically and practically, and thus legally qualified. The physician may then become convinced of these divine tools for purposes of healing, but also to give them free of charge to his patients – rich and poor.

EXPLANATION

- If the Physician prepares his homeopathic medicines himself, as he should do in order to save men from sickness.
- He may use the fresh plants itself as but little of the crude article is required, if he does not use expressed juice for purposes of healing.(larger amount is required).
- He takes a few grains in a mortar & with 100 grains of sugar of milk brings them to the one-millionth trituration three distinct times[aph -270].
- Now he further potentized a small portion of this by means of shaking [crude drugs of either dry or oily nature also same procedures is observed]

Footnote:
After having insight into the vitality of perfectly prepared homeopathic medicine, it will be given to a competent impartial person for manufacture and give them free of charge to homeopathic physician trained in homeopathic hospitals & legally qualified.

- ✦ The physician may then become convinced of these tools for purposes of healing but also to give them free of charge to his patients -rich & poor.

§ 272

ADMINISTRATION OF REMEDY

Such a globule,1 placed dry upon the tongue, is one of the smallest doses for a moderate recent case of illness. Here but few nerves are touched by the medicine. A similar globule, crushed with some sugar of milk and dissolved in a good deal of water (§ 247) and stirred well before every administration will produce a far more powerful medicine for the use of several days. Every dose, no matter how minute, touches, on the contrary, many nerves.

1 These globules (§ 270) retain their medicinal virtue for many years, if protected against sunlight and heat.

EXPLANATION

- Such a globule when placed dry upon the tongue, is one of the smallest doses for a moderate recent case of illness.
- Here few nerves are touched by the medicine,
- A similar globule which is crushed with some sugar of milk & dissolved in a good deal of water[aph 247] & stirred well before every administration will produce a more powerful medicine for the use of several days.
- Every dose touches many nerves, no matter how minute it is.

Footnote:
These globules [aph-270], retain their medicinal virtue for many years, if they are protected against sunlight & heat.

§ 273

SINGLE OR COMPLEX MEDICINE

In no case under treatment is it necessary and therefore not permissible to administer to a patient more than one single, simple medicinal substance at one time. It is inconceivable how the slightest doubt could exist as to whether it was more consistent with nature and more rational to prescribe a single, simple1 medicine at one time in a disease or a mixture of several differently acting drugs. It is absolutely not allowed in homoeopathy, the one true, simple and natural art of healing, to give the patient at one time two different medicinal substance.

1 Two substances, opposite to each other, united into neutral Natrum and middle salts by chemical affinity in unchangeable proportions, as well as sulphurated metals found in the earth and those produced by technical art in constant combining proportions of sulphur and alkaline salts and earths, for instance (natrum sulph. and calcarea sulph.) as well as those ethers produced by distillation of alcohol and acids may together with phosphorus be considered as simple medicinal substances by the homoeopathic physician and used for patients. On the other hand, those extracts obtained by means of acids of the so-called alkaloids of plants, are exposed to great variety in their preparation (for instance, chinin, strychnine, morphine), and can, therefore, not be accepted by the homoeopathic physician as simple medicines, always the same, especially as he possesses, in the plants themselves, in their natural state (Peruvian bark, nux vomica, opium) every quality necessary for healing. Moreover, the alkaloids are not the only constituents of the plants.

EXPLANATION

- We should never administer more than one single, simple medicinal substances at one time to a patient.
- It is absolutely not allowed in homeopathy, simple & natural art of healing, to give the patient two different medicinal substances at one time.
- It is more rational to prescribe a single, simple medicine at one time in a d/s.

Footnote:
Two substances, which are opposite to each other, unite into neutral Natrum & middle salts in unchangeable proportions.

- The sulphurated metals found in the earth & those produced by technical art in constant proportions of sulphur & alkaline salts & earth, e.g- natrum sulph & calcarea sulph]
- The ethers produced by distillation of alcohol & acids together with phosphorus may be considered as simple medicinal substances by the homeopathic physician & used for patients.
- But those extracts obtained by means of acids of alkaloids of plants, are exposed to great variety in their preparation, e.g- Chinin, morphine, strychine & cannot be accepted as simple medicines. Moreover, the alkaloids are not the only constituents of the plants.

§ 274

ADVANTAGE OF USE OF SINGLE MEDICINE

As the true physician finds in simple medicines, administered singly and uncombined, all that he can possibly desire (artificial disease-force which are able by homoeopathic power completely to overpower, extinguish, and permanently cure natural diseases), he will, mindful of the wise

maxim that "it is wrong to attempt to employ complex means when simple means suffice," never think of giving as a remedy any but a single, simple medicinal substance; for these reasons also, because even though the simple medicines were thoroughly proved with respect to their pure peculiar effects on the unimpaired healthy state of man, it is yet impossible to foresee how two and more medicinal substances might, when compounded, hinder and alter each other's actions on the human body; and because, on the other hand, a simple medicinal substance when used in diseases, the totality of whose symptoms is accurately known, renders efficient aid by itself alone, if it be homoeopathically selected; and supposing the worst case to happen, that it was not chosen in strict conformity to similarity of symptoms, and therefore does no good, it is yet so far useful that it promoted our knowledge of therapeutic agents, because, by the new symptoms excited by it in such a case, those symptoms which this medicinal substance had already shown in experiments on the healthy human body are confirmed, an advantage that is lost by the employment of all compound remedies.1

1 When the rational physician has chosen the perfectly homoeopathic medicine for the well-considered case of disease and administered it internally, he will leave to irrational allopathic routine the practice of giving drinks or fomentations of different plants, of injecting medicated glysters and of rubbing in this or the other ointment.

EXPLANATION

- As the true physician finds in simple medicines which is administered singly & uncombined all that he desires i.e- Artificial d/s forces which by their Homeopathic power are able to overpower, extinguish & permanently cure natural d/s.
- It is wrong to try to employ complex means when simple means suffice.
- So never think of giving any remedy but a single simple medicinal substances.
- It is also because the simple medicine were thoroughly proved with respect to their pure peculiar effects on the unimpaired healthy state of man, I.e- Medicine were proved singly.
- It is impossible to foresee how two & more medicinal substances, when compounded together, might hinder & alter each other's actions on the human body.
- Whereas a simple medicinal substances when used in d/s [the totality of whose symptoms is accurately known], provide efficient aid, if it is homeopathically selected.

Footnote:-
- When the physician has chosen the perfectly homeoapthic medicine for the case of d/s & administered it internally. He will not give irrational allopathic practice of giving drinks or fomentations of different plants, or injecting medicated glysters & of rubbing in the ointment.

§ 275

LARGE DOSE IS INJURIOUS

The suitableness of a medicine for any given case of disease does not depend on its accurate homoeopathic selection alone, but likewise on the proper size, or rather smallness, of the dose. If we give too strong a dose of a medicine which may have been even quite homoeopathically chosen for the morbid state before us, it must, notwithstanding the inherent beneficial character of its nature, prove injurious by its mere magnitude, and by the unnecessary, too strong impression which, by virtue of its homoeopathic similarity of action, it makes upon the vital force which it attacks and, through the vital force, upon those parts of the organism which are the most sensitive, and are already most affected by the natural disease.

EXPLANTATION

- The first step towards homeopathic cure includes selection of suitable medicine for any given case of d/s.
- The next step is selection of proper size or rather, smallness of the dose.
- If we give too strong a dose of a medicine which maybe homeopathically chosen for the case.
- This will prove injurious & unnecessary & too strong impression is made upon the vital force.
- Through the attack on vital force it attacks, upon those parts of the organism which are the most sensitive & are already most affected by the natural d/s.

§ 276

EFFECT OF HIGH POTENCY

For this reason, a medicine, even though it may be homoeopathically suited to the case of disease, does harm in every dose that is too large, the more harm the larger the dose, and by the magnitude of the dose and in strong doses' it does more harm the greater its homoeopathicity and the higher the potency1 selected, and it does much more injury than any equally large dose of a medicine that is unhomoeopathic, and in no respect adapted to the morbid state (allopathic).

Too large doses of an accurately chosen homoeopathic medicine, and especially when frequently repeated, bring about much trouble as a rule. They put the patient not seldom in danger of life or make this disease almost incurable. They do indeed extinguish the natural disease so far as the sensation of the life principle is concerned and the patient no longer suffers

from the original disease from the moment the too strong dose of the homoeopathic medicine acted upon him but he is in consequence more ill with the similar but more violent medicinal disease which is most difficult to destroy.2

1 The praise bestowed of late years by some homoeopathists on the larger doses is owing to this, either that they chose low dynamizations of the medicine to be administered (as I myself used to do twenty years ago, from nor knowing any better), or that the medicines selected were not homoeopathic and imperfectly prepared by their manufacturers.

2 Thus, the continuous use of aggressive allopathic large doses of mercurials against syphilis develops almost incurable maladies, when yet one or several doses of a mild but active mercurial preparation would certainly have radically cured in a few days the whole venereal disease, together with the chancre, provided it had not been destroyed by external measures (as is always done by allopathy). In the same way, the allopath gives Peruvian bark and quinine in intermittent fever daily in very large doses, where they are correctly indicated and where one very small dose of a highly potentized China would unfailingly help (in marsh intermittents and even in persons who were not affected by any evident psoric disease). A chronic China malady (coupled at the same time with the development of psora) is produced, which, if it dose not gradually kill the patient by damaging the internal important vital organs, especially spleen and liver, will put him, nevertheless suffering for years in a sad state of health. A homoeopathic antidote for such a misfortune produced by abuse of large doses of homoeopathic remedies is hardly conceivable.

EXPLANATION

- For this reason, a medicine, even though it maybe homoepathically suited to the case of d/s does harm if given in too large doses.
- It does more harm, the greater its homeopathicity & higher the potency selected in strong doses.
- It does more injury than an equally large dose of unhomeopathic medicine [allopathic]
- Too large doses of an accurately chosen homeopathic medicine, when frequently repeated, bring much trouble as a rule.
- It puts the patient in danger of life or makes his d/s almost incurable.
- They do extinguish the natural d/s & the patient no longer suffers from the original d/s but he is in consequence, more ill with the similar but more violent medicinal d/s, which is most difficult to destroy.

Footnote:
Some few homeopathic used larger doses & were praised but either they chose low dynamizations of medicine or the medicine selected were not homeopathic & imperfectly prepared by their manufactures.

- ✦ Thus, continous use of aggressive allopathic large doses of mercurials against syphilis develops almost incurable mercurial maladies.
- ✦ But the same active mercurial preparation given in one or several doses of a mild nature, would have cured the whole veneral d/s & the chancre [if it has not been destroyed by external measures, as is always done by allopathy]

- In the same way, the allopath gives peruvian bark & quinine in intermittent fever daily in very large doses. A chronic china malady is produced which gradually kill the patient by damaging the internal important vital organs, especially spleen & liver or put him suffering for years in a sad state of health. and a homeopathic antidote for such a misfortune produced by abuse of long doses of homeopathic remedies is hardly conceivable.
- Whereas when one very small dose of a highly potentized china would help the patient.

§ 277

MINIMUM DOSE

For the same reason, and because a medicine, provided the dose of it was sufficiently small, is all the more salutary and almost marvellously efficacious the more accurately homoeopathic its selection has been, a medicine whose selection has been accurately homoeopathic must be all the more salutary the more its dose is reduced to the degree of minuteness appropriate for a gentle remedial effect.

EXPLANATION

- A medicine, provided the dose of it was sufficiently small, is more salutary & almost best efficacious.
- A medicine whose selection has been accurately homeopathic must be more beneficial the more its dose is reduced.
- The dose is reduced to the degree of minuteness appropriate for a gentle remedial effect.

§ 278

POTENCY SELECTION

Here the question arises, what is this most suitable degree of minuteness for sure and gentle remedial effect; how small, in other words, must be the dose of each individual medicine, homoeopathically selected for a case of disease, to effect the best cure? To solve this problem, and to determine for every particular medicine, what dose of it will suffice for homoeopathic therapeutic purposes and yet be so minute that the gentlest and most rapid cure may be thereby obtained – to solve this problem is, as may easily be conceived, not the work off theoretical speculation; not by fine-spun reasoning, not by specious sophistry can we expect to obtain the solution of this problem. It is just as impossible as to tabulate in advance all imaginable cases. Pure experiment, careful observation of the sensitiveness of each patient, and accurate experience can alone determine this; and it were absurd to adduce the large doses of unsuitable (allopathic) medicines of the old system, which do not touch the diseased side of the organism homoeopathically, but only attack the parts unaffected by the disease, in opposition to what pure experience pronounces respecting the smallness of the doses required for homoeopathic cures.

EXPLANATION

- Now the question arises, what is this most suitable degree of minuteness for sure & a gentle remedical effect.
- How small, must be the dose of each medicine to effect the best cure?
- Pure experiment, careful observation of the sensitiveness of each patient & accurate experience can only determine the dose to effect best cure in each individual case.
- It was wrong practise to employ the large dose of unsuitable[allopathic]medicines of the old system, it only attack the parts unaffected by the d/s & don't touch the diseased side of the organisms homeopathically.

§ 279

HOMEOPATHICALLY SELECTED MEDICINE

This pure experience shows UNIVERSALLY, that if the disease do not manifestly depend on a considerable deterioration of an important viscus (even though it belong to the chronic and complicated diseases), and if during the treatment all other alien medicinal influences are kept away from the patients, the dose of the homoeopathically selected and highly potentized remedy for the beginning of treatment of an important, especially chronic disease can never be prepared so small that it shall not be stronger than the natural disease and shall not be able to overpower it, at least in part and extinguish it from the sensation of the principle of life and thus make a beginning of a cure.

EXPLANATION

- This pure experience shows UNIVERSALLY, that if the d/s, with not a considerable deterioration of an important viscus, even though it belong, to the chronic & complicated d/s.
- The dose of the Homeopathically selected & highly potentized remedy can never be prepared so small that it is not stronger than the natural d/s & small not be able to overpower it extinguish it & thus make beginning of a cure,
- During the treatment all other alien medicinal influences should be kept away from the patient.

§ 280

SIGNS OF CORRECT SELECTION IS PERFECT CURE

The dose of the medicine that continues serviceable without producing new troublesome symptoms is to be continued while gradually ascending, so long as the patient with general improvement, begins to feel in a mild degree the return of one or several old original complaints. This indicates an approaching cure through a gradual ascending of the moderate doses modified each time by succussion (§ 247). It indicates that the vital principal no longer needs to be affected by the similar medicinal disease in order to lose the sensation of the natural disease (§ 148). It indicates that the life principle now free from the natural disease begins to suffer only something of the medicinal disease hitherto known as homoeopathic aggravation.

EXPLANATION

- This dose of the medicine that is serviceable & does not produce new troublesome symptoms is to be continued.
- And the dose is gradually ascending, till the patient with general improvement, begins to feel the return of one or several old original complaints in mild degree.
- This indicates that the cure is approaching through a gradual ascending of moderate doses modified each time by succussion [aph-247].
- It also indicates that the vital principle is now free from the natural d/s & begins to suffer only something of medicinal d/s known as Homeopathic aggravation.

§ 281

SIGNS OF RESTORATION

In order to be convinced of this, the patient is left without any medicine for eight, ten of fifteen days, meanwhile giving him only some powders of sugar of milk. If the few last complaints are due to the medicine simulating the former original disease symptoms, then these complaints will disappear in a few days or hours. If during these days without medicine, while continuing good hygienic regulations nothing more of the original disease is seen, he is probably cured. But if in the later days traces of the former morbid symptoms should show themselves, they are remnants of the original disease not wholly extinguished, which must be treated with renewed higher potencies of the remedy as directed before. If a cure is to follow, the first small doses must likewise be again gradually raised higher, but less and more slowly in patients where considerable irritability is evident than in those of less susceptibility, where the advance to higher dosage may be more rapid. There are patients whose impressionability compared to that of the insusceptible ones is like the ratio as 1000 to 1.

EXPLANATION

- Now in order to be sure of this, the patient is left without any medicine for 8,10 or 15 days.
- During this period he is given some powders of sugar of milk, following conditions can occur:-

    1. If the few last complaints are due to the medicine then these complaints will disappear in a few days or hours. Here the medicine simulates the former original d/s symptoms.
    2. But if during these days without medicine & good hygienic regulations, nothing more of the original d/s is seen, he is probably cured.
    3. If in the later days former morbid symptoms traces show themselves means they are remnants of original d/s which is not, fully extinguished, this must be treated with renewed higher potencies of the remedy.
    4. The first small doses must be again gradually raised higher but less & more slowly in patient with considerable irritability & rapid in those of less susceptibility.

There are patients whose impressionability to that of the unsusceptible ones is like the ratio as 1000 to 1.

§ 282

TREATMENT OF MIASMS

It would be a certain sign that the doses were altogether too large, if during treatment, especially in chronic disease, the first dose should bring forth a so-called homoeopathic aggravation, that is, a marked increase of the original morbid symptoms first discovered and in the same way every repeated dose (§ 247) however modified somewhat by shaking before its administration (i.e., more highly dynamized).1

1 The rule to commence the homoeopathic treatment if chronic diseases with the smallest possible doses and only gradually to augment them is subject to a notable exception in the treatment of the three great miasms while they still effloresce on the skin, i.e., recently erupted itch, the untouched chancre (on the sexual organs, labia, mouth or lips, and so forth), and the figwarts. These not only tolerate, but indeed require, from the very beginning large doses of their specific remedies of ever higher and higher degrees of dynamization daily (possibly also several times daily). If this course be pursued, there is no danger to be feared as is the case in the treatment of diseases hidden within, that the excessive dose while it extinguishes the disease, initiates and by continued usage possible produces

a chronic medicinal disease. During external manifestations of these three miasms this is not the case; for from the daily progress of their treatment it can be observed and judged to what degree the large dose withdraws the sensation of the disease from the vital principle day by day; for none of these three can be cured without giving the physician the conviction through their disappearance that there is no longer any further need of these medicines.

Since diseases in general are but dynamic attacks upon the life principle and nothing material – no materia peccans – as their basis (as the old school in its delusion has fabulated for a thousand years and treated the sick accordingly to their ruin) there is also in these cases nothing material to take away, nothing to smear away, to burn or tie or cut away, without making the patient endlessly sicker and more incurable (Chron. Dis. Part 1), than he was before local treatment of these three miasms was instituted. The dynamic, inimical principle exerting its influence upon the vital energy is the essence of these external signs of the inner malignant miasms that can be extinguished solely by the action of a homoeopathic medicine upon the vital principle which affects it in a similar but stronger manner and thus extracts the sensation of internal and external spirit-like (conceptual) disease enemy in such a way that it no longer exists for the life principle (for the organism) and thus releases the patient of his illness and he is cured.

Experience, however, teaches that the itch, plus its external manifestations, as well as the chancre, together with the inner venereal miasm, can and must be cured only by means of specific medicines taken internally. But the figwarts, if they have existed for some time without treatment, have need for their perfect cure, the external application of their specific medicines as well as their internal use at the same time.

EXPLANATION

- Especially in chronic d/s, if the doses were too large, the first dose brings a so-called homeopathic aggravation.
- Here a marked increase of the original morbid symptoms first discovered occurs & in the same way at every repeated dose[aph-247], somewhat modified by shaking before its administration.

Footnote:
The exception in the above mode of treatment as discussed in above aphorisms is the treatment of the three great miasms while they still effloresce on the skin.

i.e- Recently erupted itch, the untouched chancre [on sexual organs, labia, mouth or lipsetc]& the figwarts.

- These cases require from the beginning, large doses of their specific remedies of ever higher & higher degree of dynamization daily, possibly several times daily.
- There is no danger as is the case in the treatment of d/s hidden within. In treatment of hidden d/s the excessive dose extinguishes the d/s & initiates & by continued usage possibly produces a chronic medicinal d/s.
- This is not the case during external manifestation of those three miasms because from the daily progress of their treatment it can be observed to what degree the large dose withdraws the d/s from the vital principle. Their disappearance means that there is no longer any further need of these medicines.

- D/s in general are dynamic attacks upon the life principle & nothing material -no materia pecans as their basis.
- There is nothing material to be taken away, nothing to smear away, to burn or tie or cut away, these processes make patient endlessly sicker & more incurable.
- The inner malignant miasms can be extinguished by the use of a homeopathic medicine upon the vital principle which affects the sensation of internal & external spirit -like d/s enemy & thus releases the patient of his illness & he is cured.
- However experience teaches that the itch, plus its external manifestations, as well as the chancre with the inner veneral miasm, must be cured only by means of specific medicines which are taken internally.
- BUT THE FIGWARTS, if they have existed for sometimes without treatment, for their perfect cure need external application of their specific medicines as well as their internal use at the same time.

§ 283

USEFULNESS OF SMALL DOSES

In order to work wholly according to nature, the true healing artist will prescribe the accurately chosen homoeopathic medicine most suitable in all respects in so small a dose on account of this alone. For should he be misled by human weakness to employ an unsuitable medicine, the disadvantage of its wrong relation to the disease would be so small that the patient could through his own vital powers and by means of early opposition (§ 249) of the correctly chosen remedy according to symptom similarly (and this also in the smallest dose) rapidly extinguish and repair it.

EXPLANATION

- If we want to work wholly according to nature, the true healing artist prescribe the accurately chosen homeopathic medicine in so small a dose, So that even if the medicine employed is unsuitable, the effects will be so small that the patient by his own vital powers & by means of early opposition [aph -249]of the correctly chosen remedy according to symptom similarity rapidly extinguish & repair it.

§ 284

WHAT PART OF THE BODY ARE SUSCEPTIBLE TO THE INFLUENCE OF REMEDIES

Besides the tongue, mouth and stomach, which are most commonly affected by the administration of medicine, the nose and respiratory organs are receptive of the action of medicines in fluid form by means of olfaction and inhalation through the mouth. But the whole remaining skin of the body clothed with epidermis, is adapted to the action of medicinal solutions, especially if the inunction is connected with simultaneous internal administration.1

1 The power of medicines acting upon the infant through the milk of the mother or wet nurse is wonderfully helpful. Every disease in a child yields to the rightly chosen homoeopathic medicines given in moderate doses to the nursing mother and so administered, is more easily and certainly utilized by these new world-citizens than is possible in later years. Since most infants usually have imparted to them psora through the milk of the nurse, if they do not already possess it through heredity from the mother, they may be at the same time protected antipsorically by means of the milk of the nurse rendered medicinally in this manner. But the case of mothers in their (first) pregnancy by means of a mild antipsoric treatment, especially with sulphur dynamizations prepared according to the directions in this edition (§ 270), is indispensable in order to destroy the psora – that producer of most chronic diseases – which is given them hereditarily; destroy it both within themselves and in the foetus, thereby protecting posterity in advance. This is true of pregnant women thus treated; they have given birth to children usually more healthy and stronger, to the astonishment of everybody. A new confirmation of the great truth of the psora theory discovered by me.

EXPLANATION

- Tongue, Mouth, Stomach are the most commonly affected by the administration of medicine.
- The Nose & Respiratory organs are also receptive of the action of medicines in fluid form by olfaction & inhalation through the mouth.
  But the whole remaining skin of the body covered which epidermis, is also adapted to the action medicinal solutions, especially if the rubbing of remedy is connected with simultaneous internal administration of medicine.

Footnote:
The power of medicines acting upon the infant through the milk of the mother or wet nurse is wonderfully helpful.

- ♦ If the child is diseased, the rightly chosen homeoapthic medicines given to the nursing mother in moderate doses, is utilized by the child.

- The children who don't possess psora from the mother hereditary, have psora through the milk of the nurse. This means of the milk of the nurse can be rendered medicinally in this manner.
- But the mothers in their first pregnancy by means of a mild antipsoric treatment, especially with sulphur dynamizations in order to destroy the psora -which passes to child hereditarily. This treatment destroys psora within the mother & in the foetus too.
- The pregnant women thus treated have given birth to children usually more healthy & stronger.

§ 285

EXTERNAL APPLICATION OF MEDICINE

In this way, the cure of very old disease may be furthered by the physician applying externally, rubbing it in the back, arms, extremities, the same medicine he gives internally and which showed itself curatively. In doing so, he must avoid parts subject to pain or spasm or skin eruption.1

1 From this fact may be explained those marvellous cures, however infrequent, where chronic deformed patients, whose skin nevertheless was sound and clean, were cured quickly and permanently after a few baths whose medicinal constituents (by, chance) were homoeopathically related. On the other hand, the mineral baths very often brought on increased injury with patients, whose eruptions on the skin were suppressed. After a brief period of well-being, the life principle allowed the inner, uncured malady to appear elsewhere, more important for life and health.

At times, instead, the ocular nerve would become paralyzed and produce amaurosis, sometimes the crystalline lens would become clouded, hearing lost, mania or suffocating asthma would follow or an apoplexy would end the sufferings of the deluded patient.

A fundamental principle of the homoeopathic physician (which distinguishes him from every physician of all older schools) is this, that he never employs for any patient a medicine, whose effects on the healthy human has not previously been carefully proven and thus made known to him (§§ 20,21). To prescribe for the sick on mere conjecture of some possible usefulness for some similar disease or from hearsay "that a remedy has helped in such and such a disease" – such conscienceless venture the philanthropic homoeopathist will leave to the allopath. A genuine physician and practitioner or our art will therefore never send the sick to any of the numerous mineral baths, because almost all are unknown so far as their accurate, positive effects on the healthy human organism is concerned, and when misused, must be counted among the most violent and dangerous drugs. In this way, out of a thousand sent to the most celebrated of these baths by ignorant physicians allopathically uncured and blindly sent there perhaps one or two are cured by chance more often return only apparently cured and the miracle is proclaimed aloud. Hundreds, meanwhile sneak quietly away, more or less worse and the rest remain to prepare themselves for their eternal resting place, a fact that is verified by the presence of numerous well-filled graveyards surrounding the most celebrated of these spas.*

* A true homoeopathic physician, one who never acts without correct fundamental principles, never gambles with the life of the sick entrusted to him as in a lottery where the winner is in the ratio of 1 to 500 or 1000 (blanks here consisting of aggravation or death), will never expose any one of his patients to such danger and send him for good luck to a mineral bath, as is done so frequently by allopaths in order to get rid of the sick in an acceptable manner spoiled by him or others.

their heating and intoxicating action diminished by dilution with much water.

EXPLANATION

In this way, the cure of very old d/s may be furthered by giving the medicine internally as well as applying externally by rubbing it in the back, arms & extremities.

But the parts subjected to pain or spasm or skin eruption should be avoided.

Footnote 1:

From this fact those marvellous cures (which are however infrequent) can be explained where chronic deformed patients, whose skin was sound and clean, were cured quickly and permanently after a few baths whose medicinal constituents, by chance, were homoeopathically related.

On the other hand, the mineral baths when applied on the skin whose eruptions were suppressed, very often brought on increased injury. After a brief period of well-being, the life principle allowed the inner, uncured malady to appear again but elsewhere in the more important part of life and health.

At times, the ocular nerve becomes paralyzed and produce amaurosis, or sometimes the crystalline lens of eye become clouded, or hearing is lost, mania or suffocating asthma would follow or an apoplexy occurs.

A fundamental principle of the homoeopathic physician is that he never employs a medicine to the patient, whose effects on the healthy human has not been carefully proven (aphorism 20,21).

A genuine physician and practitioner of our art will therefore never send the sick person to these numerous mineral baths because almost all such baths are unknown of their accurate, positive effects on the healthy human organism. When misused, it is counted among the most violent and dangerous drugs. In this way, out of a 1000 of sick sent to this mode of mineral baths by ignorant allopathic physician leaves them uncured. May be out of those 1000 one or two are cured by chance, they often return only apparently cured and the miracle is proclaimed aloud.

Many such sick sneak away quietly, more or less worse and the rest remain to prepare themselves for their eternal resting place (graveyard).

A true homoeopathic physician never acts without correct fundamental principles. They never gamble with the life of the sick as in a lottery where the winner is in the ratio of 1:500 or 1000. They will never expose any one of his patients to such danger and send him for good luck to a mineral bath, as is done frequently by allopaths in order to get rid of the sick in a manner spoiled by him or others.

§ 286

ELECTRICITY & GALVANISM

The dynamic force of minerals magnets, electricity and galvanism act no less powerfully upon our life principle and they are not less homoeopathic than the properly so-called medicines which neutralize disease by taking them through the mouth, or by rubbing them on the skin or by olfaction. There may be diseases, especially diseases of sensibility and irritability, abnormal sensations, and involuntary muscular movements which may be cured by those means. But the more certain way of applying the last two as well as that of the so-called electromagnetic lies still very much in the dark to make homoeopathic use of them. So far both electricity and Galvanism have been used only for palliation to the great damage of the sick. The positive, pure action of both upon the healthy human body have until the present time been but little tested.

EXPLANATION

In this aphorism we will know about dynamic forces other than so-called medicines which also have homoeopathic action.

Minerals, magnets, electricity and galvanism also act powerfully upon our life principles.

These dynamic forces are homoeopathic like medicines which are taken through mouth or by rubbing them on the skin or by olfaction to neutralize disease.

There are diseases, especially diseases of sensibility and irritability, abnormal sensations and involuntary muscular movements which may be cured by these means.

Till now electricity and galvanism have been used only for palliation of the sick.

The positive, pure action of both have been little tested upon the healthy human body.

§ 287

MAGNET AS HEALER

The powers of the magnet for healing purposes can be employed with more certainty according to the positive effects detailed in the Materia Medica Pura under north and south pole of a powerful magnetic bar. Though both poles are alike powerful, they nevertheless oppose each other in the manner of their respective action. The doses may be modified by the length of time of contact with one or the other pole, according as the symptoms of either north or south pole are indicated. As antidote to a too violent action the application of a plate of polished zinc will suffice.

EXPLANATION

The powers of the magnet can be employed for healing purposes.

They are used with more certainty according to the positive effects detailed in the Materia Medica Pura under north and south pole of a powerful magnetic bar.

Though both poles are alike powerful, they oppose each other in the manner of their respective action.

According to the symptoms either north or south pole are indicated in a case.

The doses may be modified by the length of time of contact with one or the other pole.

If a too violent action occurs then it can be treated by application of a plate of polished zinc which acts as an antidote.

§ 288

ANIMAL MAGNETISM

I find it yet necessary to allude here to animal magnetism, as it is termed, or rather Mesmerism (as it should be called in deference to Mesmer, its first founder) which differs so much in its nature from all other therapeutic agents. This curative force, often so stupidly denied and disdained for a century, acts in different ways. It is a marvellous, priceless gift of God to mankind by means of which the strong will of a well intentioned person upon a sick one by contact and even without this and even at some distance, can bring the vital energy of the healthy mesmerizer endowed with this power into another person dynamically (just as one of the poles of a powerful magnetic rod upon a bar of steel).

It acts in part by replacing in the sick whose vital force within the organism is deficient here and there, in part also in other parts where the vital force has accumulated too much and keeps up irritating nervous disorders it turns it aside, diminishes and distributes it equally and in general extinguishes the morbid condition of the life principle of the patient and substitutes in its place the normal of the mesmerist acting powerfully upon him, for instance, old ulcers, amaurosis, paralysis of single organs and so forth. Many rapid apparent cures performed in all ages, by mesmerizers endowed with great natural power, belong to this class. The effect of communicated human power upon the whole human organism was most brilliantly shown, in the resuscitation of persons who had lain some time apparently dead, by the most powerful sympathetic will of a man in full vigor of vital energy,1 and of this kind of resurrection history records many undeniable examples.

If the mesmerizing person of either sex capable at the same time of a good-natured enthusiasm (even its degeneration into bigotry, fanaticism, mysticism or philanthropic dreaming) will be

empowered all the more with this philanthropic self-sacrificing performance to direct exclusively the power of his commanding good will to the recipient requiring his help and at the same time to concentrate these, he may at times perform apparent miracles.

1 Especially of one of such persons, of whom there are not many, who, along with great kindness of disposition and perfect bodily powers, possesses but a very moderate desire for sexual intercourse, which it would give him very little trouble wholly to suppress, in whom, consequently, all the fine vital spirits that would otherwise be employed in the production of the semen, are ready to be communicated to others, by touching them and powerfully exerting the will. Some powerful mesmerisers, with whom I have become aquatinted, had all this peculiar character.

EXPLANATION

Here Hahnemann says that here he finds necessary to speak about animal magnetism, which is termed Mesmerism.

Mesmerism differs from all other therapeutic agents and acts in different ways.

It is a marvellous, priceless gift of God to mankind.

Here the strong will of a well intentioned person can bring the vital energy of the healthy mesmerizer endowed into another sick person dynamically by contact and even at some distance.

It acts by replacing the vital force within the organism which is deficient here and there and also by diminishing and distributing the vital force equally where it has accumulated too much and keeps up irritating nervous disorders.

It in general, extinguishes the morbid condition of the vital life principle of the patient and substitutes in its place, the normal of the mesmerist acting powerfully upon him.

E.g. old ulcers, amaurosis, paralysis of single organs etc.

There are many examples of such cases where the person who had been apparently dead was resuscitated by the most powerful sympathetic will of a man who is in full vigor of vital energy.1

The person who is mesmerizing the sick person can be of either sex.

He will empower his good- natured enthusiasm to the recipient requiring his help and at the same time concentrate it.

Footnote 1:

Vital energy especially of one of such persons who has great kindness of disposition and perfect bodily powers and possesses very moderate desire for sexual intercourse.

Due to which all the fine vital spirits are ready to be communicated to others and not employed in the production of semen.

It is communicated to others by touching them and powerfully exerting the will.

§ 289

MESMERISM

All the above-mentioned methods of practicing mesmerism depend upon influx of more or less vital force into the patient, and hence are termed positive mesmerism.1 An opposite mode of employing mesmerism, however, as it produces just the contrary effect, deserves to be termed negative mesmerism. To this belong the passes which are used to rouse from the somnambulic sleep, as also all the manual processes known by the names of soothing and ventilating. This discharge by means of negative mesmerism of the vital force accumulated to excess in individual parts of the system of undebilitated persons is most surely and simply performed by making a very rapid motion or the flat extended hand, held parallel to, and about an inch distant from the body, from the top of the head to the tips of the toes.2 The more rapidly this pass is made, so much the more effectually will the discharge be effected. Thus, for instance, in the case where a previously healthy woman,3 from the sudden suppression of her catamenia by a violent mental shock, lies to all appearance dead, the vital force which is probably accumulated in the precordial region, will, by such a rapid negative pass, be discharged and its equilibrium throughout the whole organism restored. So that the resuscitation generally follows, immediately.4 In like manner, a gentle, less rapid, negative pass diminishes the excessive restlessness and sleeplessness accompanied with anxiety sometimes produced in very irritable persons by a too powerful positive pass, etc.

1 When I here speak of the decided and certain curative power of positive mesmerism, I most assuredly do not mean that abuse of it, where, by repeated passes of this kind, continued for half an hour or a whole hour at a time, and, even day after day, performed on weak, nervous patients, that monstrous revolution of the whole human system is effected which is termed somnambulism, wherein the human being is ravished from the world of sense and seems to belong more to the world of spirits – a highly unnatural and dangerous state, by means of which it has not infrequently been attempted to cure chronic diseases.

2 It is a well known rule that a person who is either to be positively or negatively mesmerised, should not wear silk on any part of the body.

3 Hence a negative pass, especially if it be very rapid, is extremely injurious to a delicate person affected with a chronic ailment and deficient in vital force.

4 A strong country lad, ten years of age, received in the morning, on account of slight indisposition, from a professed female mesmeriser, several very powerful passes with the points of both thumbs, from the pit of the stomach along the lower edge of the ribs, and he instantly grew deathly pale, and fell into such a state of unconsciousness and immobility that no effort could arouse him, and he was almost given up for dead. I made his eldest brother give him a very rapid negative pass from the crown of the head over the body to the feet, and in one instance he recovered his consciousness and became lively and well.

EXPLANATION

All the above - mentioned methods of mesmerism depend upon an influx of vital force into the patient and hence are termed positive mesmerism.

An opposite mode of employing mesmerism, is termed negative mesmerism as it produces just opposite effect.

This negative mesmerism includes the passes which are used to rouse from the somnambulic sleep, also all manual processes known as soothing and ventilating.

This discharge by means of negative mesmerism of the vital force is performed by making a very rapid motion of the flat extended hand held parallel to and about an inch distance from the body, from the top of the head to the tips of the toes.

The more rapidly this pass is made, the more effectually the discharge is effected.

For e.g. in the case where a previously healthy woman, by a violent mental shock develops sudden suppression of her catamania. She lies to all appearance dead, the vital force is probably accumulated in the precordial region. So by such a rapid negative pass, the vital force is discharged and it's equilibrium is restored throughout the whole organism and resuscitation generally follows immediately.

In the same manner, a gentle, less rapid, negative pass diminishes the excessive restlessness and sleeplessness due to anxiety produced in very irritable persons by a too powerful positive pass, etc.

Footnote 1:
Here he speaks of the certain curative power of the positive mesmerism, he does not mean that abuse of it, where, repeated passes of this kind are continued for half an hour or a whole hour at a time and even day after day, on weak, nervous patients whole human system is affected which is termed somnambulism, where the human being is forced from the world of sense and goes to a highly unnatural and dangerous state.

Footnote 2:
A person who is either to be positively or negatively mesmerised, should not wear silk on any part of the body.

Footnote 3:
Hence a negative pass, especially if it be very rapid, is very injurious to delicate person affected with a chronic ailment and deficient in vital force.

Footnote 4:
A strong country lad of 10 years of age had slight indisposition.

He received several very powerful passes with the points of both thumbs, from the pit of the stomach long the lower edge of the ribs by a professed female mesmeriser.

He instantly grew deathly pale and unconscious. He could not be aroused by any means and was almost given up for dead.

Hahnemann made his eldest brother give him a very rapid negative pass from the crown of the head over the body to the feet and in one instant he recovered his consciousness and became lively and well.

§ 290

MASSAGE

Here belongs also the so-called massage of vigorous good-natured person given to a chronic invalid, who, though cured, still suffers from loss of flesh, weakness of digestion and lack of sleep due to slow convalescence. The muscles of the limbs, breast and back, separately grasped and moderately pressed and kneaded arouse the life principle to reach and restore the tone of the muscles and blood and lymph vessels. The mesmeric influences of this procedure is the chief feature and it must not be used to excess in patients still hypersensitive.

EXPLANATION

Massage of vigorous good-natured person is useful to a chronic invalid who is cured but still suffers from loss of flesh, weakness of digestion and lack of sleep due to slow convalescence.

The muscles of limbs, breast and back are separately grasped and pressed and kneaded moderately.

This arouses the life principle to reach and restore the tone of the muscles and blood and lymph vessels.

It must not be used to excess in patients who are still hypersensitive.

§ 291

BATHS

Baths of pure water prove themselves partly palliative, partly as homoeopathic serviceable aids in restoring health in acute diseases as well as in convalescence of cured chronic patients with proper consideration of the conditions of the convalescent and the temperature of the bath, its duration and repetition. But even if well applied, they may bring only physically beneficial changes in the sick body, in themselves they are no true medicine. The lukewarm baths at 25 to 27? serve to arouse the slumbering sensibility of fibre in the apparent dead (frozen, drowned, suffocated) which benumbed the sensation of the nerves. Though only palliative, still they often prove themselves sufficiently active, especially when given in conjunction with coffee and rubbing with the hands. They may give homoeopathic aid in cases where the irritability is very unevenly distributed and accumulated too unevenly in some organs as is the case in certain hysteric spasms and infantile convulsions. In the same way, cold baths 10 to 6? in persons cured medically of chronic diseases and with deficiency of vital heat, act as an homoeopathic aid. By instantaneous and later with repeated immersions they act as a palliative restorative of the tone of the exhausted fibre. For this purpose, such baths are to be used for more than momentary duration, rather for minutes and of gradually lowered temperature, they are a palliative, which, since it acts only physically has no connection with the disadvantage of a reverse action to be feared afterwards, as takes place with dynamic medicinal palliatives.

EXPLANATION

Baths of pure water proves partly palliative as homoeopathic aid in restoring health in acute diseases as well as in convalescence of cured chronic patients.

Conditions of the convalescent and temperature of bath, it's duration and repetition are to be considered during the application of bath.

But even if they are well applied, they may only bring physical beneficial changes in the sick body, they are not true medicines in themselves.

The lukewarm baths at 25-27 degree celcius arouses the sensibility of fibre in the apparent dead (frozen, drowned, suffocated person) with benumbed sensation of nerves.

When bath is given with coffee and rubbing with hands, they often prove beneficial.

They may give homoeopathic aid in cases of certain hysteric spasms and infantile convulsions where the irritability is very unevenly distributed and accumulated too unevenly in some organs.

In the same way cold baths at 10 to 6 degree celcius act as an homoeopathic aid in persons cured medically of chronic disease and with deficiency of vital heat.

By instantaneous and with repeated immersions they act as a palliative restorative of the tone of exhausted fibres.

This way they act only physically not dynamically and hence do not have disadvantage of a reverse action which occurs with dynamic medicinal palliatives.

§ 292

MOST SENSITIVE PART IS ALSO MOST SUSCEPTIBLE

Even the external surface of the body, covered as it is with skin and epidermis, is not insusceptible of the powers of medicines, especially those in a liquid form, but the most sensitive parts are also the most susceptible.1

1 Rubbing-in appears to favour the action of the medicines only in this way, that the friction makes the skin more sensitive, and the living fibres thereby more capable of feeling, as it were, the medicinal power and of communicating to the whole organism this health-affecting sensation. The previous employment of friction to the inside of the thigh makes the mere laying on the mercurial ointment afterwards quite as powerfully medicinal as if the ointment itself had been rubbed upon that part, a process which is termed rubbing-in, but it is very doubtful whether the mental itself can

penetrate in substance into the interior of the body, or be taken up by the absorbent vessels by means of this so-called rubbing-in. Homoeopathy, however, hardly ever requires for its cures the rubbing-in of any medication, nor does it need any mercurial ointment.

EXPLANATION

The external surface of the body covered as skin and epidermis is susceptible to the powers of the medicines especially those medicines in liquid form.

But the most sensitive parts are also the most susceptible.

Footnote 1:
Rubbing-in the body favours the action of medicines. During rubbing the friction makes the skin more sensitive and the living fibres are more capable of feeling the medicinal power and of communicating this health affecting sensation to the whole organism.

Homoeopathy hardly ever requires the Rubbing-in of any medication, nor it need any mercurial ointment for its cure

§ 293

MESMERISM

I find it necessary to allude here to animal magnetism, as it is termed, or rather mesmerism (as it should be called, out of gratitude to Mesmer, its first founder), which differs so much in its nature from all other therapeutic agents. This curative power, often so stupidly denied, which streams upon a patient by the contact of a well-intentioned person powerfully exerting his will, either acts homoeopathically, by the production of symptoms similar to those of the diseased state to be cured; and for this purpose a single pass made, without much exertion of the will, with the palms of the hands not too slowly from the top of the head downwards over the body to the tips of the toes,1 is serviceable in, for instance, uterine haemorrhages, even in the last stage when death seems approaching; or it is useful by distributing the vital force uniformly throughout the organism, when it is in abnormal excess in one part and deficient in other parts, for example, in rush of blood to the head and sleepless, anxious restlessness of weakly persons, etc., by means of a similar, single, but somewhat stronger pass; or for the immediate communication and restoration of the vital force to some one weakened part or to the whole organism, – an object that cannot be attained so certainly and with so little interference with the other medicinal treatment by any other agent besides mesmerism. If it is wished to supply a particular part with the vital force, this is effected by concentrating a very powerful and well-intentioned will for the purpose, and placing the hands or tips of the fingers on the chronically weakened parts, whither an internal chronic dyscrasia has transferred its important local symptom, as, for example, in the case of old ulcers, amaurosis, paralysis of certain limbs, etc.2 Many rapid apparent cures performed in all ages, by mesmerizers endowed with great natural power, belong to this class. **The effect of communicated human power upon the whole human organism was most brilliantly shown, in the resuscitation of persons who had lain some time apparently dead, by the most powerful sympathetic will of a man in full vigor of vital force,3 and of this kind of resurrection history records many undeniable examples.**

1 The smallest homoeopathic dose, which however, often effects wonders when used on proper occasions. Imperfect homoeopathists, who think themselves monstrously clever, not infrequently deluge their patients in difficult diseases with doses of different medicines, given rapidly one after the other, which, although they may have been homoeopathically selected and given in highly potentized attenuation, bring the patients into such an over-excited state that life and death are struggling for the mastery, and the least additional quantity of medicine would infallibly kill them. In such cases a mere gentle mesmeric pass and the frequent application, for a short time of the hand of a well-intentioned person to the part that is particularly affected, produce the harmonious uniform distribution of the vital force throughout the organism, and therewith rest, sleep and recovery.

2 Although by this restoration of the vital force, which ought to be repeated from time to time, no permanent cure can be effected in cases where, as has been taught above, a general internal dyscrasia lies at the root of the old local affection, as it always does, yet this positive strengthening and immediate saturation with the vital force (which no more belongs to the category of palliatives than does eating and drinking when hunger and thirst are present) is no mean auxiliary to the actual treatment of the whole disease by homoeopathic medicines.

3 Especially of one of those persons, of whom there are not many who, along with great kindness of disposition and perfect bodily powers, possesses but a very moderate desire for sexual intercourse, which it would give him very little trouble to suppress, in whom, consequently, all the fine vital spirits that would otherwise be employed in the preparation of the semen, are ready to be communicated to others, by touching them and powerfully exerting the will. Some powerful mesmerisers, with whom I have become acquainted, has all this peculiar character.

EXPLANATION

Here he says about the animal magnetism or Mesmerism in detail.

Mesmerism streams upon the patient by contact of a well-intentioned person who powerfully exerts his will over the sick.

i) He either acts homoeopathically by the production of symptoms similar to those of the diseased state to be cured, or
ii) By distributing the vital force uniformly throughout the organism, when it is in abnormal excess in one part and deficient in other parts, or
iii) For immediate communication and restoration of the vital force to some weakened part or to the whole organism by use of other medicinal treatment by any other agent besides Mesmerism.

For (i)purpose, a single pass is made without much exertion of the will, with the palms of the hands not too slowly from the top of the head downwards over the body to the tips of the toes. It is serviceable in uterine haemorrhages, even in the last stage when death seems approaching.

For (ii) purpose it is done by means of a similar, single but somewhat stronger pass.

E.g. in rush of blood to the head and sleepless, anxious restlessness of weak person etc

If we wish to supply a particular part with the vital force, this is done by concentrating a very powerful and well intentioned will and placing the hands or tips of the fingers on the chronically weakened parts.

e.g. in the case of old ulcers, amaurosis, paralysis of certain limbs etc.

This effect was the most brilliantly shown, in the resuscitation of persons who had lain sometime apparently dead, by the most powerful sympathetic will of a man in full vigor of the vital force and there are many examples of this kind.

Footnote 1:

The smallest homoeopathic dose, often acts wonder when used on proper occasions. Imperfect homoeopathists often give patients doses of different medicines in difficult diseases. These medicines are given rapidly one after the other.

Although they may be homoeopathically selected and given in highly potentized attenuation, it brings patient into such an over-excited state that life and death are struggling for the mastery. Now the least additional quantity of medicine would kill them.

In such cases a mere gentle mesmeric pass and the frequent application of the hand of a well-intentioned person, for a short time to the part particularly affected produce the uniform distribution of the vital force throughout the organism and produces rest, sleep and recovery.

Footnote 2:

By this restoration of the vital force, which is repeated from time to time, no permanent cure can be effected in those cases where a general internal dyscrasia lies at the root of the old local affection. This requires actual treatment of the whole disease by homoeopathic medicines.

Footnote 3:

Vital energy especially of one of such persons who has great kindness of disposition and perfect bodily powers and possesses very moderate desire for sexual intercourse.

Due to which all the fine vital spirits are ready to be communicated to others and not employed in the production of semen.

It is communicated to others by touching them and powerfully exerting the will.

§ 294

POSITIVE MESMERISM

All the above-mentioned methods of practicing mesmerism depend upon an influx of more or less vital force into the patient, and hence are termed positive mesmerism.1 An opposite mode of employing mesmerism, however, as it produces just the contrary effect, deserves to be termed

negative mesmerism. To this belong the passes which are used to rouse from the somnambulic sleep, as also all the manual processes known by the names of soothing and ventilating. This discharge by means of negative mesmerism of the vital force accumulated to excess in individual parts of the system of undebiliated persons is most surely and simply performed by making a very rapid motion of the flat extended hand, held parallel to, and about an inch distant from the body, from the top of the head to the tips of the toes.2 The more rapidly this pass is made, so much the more effectually will the discharge be effected. Thus, for instance, in the case where a previously healthy woman,3 from the sudden suppression of her catamenia by a violent mental shock, lies to all appearance dead, the vital force which is probably accumulated in the precordial region, will by such a rapid negative pass, be discharged and its equilibrium throughout the whole organism restored, so that the resuscitation generally follows immediately.4 In like manner, a gentle, less rapid, negative pass diminishes the excessive restlessness and sleeplessness accompanied with anxiety sometimes produced in very irritable persons by a too powerful positive pass, etc.

* **This Section corresponds to § 289 of the Sixth Edition.**

1 When I here speak of the decided and certain curative power of positive mesmerism, I most assuredly do not mean the abuse of it, where, by repeated passes of this kind, continued for half an hour or a whole hour at a time, and, even day after day, performed on weak, nervous patients, that monstrous revolution of the whole human system is effected which is termed somnambulism, wherein the human being is ravished from the world of sense and seems to belong more to the world of spirits – a highly unnatural and dangerous state, by means of which it has not infrequently been attempted to cure chronic diseases.

2 It is a well known rule that a person who is either to be positively or negatively mesmerised, should not wear silk on any part of the body.

3 Hence a negative pass, especially if it be very rapid, is extremely injurious to a delicate person affected with a chronic ailment and deficient in vital force.

4 A strong country lad, ten years of age, received in the morning, on account of slight indisposition, from a professed female mesmeriser, several very powerful passes with the points of both thumbs, from the pit of the stomach along the lower edge of the ribs, and he instantly grew pale, and fell into such a state of unconsciousness and immobility that no effort could arouse him, and he was almost given up for dead. I made his eldest brother give him a very rapid negative pass from the crown of the head over the body to the feet, and in one instant he recovered his consciousness and became lively and well.

EXPLANATION

Aphorism 294 is same as aphorism 289 of the 6th edition

All the above - mentioned methods of mesmerism depend upon an influx of vital force into the patient and hence are termed positive mesmerism.

An opposite mode of employing mesmerism, is termed negative mesmerism as it produces just opposite effect.

This negative mesmerism includes the passes which are used to rouse from the somnambulic sleep, also all manual processes known as soothing and ventilating.

This discharge by means of negative mesmerism of the vital force is performed by making a very rapid motion of the flat extended hand held parallel to and about an inch distance from the body, from the top of the head to the tips of the toes.

The more rapidly this pass is made, the more effectually the discharge is effected.

For e.g. in the case where a previously healthy woman, by a violent mental shock develops sudden suppression of her catamania. She lies to all appearance dead, the vital force is probably accumulated in the precordial region. So by such a rapid negative pass, the vital force is discharged and it's equilibrium is restored throughout the whole organism and resuscitation generally follows immediately.

In the same manner, a gentle, less rapid, negative pass diminishes the excessive restlessness and sleeplessness due to anxiety produced in very irritable persons by a too powerful positive pass, etc.

Footnote 1:
Here he speaks of the certain curative power of the positive mesmerism, he does not mean that abuse of it, where, repeated passes of this kind are continued for half an hour or a whole hour at a time and even day after day, on weak, nervous patients whole human system is affected which is termed somnambulism, where the human being is forced from the world of sense and goes to a highly unnatural and dangerous state.

Footnote 2:
A person who is either to be positively or negatively mesmerised, should not wear silk on any part of the body.

Footnote 3:
Hence a negative pass, especially if it be very rapid, is very injurious to delicate person affected with a chronic ailment and deficient in vital force.

Footnote 4:
A strong country lad of 10 years of age had slight indisposition.

He received several very powerful passes with the points of both thumbs, from the pit of the stomach long the lower edge of the ribs by a professed female mesmeriser.

He instantly grew deathly pale and unconscious. He could not be aroused by any means and was almost given up for dead.

Hahnemann made his eldest brother give him a very rapid negative pass from the crown of the head over the body to the feet and in one instant he recovered his consciousness and became lively and well.

Believe in yourself! Have faith in your abilities!
Without a humble but reasonable confidence in your own powers
you cannot be successful or happy.

GLOSSARY

1. *Aggravation- A noticeable intensification of the disease symptoms previously observed. Often associated with the action of the correct homeopathic remedy.*
2. *Antidote - A substance, or a remedy, that counteracts the effect of a homeopathic remedy. High temperatures are thought to antidote remedies. Mint is said to be an antidote of Natrum muriaticum. Many feel that coffee antidotes homeopathic remedies. When a person is reacting incorrectly to a homeopathic remedy, an antidote may be given to neutralize the effects.*
3. *Anti-psoric -- The group of homeopathic medicines, identified by Hahnemann, that cure the psoric miasm and associated diseases.*
4. *Allopathy -- The treatment of disease by using medicines that oppose the presenting symptoms.*
5. *Avagadro's Number -- 6.03×10 to the 23rd power. The number of molecules contained in 1 mole of a substance. Potencies greater than 12c or 24x no longer contain any molecules of the original substance.*
6. *Boenninghausen's Concordances -- Boenninghausen's lists of remedy relationships.*
7. *Causation rubric -- A rubric that reflects the cause of the disease.*
8. *Cell salts (biochemic remedies, tissue salts) - A homeopathic physician, W. H. Schuessler, developed the Biochemic system using 12 different 'cell salts'. Schuessler felt these were fundamental to the proper function of the human body. Prepared in low potency (3x or 6x) and used based on homeopathic indications.*
9. *Centesimal - One of three potency scales used in homeopathic pharmacy. It was the first potency developed by Hahnemann. 1 part medicinal substance (dry or tincture), mixed with 99 parts diluent (lactose or alcohol), and then succussed (shaken), yields the 1c potency. Taking 1 part of that potency mixed with 99 parts diluent, then succussed, yields the 2c potency. This is continued until the desired potency is reached. A 200c has gone through this process 200 times. A 1M potency has gone through this process 1,000 times. The higher the potency, the stronger the stimulation of the vital force.*
10. *Centrifugal - Moving away from the center*
11. *Centripetal - Moving towards the center*
12. *Characteristic symptom - A symptom that is 'striking, strange, unusual, peculiar' in the case. Close attention is paid to characteristic symptoms as they must correspond to symptoms of the remedy if it is to cure. For example, burning pain better heat, or better lying on the painful side.*
13. *Chronic Disease -- Disease that arise from the dynamic contagion of a chronic miasm. Left to themselves without their specific remedy, they continue to increase indefinitely, despite the best mental and dietary habits.*

14. *collective disease -- In epidemics, the collective disease reveals itself in the totality of the signs and symptoms of several cases.*
15. *Common symptoms - Symptoms that are common to a specific disease, for example, stiff joints in arthritis, or yellow skin in jaundice.*
16. *Complementary - Complementary remedies enhance or augment the action of the previous remedy.*
17. *Complete symptom - Etiology, location (including radiation or extension of sensation), sensation, modalities, and concomitants all together give a complete symptom.*
18. *Concomitant - Occurring simultaneously. Refers to symptoms that happen at the same time as the chief complaint. One of the parts of a complete symptom.*
19. *Constitution -- The physical body and mental temperament that is expressive of the natural traits and predisposition of the individual.*
20. *Contagion -- An infectious state transferred by contact.*
21. *Decimal - The first experiments with the decimal scale were performed by Constantine Hering in 1833. 1 part medicinal substance (dry or tincture), mixed with 9 parts diluent (lactose or alcohol), and then succussed (shaken), yields the 1X (D) potency. Taking 1 part of that potency mixed with 9 parts diluent, then succussed, yields the 2X (D) potency. This is continued until the desired potency is reached.*
22. *Degree -- A combination of the frequency with which a remedy cures a symptom in provings or clinical practice. A numerical value is assigned to a remedy in a rubric in a repertory. In the Synthesis Repertory, this is a range from 1-4.*
23. *Diathesis -- A mental or physical [inherited or acquired] chronic predisposition or disease state.*
24. *Doctrine of Signatures -- The concept that any organic substance carries within itself the likeness of some organ or part of the human economy, as a sign that this particular substance was applicable to disturbances of that organ.*
25. *Drainage remedies -- Remedies used to balance, nourish, or detoxify the system.*
26. *dyscrasia -- An illness or sickness.*
27. *Elimination rubric -- A rubric used in a repertorization to eliminate consideration of any remedy that is not found within.*
28. *Etiology - The cause of disease. One of the aspects of a complete symptom.*
29. *Families -- Looking at remedies from the standpoint of botanical relationships, animal groupings, or place in the Periodic Table.*
30. *Fluxion -- Method of homeopathic pharmacy that does not succuss past a 30c potency. The pressure of water is used instead.*
31. *Geginwirking (counter action) -- Hahnemann divides the symptoms we see into two different types: those which result from the first encounter between the vital force and the external agent, and the ones which are a result of the vital force's reaction to the symptoms of that primary encounter-counter action.*
32. *Gemut -- Emotions, emotional mind.*
33. *Genus Epidemicus -- A remedy which is found to be curative in the majority of cases of the same disease (eg., epidemics). Hahnemann taught that the genus epidemicus remedies should*

be chosen by the uncommon characteristic symptoms of all the patients not the common symptoms of the epidemic disease.

34. *Grafting* -- Method of making medicated pellets by placing non-medicated pellets in contact with medicated ones. Also done with liquid potencies.
35. *Heilkunst* -- Complete medical system
36. *Hering's Law* -- A true cure takes place from within to without; from the more important organs to the lesser important; from above to below; heals the symptoms in the reverse order of their development.
37. *Homeopathy* - System of natural medicine developed by Samuel Hahnemann. Based on the Law of Similars.
38. *Homeoprophylaxis* -- Use of homeopathic medicines to prevent the occurrence of a disease.
39. *Inimical* -- These are remedies that have been shown to have an adverse effect on following one another.
40. *Intercurrent* -- Remedy used to provide renewed activity in a stalled case.
41. *Isopathy* - The treatment of a disease with the identical disease agent.
42. *Keynote* - A unique feature or fundamental aspect of a remedy.
43. *Lebenskraft* -- Life force or life power
44. *LM (50 millesimal, Q)* - The second potency scale developed by Hahnemann, introduced in the sixth edition of the Organon. Start with a 3c triturate of a remedy. One part is placed into 500 drops liquid (400 drops water, 100 drops alcohol). One drop is placed into 100 drops of alcohol. This is succussed by hand 100 times. One drop of this mixture is used to medicate 500@10 pellets. This is the Q1 potency(sometimes written 0/1).
45. The Q2 is made by taking 1 of these medicated pellets, putting it into 1 drop of water, and then mixing into 100 drops of alcohol. This mixture is succussed 100 times by hand."LM (50 millesimal, Q) - the second potency scale developed by Hahnemann, introduced in the sixth edition of the Organon. Start with a 3c triturate of a remedy. One part is placed into 500 drops liquid (4 parts water, 1 part alcohol 95% v/v). One drop is placed into 2 ml alcohol 95% v/v. This is succussed by hand 100 times. One drop of this mixture is used to medicate 500@10 pellets. This is the Q1 potency (sometimes written 0/1). The Q2 is made by taking 1 of these medicated pellet and placing it into 2 ml alcohol 95% v/v. This mixture is succussed 100 times by hand."
46. *Location* - Where the symptom is experienced. Location is one of the parts of a complete symptom.
47. *Magnetism* -- Rubbing or stroking.
48. *Materia medica* - "Materials of medicine" in Latin. A reference that lists the curative indications and therapeutic actions of homeopathic medicines. This information is derived from provings and clinical experience
49. *Mesmerism* -- Healing force by which a well-intentioned man exerts his strong will over a patient with or without touching him, or even at some distance, in such a way that the vital force of the healthy mesmerizer gifted with this power dynamically flows into the patient.
50. *Miasm* -- A diathesis based on an infection, its sequellae, or inherited effects.

51. *Modality* - A condition that makes a person or their symptom better or worse. For example, better in a hot bath, abdominal pain better bending over, worse rainy weather, etc. Modalities are one of the parts of a complete symptom.
52. *Nosode* - A homeopathic remedy prepared from diseased tissue or the product of disease.
53. *One-sided diseases* -- Diseases that seem less amenable to cure because of an apparent paucity of symptoms, one or two symptoms predominate, obscuring almost all the others.
54. *Organon* - The Organon of Medicine, by Samuel Hahnemann, the founder of homeopathy. This book describes the principles and practice of homeopathy. Hahnemann wrote 6 editions of the Organon from 1810-1842. The sixth edition, though finished in 1842, was not published until 1921.
55. *Originating cause* -- The factor responsible for the genesis of something.
56. *Potency* - The strength of a homeopathic remedy. Determined by how many times the remedy has been succussed and diluted during preparation. A number and a letter are associated with the remedy name to indicate which potency scale has been used. An example of the decimal scale would be Arnica 6x. An example of the centesimal scale would be Arnica 30c. An example of the 50 millesimal scale (LM) would be Arnica LM1. These are the 3 potency scales currently in use.
57. *Potentized* - Usually refers to a substance prepared according to homeopathic pharmaceutical standards. This means that it has gone through serial dilution and succussion.
58. *Plussing* -- Extension of a dose by adding water to the remedy solution and succussing further.
59. *Primary effects* -- Every power that acts on life, every medicine, alters the vital force more or less and brings about in human health certain modifications of greater or lesser duration. Although it is a product of both the medicinal and the vital force, this primary action nevertheless belongs more to the domain of the former.
60. *Proving* - The most accurate method of ascertaining the action of medicines on human health. Medicines (usually potentized) are administered to healthy people to discover the symptoms they are capable of producing and thereby able to cure.
61. *Psora* -- The 'itch dyscrasia'. One of the three major miasms described by Hahnemann. Deficiency is a key element.
62. *Remedy* - Medicine, as in homeopathic remedy.
63. *Repertorize* - To repertorize a case one looks up symptoms in a repertory.
64. *Repertory* - An index of the homeopathic materia medica by symptom. A list of remedies is indicated for each symptom. All modern day repertories use Kent's Repertory as their starting point.
65. *Rubric* - A symptom as written in a homeopathic repertory.
66. *Rarcode* - A tissue or glandular extract made into a homeopathic remedy.
67. *Scrofula* -- Tuberculosis of the lymph glands.
68. *Secondary effects* -- Our vital force strives to oppose its energy to this influence. This, its life-preserving reaction, is an automatic activity called secondary effects.
69. *Sensation* - The experience of a symptom, what it feels like. One of the parts of a complete symptom.

70. *Similia Similibus Currentur ["Likes are cured by Likes"]* -- The homeopathic doctrine stating that any substance which is capable of producing morbid symptoms in the healthy will remove similar symptoms occurring as an expression of disease.
71. *Simillimum* - The most similar remedy corresponding to a case. As such, the remedy most likely to cure.
72. *Simple substance* -- The basic material from whence all force and forms in the universe have their origin.
73. *Stimmung* -- Tuning, mood, pitch. Health is harmony, tone, and perfect pitch [Stimmung].
74. *Succussion* - The process of forcefully striking a homeopathic remedy against a firm surface.
75. *Sycosis* -- Hahnemann's term for the chronic effects of the gonorrheal miasm. Excess is a key element.
76. *Syphilis* -- Chronic effects of the syphilitic miasm as described by Hahnemann. Destruction is a key element.
77. *Verstimmung* -- Disease is a mistuning [Verstimmung] of this healthy tone causing dissonance in life.
78. *Susceptibility* -- The degree to which a person is sensitive to a remedy or a disease.
79. *Symptom complex* -- The group of symptoms pertaining to a particular remedy.
80. *Totality* -- The aggregate of the characteristic symptoms in a case. The totality of a single symptom refers to a complete symptom.
81. *Underlining* -- Method of recording the intensity of a symptom.
82. *Vigor vitae* -- Life force
83. *Vis Medicatrix Naturae* -- The healing power of nature.
84. *Vital force* - The energy that maintains life in the individual. See aphorisms 9-12 of the Organon.
85. *Wesen* -- Essence, nature, substance.
86. *Dynamis* - Life energy, vital force.
87. *Potentized* - Usually refers to a substance prepared according to homeopathic pharmaceutical standards. This means that it has gone through serial dilution and succussion.
88. *Remedy* - Medicine, as in homeopathic remedy.
89. *Succussion* - The process of forcefully striking a homeopathic remedy against a firm surface.
90. *Vital force* - The energy that maintains life in the individual.
91. *Soul of the organon* -- Given by Dr. Jyoti joshi, it is theory book of organon of medicine.

Focus on your goal, don't look in any direction but ahead.

This book is arranged according to syllabus of B+
It will guide BHMS students for examination purpose as an Organon teacher. With best wishes..

Dr. Goutam Mandal.
(DR. GOUTAM MANDAL)
MD (Repertory)
Asst. Professor. Community Med
Chandola Hom. Medical Coll
& Hospital Rudrapur.

(1) It fullfill all the necessary content that will clear the basics of the students.

Dr. Vinita Bashna
Lecturer (Surgery)

(1) The book is explained in very simple language so it will be easy for students to understand.

Dr. Archana Srivastava
(Lecturer (Hom. Pharmac

(1) Each aphorism is explained in details so it will be ea for student to get each and every point at one place and there is no need to refer any other organon book.

Vandana
(Dr. Vandana Gangwa
Lecturer.

Some Written Comments of Teachers/Professors on the first book "SOUL OF THE ORGANON"

Some Written Comments of Teachers/Professors on the first book "SOUL OF THE ORGANON"

www.ingramcontent.com/pod-product-compliance
Lightning Source LLC
Chambersburg PA
CBHW081423220526
45466CB00008B/2251